Insights Into Incontinence and the Pelvic Floor

Fulya Dökmeci • Diaa E. E. Rizk
Editors

Insights Into Incontinence and the Pelvic Floor

MIPS Mediterranean Incontinence and Pelvic Floor Society

Springer

Editors
Fulya Dökmeci
Obstetrics and Gynecology
Ankara University School of Medicine
Ankara, Turkey

Diaa E. E. Rizk
Obstetrics and Gynecology
College of Medicine and Medical
Sciences, Arabian Gulf University
Manama, Bahrain

ISBN 978-3-030-94173-4 ISBN 978-3-030-94174-1 (eBook)
https://doi.org/10.1007/978-3-030-94174-1

This Springer imprint is published by the registered company Springer Nature Switzerland AG
The registered company address is: Gewerbestrasse 11, 6330 Cham, Switzerland

Preface

We aim to provide the readership of this book with a better understanding of pelvic floor medicine and incontinence by including original and scholarly research studies presented at the annual scientific meetings of *the Mediterranean Incontinence and Pelvic Floor Society (MIPS).* MIPS was founded in Palermo, Sicily, Italy, on 17 November 2012 based on a belief for the need of a professional organization that represents healthcare providers interested in male and female incontinence and pelvic floor health from the Mediterranean region. MIPS is a registered, nonprofit organization based in Milan, Italy, that is open to membership from all countries. The mission of MIPS is to facilitate the exchange of clinical experience and scientific knowledge between incontinence caregivers and researchers working in Mediterranean countries with close geographical and historical ties and a similar sociocultural background. This endeavor will have a positive impact on health care, service delivery, and community awareness of pelvic floor disorders.

The inaugural meeting of MIPS was held in Noto, Sicily, Italy, on 29–30 November 2013 followed by seven subsequent annual meetings in different Mediterranean countries. Over the past 9 years, the Executive Board of MIPS has been working hard to establish the society as a leader in professional education, scientific research, and clinical care of male and female pelvic floor dysfunctions in the Mediterranean region. We dedicate this book, whose publication coincides with the tenth anniversary of founding the society, to all our members who significantly participated in the success of MIPS. We are also grateful to all authors of this book for their scientific contributions. Without their efforts, this book would not have been possible particularly during the recent challenging times of the Covid-19 pandemic.

The primary goal of MIPS is to disseminate scientific knowledge and improve awareness regarding male and female urinary and fecal incontinence and diseases of the pelvic floor. As such, this book collates seminal research from the annual scientific meetings of MIPS with the objective of sharing research findings related to those topics from Mediterranean countries. Our intention was to write a book with a slightly different focus than other textbooks written in the field of pelvic floor medicine and incontinence. Hence, we included information from a Mediterranean perspective that simply describes the research experience of incontinence care providers working in the region and supplemented this with detailed case studies at the end of each chapter. We believe that the message of the book is clear and hope that our contribution will add to the body of scientific knowledge as well as to evidence-based clinical practice of pelvic floor medicine and incontinence.

Ankara, Turkey — Fulya Dökmeci
Manama, Bahrain — Diaa E. E. Rizk

Contents

About the Authors

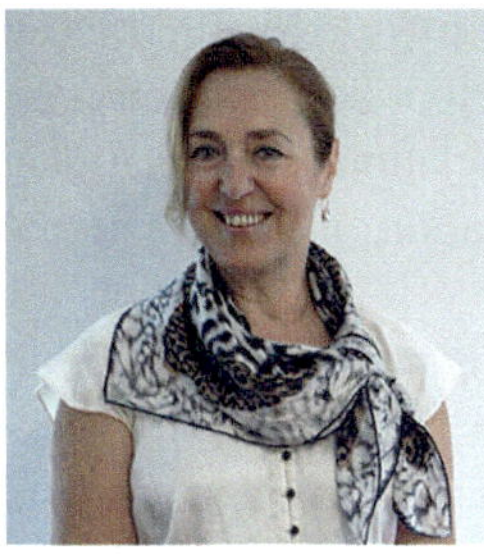

Fulya Dökmeci graduated from Ankara University School of Medicine in 1985 and was qualified as an obstetrician and gynecologist in 1991.

She studied transvaginal ultrasonography as well as clinical gynecology at Chiba University School of Medicine, Chiba, Japan, in 1988.

She was involved in the project JHPIEGO, Johns Hopkins Program for International Education in Gynecology and Obstetrics, and was certificated as the national trainer in "Standardization and Training of Clinical Skills" as well as "Advanced Clinical Training Skills and Group Dynamics" in 1998.

She received the "Advanced Gynecological Laparoscopy Skill" equivalency certificate by the "Accreditation Council for Gynecologic Endoscopy" board, USA, in 1999.

She completed her fellowship program for "Teaching and Learning" and "Educational Leadership" in the Division of Medical Education as a scholar of ECFMG/FAIMER and studied as a visiting professor in the Division of Pelvic Medicine and Reconstructive Surgery in Keck School of Medicine, University of Southern California, USA, for 1 year from 2002 to 2003.

She was subsequently appointed as an associate professor in 1996 and as a professor in 2003.

She has worked as the coordinator of the Postgraduate Medical Education of Ankara University School of Medicine for more than 10 years. She served as the pioneer academic staff of the Department of Medical Education and Informatics between 1999 and 2010.

She pioneered the establishment of the "Urogynecology Unit" in the Department of Obstetrics and Gynecology in Ankara School of

Medicine. She also played a pioneer role with her colleagues in the establishment of the "English Urogynecology Doctorate Program," which is the first in its field in Turkey, within the body of Ankara University in 2018.

She is a member of many national and international societies, such as Turkish Society of Gynecology and Obstetrics, Turkish Urogynecology and Pelvic Reconstructive Surgery, Turkish Society of Gynecological Endoscopy, Accreditation Council of Gynecologic Endoscopy, Mediterranean Incontinence and Pelvic Floor Society, European Urogynecological Association, International Urogynecological Association, and International Continence Society.

She has organized many national and international scientific meetings, courses, and workshops as well as attended as invited lecturer and moderator and has also been serving as the trainer of many undergraduate and graduate students in the fields of "obstetrics and gynecology," "development of medical education," and "pelvic floor health and urogynecology."

She has contributed to more than 100 scientific publications in English or Turkish, including original articles, projects, editorials, reviews, and book chapters.

Currently, she is a professor at the Department of Obstetrics and Gynecology and has been serving as the chief of the "Gynecology and Urogynecology" section of this department in Ankara University School of Medicine since 2009. She is the President of Turkish Urogynecology and Pelvic Floor Reconstructive Surgery Association and is also running as a member of the Executive Board and Chair of the Educational Committee of Mediterranean Incontinence and Pelvic Floor Society.

She is married and has one daughter.

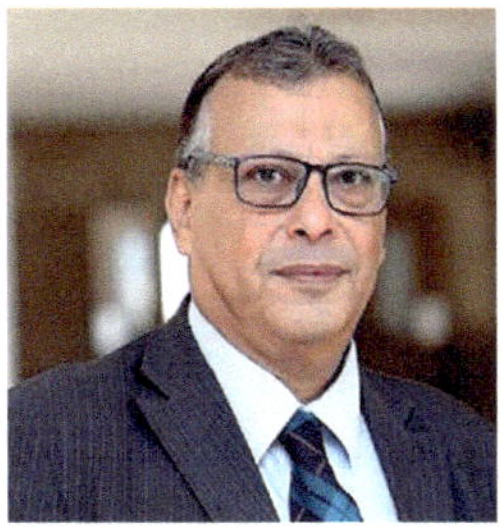

Diaa E. E. Rizk is the Professor and Chairman of Obstetrics and Gynecology, College of Medicine and Medical Sciences, Arabian Gulf University, Manama, Bahrain. He has completed training in obstetrics and gynecology and then in urology and colorectal surgery. He has published over 160 original articles, special contributions, editorials, reviews, and case reports and over 70 abstracts in peer-reviewed indexed scientific journals. He has been one of the editors of the International Urogynecology Journal from 2007 to 2021. He serves on the editorial board of many medical journals and is currently a member of the editorial board of Female Pelvic Medicine & Reconstructive Surgery. He has extensive experience in clinical practice and has made important contributions to training and service provision in obstetrics and gynecology, women's health, and urogynecology. He has served on several national, regional, and international committees for the International Urogynecology Association (IUGA), International Continence Society (ICS), International Federation of Gynecology and Obstetrics (FIGO), World Federation of Medical Education (WAME), and World Health Organization (WHO). In 2013, he co-founded the Mediterranean Incontinence and Pelvic Floor Society (MIPS), where he has been serving as President since 2016 until present.

Contributors

Fernando Diez-Caballero Alonso Clínica Universidad de Navarra, Pamplona, Spain

José Luis Álvarez-Ossorio Hospital Universitario Puerta Del Mar, Urology, Cádiz, Spain

Enrico Ammirati Città Della Salute E Della Scienza Di Torino, Unità Spinale Unipolare-CTO-SC Neuro-Urologia, Torino, Italy

Alfredo Rodríguez-Antolín Hospital Universitario 12 de Octubre, Urología, Madrid, Spain

Laura Mateu Arrom Fundació Puigvert, Barcelona, Spain

Douskos Athanasios Urogynecology Unit, National and Kapodistrian University, Athens, Greece

Felipe Villacampa Aubá Clínica Universidad de Navarra, Madrid, Spain

Virginia Martinez Fundació Puigvert, Barcelona, Spain

Emilio Blanco-Tarrío Grupo De Investigación Multidisciplinar Urológico Renal (GRUMUR), Instituto de Investigación Biomédica De Salamanca (IBSAL), Salamanca, Spain

A. Botter Laboratory for Engineering of the Neuromuscular System (Lisin), Dept Electronics and Telecommunications-Politecnico, Torino, Italy

Serpil Bozkurt Private Clinic, Istanbul, Turkey

Jose María Velis Campillo Clínica Universidad de Navarra, Pamplona, Spain

Giorgio Canepa Ente Ospedaliero Ospedali Galliera, Dipartimento Di Urologia, Genova, Italy

Roberto Carone Città Della Salute E Della Scienza Di Torino, Unità Spinale Unipolare-CTO-SC Neuro-Urologia, Torino, Italy

Alice Carvalhais LAETA, INEGI, CESPU, Escola Superior de Tecnologias da Saúde do Tâmega e Sousa, Porto, Portugal

Cristina Gutiérrez Castañé Clínica Universidad de Navarra, Pamplona, Spain

Aygen Celik Department of Obstetrics and Gynecology, Maltepe University Faculty of Medicine, Istanbul, Turkey

Corrado Cescon Independent Researcher, Vacallo, Switzerland

Elif Nazlı Çetindağ Department of Obstetrics and Gynecology, Lösante Children's and Adult Hospital, Ankara, Turkey

Şerife Esra Çetinkaya Department of Obstetrics and Gynecology, Ankara University School of Medicine, Cebeci Hospital, Ankara, Turkey

Department of Obstetrics and Gynecology, Ankara University School of Medicine, Ankara, Turkey

Faculty of Health Science, Physiotherapy and Rehabilitation Department, Atılım University, Ankara, Turkey

Fernando Ramón De Fata Chillón Clínica Universidad de Navarra, Madrid, Spain

Kalantzis Christos Urogynecology Unit, National and Kapodistrian University, Athens, Greece

Vanessa Talavera Cobo Universidad de Navarra, Pamplona, Spain

Mónica Paola Coderque-Mejía Department of Urology, Complejo Asistencial Universitario de Salamanca, Salamanca, Spain

Beatriu Roca Comella Department of Obstetrics and Gynecology, Consorci Sanitari de Terrassa, Terrassa, Spain

Ángel García Cortés Clínica Universidad de Navarra, Pamplona, Spain

David Rosell Costa Clínica Universidad de Navarra, Pamplona, Spain

Martin Costal Urology Department, Hospital La Princesa, Madrid, Spain

Maria Luisa Bayo Delgado Universidad de Navarra, Pamplona, Spain

Zacharakis Dimitrios Urogynecology Unit, National and Kapodistrian University, Athens, Greece

Valsamidis Dimitris Urogynecology Unit, National and Kapodistrian University, Athens, Greece

José María De Dios-Hernández Grupo De Investigación Multidisciplinar Urológico Renal (GRUMUR), Instituto de Investigación Biomédica De Salamanca (IBSAL), Salamanca, Spain

Fulya Dökmeci Department of Obstetrics and Gynecology, Ankara University School of Medicine, Ankara, Turkey

Department of Obstetrics and Gynecology, Ankara University School of Medicine, Cebeci Hospital, Ankara, Turkey

Faculty of Health Science, Physiotherapy and Rehabilitation Department, Atılım University, Ankara, Turkey

K. Drusany-Staric Gynec and Obst Dept Div., University of Ljubljana, Ljubljana, Slovenia

Pitsouni Elieni Urogynecology Unit, National and Kapodistrian University, Athens, Greece

Andreea Enache Clinical Hospital of Obstetrics and Gynecology "Prof. Dr. Panait Sarbu", Bucharest, Romania

Traian Enache Clinical Hospital of Obstetrics and Gynecology "Prof. Dr. Panait Sarbu", Bucharest, Romania

Carlos Errando Fundació Puigvert, Barcelona, Spain

Cristina Margarita Fernández-Ávila Hospital Universitario Puerta Del Mar, Urology, Cádiz, Spain

Rodrigo García-Baquero Hospital Universitario Puerta Del Mar, Urology, Cádiz, Spain

María Begoña García-Cenador Department of Surgery, University of Salamanca, Salamanca, Spain

Jose Enrique Robles García Clínica Universidad de Navarra, Pamplona, Spain

Paolo Geretto Città Della Salute E Della Scienza Di Torino, Unità Spinale Unipolare-CTO-SC Neuro-Urologia, Torino, Italy

Alessandro Giammò Città Della Salute E Della Scienza Di Torino, Unità Spinale Unipolare-CTO-SC Neuro-Urologia, Torino, Italy

Antonella Giannantoni Functional and Surgical Urology Unit, Department of Medical and Surgical Sciences and Neurosciences, University of Siena, Siena, Italy

Borja Garcia Gomez Urology Department, Hospital Universitario 12 De Octubre, Madrid, Spain

Gemma López Gómiz Department of Obstetrics and Gynecology, Consorci Sanitari de Terrassa, Terrassa, Spain

Ignacio González-Casado Grupo De Investigación Multidisciplinar Urológico Renal (GRUMUR), Instituto de Investigación Biomédica De Salamanca (IBSAL), Salamanca, Spain

Javier Gonzalvez Urology Department, Hospital La Princesa, Madrid, Spain

Marilena Gubbiotti Department of Urology, Pelvic Unit, San Donato Hospital, Arezzo, Italy

Ali Gursoy Department of Obstetrics and Gynecology, Maltepe University Faculty of Medicine, Istanbul, Turkey

Filomena Herrera-Criado Grupo De Investigación Multidisciplinar Urológico Renal (GRUMUR), Instituto de Investigación Biomédica De Salamanca (IBSAL), Salamanca, Spain

Erdin Ilter Department of Obstetrics and Gynecology, Maltepe University Faculty of Medicine, Istanbul, Turkey

Carlo Introini Ente Ospedaliero Ospedali Galliera, Dipartimento Di Urologia, Genova, Italy

Mihai Ionica Clinical Emergency Hospital "Floreasca", Bucharest, Romania

Manuel Alonso Isa Urology Department, Hospital Universitario 12 De Octubre, Madrid, Spain

Svetlana Jankovic Department of Obstetrics and Gynecology, "Narodni Front", Belgrade, Serbia

Belgrade University Medical School, Belgrade, Serbia

Miguel Jiménez Urology Department, Hospital Ramón y Cajal, Madrid, Spain

Renato Natal Jorge LAETA, INEGI, Faculdade de Engenharia, Universidade do Porto, Porto, Portugal

Ahkam Göksel Kanmaz Tepecik Education and Research Hospital, Obstetrics and Gynecology Clinic, İzmir, Turkey

Fuat Kaplan WCHN Rudy Ruggles Biomedical Research Institute Danbury, Danbury, CT, USA

Kazibe Koyuncu Department of Obstetrics and Gynecology, Istanbul Kartal Dr. Lütfi Kırdar City Hospital, Istanbul, Turkey

Esther Gómez Lanza Urology Department, Hospital Moisés Broggi de Sant Joan Despí, Barcelona, Spain

Bernardino Miñana López Clínica Universidad de Navarra, Madrid, Spain

Luis López-Fando Urology Department, Hospital La Princesa, Madrid, Spain

Pablo Doménech López Clínica Universidad de Navarra, Pamplona, Spain

Javier Lorca Urology Department, Hospital Ramón y Cajal, Madrid, Spain

María Fernanda Lorenzo-Gómez Department of Surgery, University of Salamanca, Salamanca, Spain

Department of Urology, Complejo Asistencial Universitario De Salamanca, Salamanca, Spain

Grupo De Investigación Multidisciplinar Urológico Renal (GRUMUR), Instituto de Investigación Biomédica De Salamanca (IBSAL), Salamanca, Spain

Adolf Lukanović Department of Gynecology, University Medical Centre Ljubljana, Ljubljana, Slovenia

Division of Gynecology and Obstertrics, Department of Gynecology, Medical Faculty, University Medical Centre Ljubljana, University of Ljubljana, Ljubljana, Slovenia

Gynec and Obst Dept Div., University of Ljubljana, Ljubljana, Slovenia

Univerzitetni Klinicni Center Ljubljana, Ginekološka Klinika, Ljubljana, University of Ljubljana, Medical Faculty, Ljubljana, Slovenia

Univerzitetni Klinicni Center Ljubljana, Ginekološka Klinika, Ljubljana, Slovenia

Jan Lužnik University Medical Centre, Maribor, Slovenia

Marijan Lužnik General Hospital Slovenj Gradec, Slovenj Gradec, Slovenia

Juan Llopis Manzanera Urology Department, Hospital de Mataró, Barcelona, Spain

Francisco Javier Ancizu Marckert Clínica Universidad de Navarra, Pamplona, Spain

Misericordia Martínez-Huélamo Grupo De Investigación Multidisciplinar Urológico Renal (GRUMUR), Instituto de Investigación Biomédica De Salamanca (IBSAL), Salamanca, Spain

Juan Antonio Romero Martin Urology Department, Hospital de Mataró, Barcelona, Spain

Roberto Merletti Lisin, Politecnico Di Torino, Torino, Italy

José Antonio Mirón-Canelo Department of Public Health, University of Salamanca, Salamanca, Spain

Marcel Moisa Clinical Hospital of Obstetrics and Gynecology "Prof. Dr. Panait Sarbu", Bucharest, Romania

Javier Gil-Moradillo Hospital Universitario 12 de Octubre, Urología, Madrid, Spain

Giuseppe Morgia Azienda Ospedaliera Universitaria Policlinico Vittorio Emanuele, Dipartimento Di Urologia, Catania, Italy

Cristina Mozzi ASL Alessandria, Ospedale San Giacomo Di Novi Ligure, Dipartimento Di Urologia, Novi Ligure, Italy

Carlos Müller-Arteaga Department of Urology, Hospital Universitario De Ourense, Ourense, Spain

Gregor Norčič Division of Surgery, Department of University of Ljubljana, University Medical Centre Ljubljana, Ljubljana, Slovenia

Department of Abdominal Surgery, University Medical Centre Ljubljana, Ljubljana, Slovenia

Jose Manuel Duarte-Ojeda Hospital Universitario 12 de Octubre, Urología, Madrid, Spain

Javier Romero Otero Urology Department, Hospital Universitario 12 De Octubre, Madrid, Spain

Umit Ozekici Department of Obstetrics and Gynecology, Maltepe University Faculty of Medicine, Istanbul, Turkey

Tülin Özkan Department of Medical Biology, Ankara University School of Medicine, Ankara, Turkey

Daniel Gonzalez Padilla Urology Department, Hospital Universitario 12 De Octubre, Madrid, Spain

Bárbara Padilla-Fernández Departamento de Cirugía, Facultad de Medicina, Universidad de La Laguna, Tenerife, Spain

Ana Arrébola-Pajares Hospital Universitario 12 de Octubre, Urología, Madrid, Spain

Sherrie Palm Association for Pelvic Organ Prolapse Support, Mukwonago, WI, USA

Joan Palou Fundació Puigvert, Barcelona, Spain

Blanca Madurga-Patuel Hospital Universitario Puerta Del Mar, Urology, Cádiz, Spain

Berna Haliloglu Peker Department of Obstetrics and Gynecology, Maltepe University Faculty of Medicine, Istanbul, Turkey

Hakan Peker Nisantasi Vocational School, Nisantasi University, Istanbul, Turkey

Juan Ignacio Pascual Piédrola Clínica Universidad de Navarra, Pamplona, Spain

José Medina-Polo Hospital Universitario 12 de Octubre, Urología, Madrid, Spain

Juan Justo-Quintas Hospital Universitario 12 de Octubre, Urología, Madrid, Spain

E. Raimondi General Practitioner, Obstet Gynec Dept-Università, Varese, Italy

Marino Romero Ramírez Department of Obstetrics and Gynecology, Consorci Sanitari de Terrassa, Terrassa, Spain

Diego Riva IRCCS Humanitas Research Hospital, Humanitas San Pio X, Milan, Italy

Ana Teresa Roberto-Alcacer Department of Surgery, University of Salamanca, Salamanca, Spain

Marcos Torres Roca Clínica Universidad de Navarra, Pamplona, Spain

Esther García Rojo Urology Department, Hospital Universitario 12 De Octubre, Madrid, Spain

Santiago Chiva San Román Clínica Universidad de Navarra, Pamplona, Spain

Stefano Rosadi Department of Urology, Pelvic Unit, San Donato Hospital, Arezzo, Italy

Cristina Rossi ASL Alessandria, Ospedale San Giacomo Di Novi Ligure, Dipartimento Di Urologia, Novi Ligure, Italy

Thuane Da Roza Laboratory of Biomechanics, Center for Health and Sports Sciences (CEFID), Universidade do Estado de Santa Catarina (UDESC), Florianópolis, Brazil

Laia Sabiote Rubio Fundació Puigvert, Barcelona, Spain

Cristina Gutierrez-Ruiz Fundació Puigvert, Barcelona, Spain

Mercedes Ruiz Urology Department, Hospital Ramón y Cajal, Madrid, Spain

Urška Eržen Rupnik Community Health Centre Idrija, Idrija, Slovenia

Department of Gynecology, University Medical Centre Ljubljana, Ljubljana, Slovenia

Cristina Salvatierra-Pérez Department of Urology, Hospital Universitario San Pedro, Logroño, Spain

Andrew Sammut Department of Obstetrics and Gynaecology, Mater Dei, Hospital, Triq Dun Karm, Msida, MSD, Malta

Alvaro Sánchez Urology Department, Hospital Ramón y Cajal, Madrid, Spain

Alfonso Sánchez-Escudero Grupo De Investigación Multidisciplinar Urológico Renal (GRUMUR), Instituto de Investigación Biomédica De Salamanca (IBSAL), Salamanca, Spain

Jordi Moreno Sánchez Department of Obstetrics and Gynecology, Consorci Sanitari de Terrassa, Terrassa, Spain

Sandro Sandri Asst Ovest Milanese, Ospedale Fornaroli Di Magenta, Magenta, Italy

Marta Santiago Urology Department, Hospital Ramón y Cajal, Madrid, Spain

Miguel Ángel Barranco Sanz Urology Department, Hospital de Mataró, Barcelona, Spain

Alejandro Sanz-Ruiz Department of Urology, Complejo Asistencial Universitario de León, León, Spain

Mehmet Murat Seval Department of Obstetrics and Gynecology, Ankara University School of Medicine, Cebeci Hospital, Ankara, Turkey

Department of Obstetrics and Gynecology, Ankara University School of Medicine, Ankara, Turkey

Faculty of Health Science, Physiotherapy and Rehabilitation Department, Atılım University, Ankara, Turkey

Cristóbal Ramírez Sevilla Urology Department, Hospital de Mataró, Barcelona, Spain

Emel Sönmezer Faculty of Health Science, Physiotherapy and Rehabilitation Department, Atılım University, Ankara, Turkey

Hatzilia Sophia Urogynecology Unit, National and Kapodistrian University, Athens, Greece

Alejandro Sousa-Escandón Department of Urology, Hospital de Monforte de Lemos, Lugo, Spain

Kristina Drusany Starič Division of Gynecology and Obstertrics, Department of Gynecology, Medical Faculty, University Medical Centre Ljubljana, University of Ljubljana, Ljubljana, Slovenia

Univerzitetni Klinicni Center Ljubljana, Ginekološka Klinika, Ljubljana, University of Ljubljana, Medical Faculty, Ljubljana, Slovenia

Univerzitetni Klinicni Center Ljubljana, Ginekološka Klinika, Ljubljana, Slovenia

Athanasiou Stavros Urogynecology Unit, National and Kapodistrian University, Athens, Greece

Mateo Hevia Suárez Clínica Universidad de Navarra, Pamplona, Spain

Raquel Sopeña-Sutil Hospital Universitario 12 de Octubre, Urología, Madrid, Spain

Fulya Tekşen Department of Medical Biology, Ankara University School of Medicine, Ankara, Turkey

Grigoriadis Themos Urogynecology Unit, National and Kapodistrian University, Athens, Greece

Luca Timossi Ospedale Evangelico Internazionale, Dipartimento Di Urologia, Genova, Italy

Merve Toy Department of Obstetrics and Gynecology, Ankara University School of Medicine, Ankara, Turkey

Bulut Varlı Department of Obstetrics and Gynecology, Ankara University School of Medicine, Cebeci Hospital, Ankara, Turkey

Department of Obstetrics and Gynecology, Ankara University School of Medicine, Ankara, Turkey

Alberto Vella Department of Obstetrics and Gynaecology, Mater Dei, Hospital, Triq Dun Karm, Msida, MSD, Malta

Manuel José Vicente-Arroyo Grupo De Investigación Multidisciplinar Urológico Renal (GRUMUR), Instituto de Investigación Biomédica De Salamanca (IBSAL), Salamanca, Spain

Vanessa Viegas Urology Department, Hospital La Princesa, Madrid, Spain

Albert Font Vilamitjana Department of Obstetrics and Gynecology, Consorci Sanitari de Terrassa, Terrassa, Spain

Erdal Yucel Department of Obstetrics and Gynecology, Zeynep Kamil Women and Children Diseases Training and Research Hospital, Istanbul, Turkey

Erdal Yucel Department of Obstetrics and Gynecology, Zeynep Kamil Women and Children Diseases Training and Research Hospital, Istanbul, Turkey

Vita Zacesta Riga Stradins University, Riga, Latvia

Dipartimento di Ginecologia e Ostetricia, Ente Ospedaliero Cantonale, Bellinzona, Switzerland

Part I

Female Incontinence

Impact of Urinary Incontinence on Quality of Life

1

Andrew Sammut and Alberto Vella

1.1 Literature Review

UI has been estimated to affect approximately 21.6% of the worldwide population by 2018 [1]. The association between obesity, DM, and LUTS has been implicated not only in humans but also in animal models [2–4]. In the latter, the underlying pathophysiology was found to be related to vesical urothelial proliferation and urethral fibrosis [2, 5]. Further supporting the link between obesity and UI is the fact that surgical and nonsurgical weight loss has been shown to subjectively and objectively improve SUI and/or UUI [6–8]. The associations between various metabolic abnormalities and LUTS and their effect on quality of life (QoL) have not been adequately researched until recent years. More research is needed in these fields in order to put more light on these associations. A literature search was conducted using PubMed. The following keywords were used: 'ICIQ short form', 'menopause', 'metabolic syndrome', 'urinary incontinence', and 'quality of life'. No date or language limits were included. The collated literature was analysed and separated into two groups: literature pertaining to biochemical variables in relation to UI in women and literature pertaining to QoL in relation to UI in women. Numerous studies were published in relation to different metabolic factors, QoL, and UI.

1.1.1 The Metabolic Syndrome

Obesity is a well-known risk factor for multiple medical conditions, including DM; ischaemic heart disease; cerebrovascular accidents; malignancies; respiratory conditions, such as sleep apnoea; musculoskeletal conditions; and LUTS [9–13]. The MetS is a constellation of abnormal anthropometric and biochemical markers of which insulin resistance of varying degrees forms the common underlying pathophysiology [14]. Other abnormalities include central obesity, atherogenic dyslipidaemia, hypertension (HT), hyperuricaemia, as well as pro-inflammatory and prothrombotic states [10, 15]. This constellation of abnormalities is well-known to predispose to cardiovascular disease and DM [14, 15]. The MetS has also been linked to various urologic conditions, such as urolithiasis, LUTS, and female incontinence [16–20]. In recent years, the MetS has been assigned different diagnostic criteria by various expert groups. The three most accepted worldwide definitions of the MetS have been formulated by the World Health Organization (WHO); the European Group for the Study of Insulin Resistance (EGIR); and the National Cholesterol Education Programme—Adult Treatment Panel III (NCEP-ATP III) [21]. Whilst

A. Sammut (✉) · A. Vella
Department of Obstetrics and Gynaecology, Mater Dei, Hospital, Triq Dun Karm, Msida, MSD, Malta
e-mail: andrew-paul.sammut@gov.mt; alberto.vella@gov.mt

F. Dökmeci, D. E. E. Rizk (eds.), *Insights Into Incontinence and the Pelvic Floor*,
https://doi.org/10.1007/978-3-030-94174-1_1

the definitions formulated by the WHO and the EGIR have insulin resistance of varying degrees as a pre-requisite for the initial diagnosis of the MetS in their definition, the same cannot be said for the definition of the MetS by the NCEP-ATP III. The criteria to diagnose the MetS as defined by the NCEP-ATP III includes any three of the following metabolic variables: raised fasting plasma glucose (≥5.6 mmol/L), HT, low HDL cholesterol levels, hypertriglyceridemia, and increased waist circumference. Notes are made of the lower thresholds given by the NCEP-ATP III for DM (≥5.6 mmol/L), hyperlipidaemia, and HT, compared to those of the WHO. Conversely, a higher threshold for waist circumference is provided by the WHO compared to the NCEP-ATP III. Moreover, the WHO is the only organisation which includes a raised urinary albumin-creatinine excretion ratio as a possible criterion to diagnose the MetS. With all these different diagnostic criteria by different working groups, the International Diabetes Federation (IDF) decided to come out with a single worldwide definition of the MetS. A workshop was convened in London, UK, in May 2004 where experts and representatives from the five continents formulated a worldwide definition. A consensus was reached and the following were the agreed criteria on which to diagnose the MetS: ethnic- and gender-specific waist circumferences, or a BMI of ≥30 kg/m^2, and any other two metabolic abnormalities which include HT, hypertriglyceridemia, low HDL cholesterol, or a raised fasting plasma glucose level.

1.1.2 The Metabolic Syndrome and Lower Urinary Tract Dysfunction

Irwin et al. [22] in the EPIC study, a population-based study involving Canada, Germany, Italy, Sweden, and the UK, pointed out the high prevalence of LUTS. In a random sample of men and women aged ≥18 years living in one of these countries, the prevalence of storage, voiding, and post-voiding LUTS was calculated. LUTS was highly prevalent in women of ≥40 years (66.6%). In this study, nocturia was highly prevalent in women (54.5%), whilst the prevalence of storage LUTS in women stood at a staggering 59.2%. The high prevalence of nocturia in women in this study was related to the definition used in this study as outlined by the International Continence Society (ICS). The ICS defines nocturia as the complaint of waking up one or more times at night [23]. Upon changing the definition of nocturia from one to two micturitions per night, the prevalence of LUTS in women fell down to 24%. Conversely, the prevalence of voiding LUTS in women stood at 19.5%. The prevalence of LUTS was found to increase with age. The limitations of this study included the use of self-reports, the mode of administration of the questionnaire, and the rate of response by invitees to the questionnaire.

The Look AHEAD study was a large-scale cross-sectional study conducted by Phelan et al. [24]. In this randomised clinical trial, 2994 overweight or obese women with type 2 DM, between 45 and 76 years, were enrolled. The prevalence of weekly UI was as high as 27%, superseding the prevalence of common complications of DM, such as retinopathy (7.5%), microalbuminuria (2.2%), and neuropathy (1.5%). Women with a BMI of ≥35 kg/m^2 had a higher prevalence of UI, particularly SUI, when compared to non-obese women. Women with a higher BMI were more likely to be postmenopausal or on oestrogen replacement or had undergone a hysterectomy. Moreover, incontinent women showed a tendency to be older and poor in their physical and psychological well-being. They were also more likely to be current or former smokers. Parity, BP, and cardiovascular disease were not shown to be any different in the prevalence of UI in women. Multivariable logistic regression models were used to analyse risk factors. Non-Hispanic white women, prior hysterectomy, and urinary tract infections increased the odds of UI. BMI of 35–39 kg/m^2 and of ≥40 kg/m^2 were associated with an odds ratio (OR) of 1.65 and 1.84, respectively. Risk factors for UI and UUI included age >70, sleep apnoea, asthma, poor health quality, high waist circumference, and smoking.

Obesity was a key risk factor for SUI in another study conducted by Demir et al. [25].

The study involved 719 women suffering from UI. The participants were compared to risk factors, QoL scores, severity of incontinence, as well as other demographics. Risk factors for SUI in this study included HT, multiparity, a high BMI, and a lower educational level. Mommsen et al. [26] also highlighted the close association between UI and BMI, particularly SUI. In this study, risk factors for UUI were HT and DM.

In the EPICONT study, a cross-sectional, population-based study conducted by Hannestad et al. [27], all women aged ≥20 were invited ($N = 47{,}313$). The participation rate in this study stood at 80% ($n = 27{,}936$). A questionnaire was given to elucidate whether the participants had any form of involuntary urine loss. The participants were also given a severity index scale to classify the severity of urinary incontinence. Formal urodynamics was carried out. Urodynamics has been considered as the 'gold standard' for diagnosing lower urinary tract complaints [28]. The prevalence of UI was 27.6%. BMI; smoking habit status; tea, coffee, and alcohol intake; and the degree of physical exercise were recorded. Cigarette smoking (>20 per day), increasing BMI, and tea-drinking were associated with a higher prevalence of UI. Severe UI was closely related to cigarette smoking, irrespective of the number of cigarettes consumed. In the same study, low-intensity exercise was negatively correlated with UI and therefore beneficial. Conversely, high-intensity exercise, alcohol, and coffee were not found to have a statistically significant effect on the prevalence of UI.

Townsend et al. [29], in a prospective study analysing the relationship between BMI, weight gain, and new-onset UI, found that weight gain and high BMI were strong independent risk factors for the development of UI in middle-aged women of between 37 and 54 years ($p = <0.001$). Women who gained >30 kg compared to those who gained 5.1–10 kg were found to have higher odds for UI (4.04 vs. 1.44). Women with a BMI of ≥35 kg/m^2 were found to have a greater risk of developing at least monthly incontinence when compared to women with a BMI of between 21 and 22.9 kg/m^2 (OR 2.11). Suskind et al. [7], in a prospective observational cohort study involving 1475 elderly women aged between 70 and 79, estimated the prevalence of UI, BMI, and other factors. At 3 years, 28% of women had persistent or new-onset UUI compared to the prevalence of 16% at the onset of the study. On the other hand, the prevalence of SUI remained constant at 14%. Of interest in this study, similar to the study by Townsend et al. [29] but from a different perspective, was the association between weight loss and SUI. The researchers found lower adjusted odds for SUI with a ≥5% loss of BMI (AOR 0.46, $p = 0.1$) or ≥5% fat mass (AOR 0.53, $p = 0.1$).

In another study conducted by Townsend et al. [30], increasing BMI and waist circumference were associated with UI. Raised BMI was associated with UUI and MUI ($p = 0.003$ vs. 0.03), but not SUI ($p = 0.77$). On the other hand, waist circumference was associated with SUI ($p = <0.001$). Elia et al. [9], in a study involving 553 women with LUTS, found that BMI was associated with UI (AOR 1.95; 95% CI 1.18–3.19). Peyrat et al. [31], in a study involving 1700 women, found that UI was highly prevalent in young and middle-aged women (27.5%; 95% CI 25.4–29.7). This prevalence was found to be higher at the age of ≥40 (RR 2.16; 95% CI 1.86–2.57). Other risk factors for UI, particularly SUI, were pregnancy (RR 2.22), previous hysterectomy (RR 1.52), previous vaginal birth (RR 2.15), and postpartum UI (2.57). However, contrary to other studies, obesity and previous caesarean delivery were not found to significantly increase the overall risk of UI.

Danforth et al. [32], in a large-scale study involving participants from two pooled cohorts of women ($N = 71{,}650$) between the ages of 37 and 79, found a significant association between DM and UUI (OR 1.4, 95% CI 1.0–1.9, $p = 0.03$). This association was, however, limited to UUI and not to other types of UI. Moreover, the adjusted odds of incidence of UI in women with DM was found to be 20% more (OR 1.2, 95% CI 1.0–1.3, $p = 0.01$) than in women without DM. Similar to this, in a case-control study conducted by Izci et al. [33] on 1381 women in Turkey, UI was found to be more prevalent in diabetic women (OR 2.5, 95% CI 1.8–3.3; $p = 0.000$). Age (OR 1.02; 95% CI 1.00–1.04;

$p = 0.016$) and BMI (OR 1.07; 95% CI 1.04–1.11; $p = 0.000$) were found to be independent determinants of UI. A significant association was found between diabetes and obese women ($p = 0.003$). Similarly, in a study involving 362 women, Park et al. [34] found that women with the MetS had a 2.5-fold risk for SUI when compared to those without the MetS ($p = <0.001$). Independent risk factors for SUI were found to be BMI (OR 3.574; 95% CI 0.09–0.31, $p < 0.001$) and insulin resistance (OR 2.563; 95% CI 0.04–0.31, $p = 0.011$). Similar findings were noted by Otunctemur et al. [35] in a study involving 400 equally divided pre- and postmenopausal women, with and without the MetS. In this study, once again, SUI was more prevalent in both pre- and postmenopausal women ($p = 0.001$ vs. $p = <0.001$) with the MetS. Elevated glucose levels and waist circumference were significantly associated with SUI ($p < 0.05$).

Diabetic cystopathy is a form of bladder dysfunction in patients with DM. It is characterised by voiding dysfunction, lower urine peak flow rates, high post-residual volumes, decreased bladder compliance, and a higher percentage of bladder-outflow obstruction resulting in overflow incontinence [36]. Karoli et al. [37] studied 102 women with DM and LUTS in a cross-sectional study. Storage and voiding scores in women with DM were found to be higher when compared to age- and BMI-matched controls. In this study, the presence of the MetS was correlated to LUTS (OR 2.6, 95% CI 0.98–1.12; $p = 0.02$) and OAB (OR 3.2, 95% CI 1.60–5.80; $p = 0.01$). However, only HT was found to be associated with these urological conditions. In the study conducted by Tai et al. [38], the relationship between the MetS, LUTS, and OAB was further strengthened. In their study, involving 518 women divided into MetS and non-MetS groups, the MetS group had a higher post-void residual urine volume compared to the non-MetS group. The MetS was strongly correlated to LUTS and OAB. HT, hypertriglyceridemia, and low HDL cholesterol were independently associated with LUTS and OAB. Furthermore, peripheral neuropathy was associated with LUTS in women with DM. In a community-based, cross-sectional, nationwide study involving 2025 women in Sri Lanka, Pathiraja et al. [39] found that DM (OR 1.97; 95% CI 1.19–3.23) and parity (OR 1.1; 95%CI 1.02–1.21) were risk factors for UI. Jackson et al. [40], in a cross-sectional analysis of a population-based study involving 1017 women aged 55–75 years, found that diabetic women reported more severe incontinence, particularly MUI. Moreover, the duration of diabetes, treatment type, peripheral neuropathy, and retinopathy were correlated with severe incontinence. However, the strength of this observation was weakened upon introducing BMI on multiple regression. In a study conducted by Hong et al. [41], a strong correlation between age and LUTS was found. Congruent to the study conducted by Tai et al. [38], an association between hypertriglyceridemia and LUTS was noted.

Schreiber Pedersen et al. [42] further supported the link between MetS and UI in a large-scale study involving 8000 women in two regions in Germany and Denmark. The prevalence of SUI was more common in younger women. On the other hand, UUI and MUI were found to be more common in women over 80 years of age. The prevalence of UI, mostly of the mixed type, was found to be the highest (67.3%) in women with a BMI of ≥ 35 kg/m^2. Once more, age, BMI, and vaginal deliveries were significantly associated with UI.

1.1.3 Urinary Incontinence and Menopause

Postmenopausal women are known to be more prone to LUTS, including recurrent urinary tract infections and UI [43]. In the HERS study, a large-scale study involving 2763 postmenopausal women with a mean age of 67 years, Brown et al. [44] reported a prevalence of 56% of women experiencing weekly UI. In this study, SUI was significantly more common in obese postmenopausal women. Conversely, older and diabetic women reported a higher prevalence of UUI. In another study involving 1584 women with different racial backgrounds, Jackson et al. [45] found that UUI was associated with oral oestrogen use,

Caucasian women, arthritis, as well as decreased physical activity. Factors for SUI included Caucasian women, arthritis, chronic obstructive airway disease, oral oestrogen use, as well as a high BMI. Oral and vaginal oestrogens were reported to be associated with any type of UI in the study by Jackson et al. [40]. This is in contrast to the latest guidelines issued by the EAU, who advocate the use of vaginal oestrogens in women with urinary incontinence secondary to vulvovaginal atrophy [19].

1.1.4 Quality of Life in Women with Urinary Incontinence

UI is a multifactorial, complex medical condition which can exert psychological, social, and emotional sequelae, thus affecting patients' QoL [46, 47]. In 1998, the first International Consultation on Incontinence meeting, organised by the ICS and the International Consultation on Urological Diseases, was held in Monaco [48]. The rationale behind this meeting was to develop a universally acceptable tool in the form of a questionnaire to be used in the clinical and research fields pertaining to the field of UI. The scientific committee developed the first modular questionnaire: the ICIQ-UI Short Form questionnaire [49] (see Appendix). The ICIQ-UI Short Form questionnaire is a concise and robust questionnaire which can be easily completed by physicians and patients alike [50, 51]. When compared to the King's Health Questionnaire, which is another tool used to assess QoL of patients with UI, the ICIQ-UI Short Form was found to be more feasible and easy to use [52, 53]. It specifically focuses on the frequency, severity, and impact on QoL of male and female patients with UI. Further, the questionnaire can be used in both clinical and research fields. It consists of four sets of questions. The first three questions of this self-administered tool cover the following areas: frequency of incontinence, perceived amount of incontinence, and the degree of interference in life. The fourth question defines the type of UI: SUI, UUI, and MUI. The sum of the first three questions contributes towards the final score with the possible minimum score being 0 and the maximum being 21. A score of 1–5 denotes slight interference; a score of 6–12 denotes moderate interference; a score of 13–18 denotes severe interference; whilst a score of 19–21 denotes very severe interference in activities of daily living [54]. The English version of the ICIQ-UI short form questionnaire underwent rigorous testing in order to ensure its validity and reliability [49].

The ICIQ-UI Short Form questionnaire has been used in numerous studies evaluating patient urinary symptoms, severity, and QoL, as well as to outline the effect of conservative and surgical urogynaecological treatments. In a prospective study involving 18 male and 42 female patients, Seckiner et al. [55] found that the ICIQ-UI Short Form compared to formal urodynamics was practical and reliable in evaluating patients with UUI. In another study conducted by Karantanis et al. [56], the ICIQ-UI Short Form questionnaire was compared to the 24-h pad test diary loss and other tests in women with USI. Strong correlations were observed between the questionnaire and the 24-h pad test, thus providing evidence of the possible widespread use of the questionnaire to measure outcomes in patients with SUI. In a study conducted by Simsek et al. [57], the QoL and sexual function of women with SUI pre- and post-transobturator tape insertion were assessed. The study found significant improvement in the ICIQ-UI Short Form scores, thus better QoL. Conversely, women who sustained UI post-procedure reported higher scores, thus a reduction in overall QoL. Another study parallel to this was carried out in Italy by Meschia et al. [58]: 206 women who underwent the insertion of a single-incision mid-urethral sling were assessed post-procedure. At 1-year post-procedure, the ICIQ-UI Short Form questionnaire was used to assess the mean improvement of symptoms post-procedure. In this study, procedure failure was found to be significantly more in obese women. The ICIQ-UI Short Form questionnaire was used in yet another study analysing outcome measures post-surgical procedures for women with SUI and MUI. In a multicentre prospective cohort study involving 277 women, Diez-Itza et al. [59]

Initial number

ICIQ-UI Short Form

CONFIDENTIAL

DAY MONTH YEAR

Today's date

Many people leak urine some of the time. We are trying to find out how many people leak urine, and how much this bothers them. We would be grateful if you could answer the following questions, thinking about how you have been, on average, over the PAST FOUR WEEKS.

1 Please write in your date of birth: DAY MONTH YEAR

2 Are you *(tick one)***:** Female ☐ Male ☐

3 How often do you leak urine? *(Tick one box)*

never	☐	0
about once a week or less often	☐	1
two or three times a week	☐	2
about once a day	☐	3
several times a day	☐	4
all the time	☐	5

4 We would like to know how much urine you think leaks.
How much urine do you usually leak (whether you wear protection or not)?
(Tick one box)

none	☐	0
a small amount	☐	2
a moderate amount	☐	4
a large amount	☐	6

5 Overall, how much does leaking urine interfere with your everyday life?
Please ring a number between 0 (not at all) and 10 (a great deal)

0 1 2 3 4 5 6 7 8 9 **10**
not at all — a great deal

ICIQ score: sum scores 3+4+5 ☐☐

6 When does urine leak? *(Please tick all that apply to you)*

- never – urine does not leak ☐
- leaks before you can get to the toilet ☐
- leaks when you cough or sneeze ☐
- leaks when you are asleep ☐
- leaks when you are physically active/exercising ☐
- leaks when you have finished urinating and are dressed ☐
- leaks for no obvious reason ☐
- leaks all the time ☐

Thank you very much for answering these questions.

found that the change in ICIQ scores positively correlated with the degree of satisfaction.

In a classic study conducted by Abrams et al. [60], 1203 women with UI in the UK, France, Germany, and the USA participated in a survey which assessed symptoms and impact of UI on activities of daily living, QoL, and psychological well-being. Results showed that the amount of urine leaks as perceived by the respondents positively associated with the ICIQ-UI Short Form scores. Psychological well-being was found to be negatively associated with QoL scores.

Martinez Franco et al. [61] used the ICIQ-UI Short Form questionnaire to calculate the prevalence of UI in pregnant women in their first and third trimester, as well as to figure out which type of UI was the most common. The study revealed that over a third of pregnant women who participated in the study complained of UI, mainly SUI (48.05%). Two hundred and eighteen women with SUI participated in a study which involved the use of pelvic floor muscle therapy (PFMT). Nystrom et al. [62] reported improved ICIQ scores by women with SUI after 4 months of PFMT.

Timmermans et al. [63] utilised the ICIQ-UI Short Form questionnaire to formulate a way on how to rate a patient's permanent impairment. This was done by comparing ICIQ scores of 120 patients to their actual urodynamic diagnosis. The researchers found that the ICIQ score and age were independent predictors of urodynamic incontinence, thus further strengthening the validity of the ICIQ-UI Short Form questionnaire as an impairment-rating tool.

1.2 Case Study: Anthropometric and Psychosocial Impacts on Maltese Women with Urinary Incontinence

(a) **Aim and Scope**

The aims of this study are to assess whether there is any relationship between various metabolic parameters, such as HT, DM, and BMI, and the different types of UI in women referred to the urodynamics' clinic at Mater Dei Hospital, Msida, Malta. Moreover, the severity of UI in this cohort of women was also studied.

(b) **Study Design and Material Methods**

A cross-sectional design was chosen for this study. The scope behind this study design was to take a snapshot of the women referred for urodynamic studies at the urodynamics clinic situated at the Antenatal and Gynaecology Outpatients' department of Mater Dei Hospital. All women who were referred for urodynamic studies between February 2016 and July 2016 were invited to participate. Participants with a history of neurological problems, such as cerebrovascular accidents or multiple sclerosis, mobility problems, or evidence of a urinary tract infection were excluded from the study, with the latter being prescribed empirical antibiotic therapy. Participants who were already on oral treatment for OAB, such as oxybutynin, or SUI, such as duloxetine, were excluded from the study. These drugs are known to affect the results of invasive urodynamics. The total number of women who met a pre-defined set of criteria, and who were subsequently invited to participate in the study, stood at 120 ($N = 120$). The percentage of women who met the criteria and accepted the invitation to participate in this study was 85% ($n = 102$).

(c) **Results of the Study**

In this study, the total number of women who were invited to participate was 120 ($N = 120$). The percentage of women who accepted the invitation to participate in this study following informed consent stood at 85% ($n = 102$). The mean age was 55 years with a range of between 31 and 87 years.

1.2.1 Types of Urinary Incontinence

Out of 102 women ($n = 102$) who accepted to participate in this study, 23.5% ($n = 24$) had OAB syndrome, 33.3% ($n = 34$) had SUI, 41.2% ($n = 42$) had MUI, whilst 2% had other diagnoses. The definitions used were those outlined by the ICS. The diagnoses were obtained from the history and clinical examination at the time of the urodynamic investigation.

1.2.2 Components of the Metabolic Syndrome

The weight and height of the participants were taken using a stadiometer combined with a digital weighing scale. The BMI was calculated using the following formula: weight (Kg) divided by the height $(m)^2$. A body mass index ≥ 30 kg/m^2 was taken as a major pre-requisite to diagnose the MetS, as defined by the new worldwide definition of the MetS by the International Diabetes Federation [21]. The number of women who met this criteria ($n = 67$) stood at 65.7% of the women participating in the study. The rest of the population under study ($n = 35$; 34.33%) had a BMI of <30 kg/m^2.

1.2.3 Hyperlipidaemia

Fasting serum samples were taken to assess for the presence of hyperlipidaemia. Fasting was defined as no caloric intake for 12 h [64]. Women who were already on lipid-lowering agents, such as statins or fibrates, were considered as having satisfied this criteria. Hyperlipidaemia was defined as either a low serum HDL cholesterol or the presence of hypertriglyceridemia. The cut-off values for diagnosis were as those listed in the worldwide consensus definition issued by the International Diabetes Federation [21]. The study population consisted of 29 ($n = 29$; 28.4%) women who had either hyperlipidaemia or were already on lipid-lowering agents. The number of women who had normal serum HDL cholesterol and/or triglyceride level stood at 71.6% ($n = 73$).

1.2.4 Diabetes

Fasting plasma samples were withdrawn to screen for the presence of DM. Fasting was defined as no caloric intake for at least 8 h. A plasma glucose level of ≥ 5.6 mmol/L was considered to be a pre-requisite to diagnose the MetS [21]. Participants who were either on oral hypoglycaemic agents, such as metformin, and/or insulin, and/or diet in view of a known diagnosis of DM, were considered as having satisfied the criteria for the MetS. The number of women who had DM stood at 38.2% of the population under study ($n = 39$). The number of women who were euglycaemic stood at 61.7% of the population under study ($n = 63$).

1.2.5 Hypertension

The blood pressure of the participants was measured using an aneroid sphygmomanometer, using the appropriate cuff size according to the circumference of the participant's arm, with the arm well-supported and at the level of the heart. Participants who were already on any antihypertensive treatment were considered to satisfy the criteria of the MetS. The ratio of women who were found to be hypertensive ($n = 51$) to the proportion who were normotensive ($n = 51$) was equal.

1.2.6 The Metabolic Syndrome

The number of women who had a high BMI and two or more other metabolic disturbances was considered as having met the criteria to diagnose the MetS. This population stood at 35.3% ($n = 36$) of the population under study. The number of women who had less than two biochemical abnormalities, irrespective of their BMI, were considered not to have the MetS. This population stood at 64.7% ($n = 66$) of the population under study.

1.2.7 Menopausal Status

The menopausal status of the participants was also studied. The participants ($n = 102$) were stratified according to whether they were premenopausal or menopausal. The menopause was defined as secondary amenorrhoea for 12 consecutive months. In this study, 29.4% ($n = 30$) of participants were pre-menopausal, whilst 70.6% ($n = 72$) were postmenopausal.

1.2.8 Normal and Instrumental Vaginal Deliveries

The proportion of women under study who gave a history of a previous normal vaginal delivery stood at 80.4% ($n = 82$). The proportion of women who did not give a history of a previous normal vaginal delivery stood at 19.6% ($n = 20$). The proportion of women under study who gave a history of a previous instrumental delivery in their reproductive years stood at 2.9% ($n = 3$), whilst the proportion of women who did not give a history of a previous instrumental delivery stood at 97.1% ($n = 99$).

1.2.9 ICIQ-UI Short Form Scores

The participants in this study were asked to grade the perceived severity of UI as per questions 3–5 of the ICIQ-UI Short Form questionnaire. The majority of women, 40.2% ($n = 41$), experienced moderate interference in life secondary to UI, with a score of between 6 and 12 on the questionnaire. The number of women who classified the degree of interference of UI as being severe amounted to 27.5% ($n = 28$). Slight interference was reported by 20.6% ($n = 21$) of women, whilst 11.7% ($n = 12$) of women reported very severe interference by their condition.

1.3 Statistical Analysis

The data in this study was analysed using the following statistical tests: Chi-squared test, Fisher's exact test, Kappa, Mann-Whitney U test, and the T-test for univariate analyses. Multiple linear regression models were used to assess for multiple variables which were found to be statistically significant. SPSS version 20 was used. Statistical significance was set at 0.05 level.

The level of agreement between clinical diagnosis of the participants and the urodynamic diagnosis was analysed using Kappa statistics. Patients who complained of mixed-urinary symptoms had a very good level of agreement when compared to the urodynamic diagnosis (Kappa coefficient 0.960). On the other hand, there was a fair level of agreement in patients who presented with SUI (Kappa coefficient 0.329) and a moderate level of agreement in patients who presented with OAB symptoms (Kappa coefficient 0.430). The presence of the different types of UI in women in this study was analysed according to whether women were pre- or postmenopausal. The prevalence of OAB syndrome was not found to be significantly more in postmenopausal women. Contrary to this, the prevalence SUI and MUI was found to be significantly more in postmenopausal women (Fisher's exact 0.000 vs. 0.041).

The presence of SUI was analysed against the different constituents of the MetS. HT and hyperlipidaemia were not significantly higher in women with SUI. Contrary to this, DM was found to be significantly higher in women with SUI (Fisher's exact test 0.000; p value <0.000).

The presence of OAB syndrome was analysed against metabolic factors of the MetS. HT and hyperlipidaemia were once again not found to be statistically significant in women with OAB syndrome. However, DM was once again found to be statistically more prevalent in women with OAB syndrome (Pearson Chi-square 0.005; p value 0.004). The presence of various metabolic parameters of the MetS was then analysed in women with MUI type of UI. However, no statistical significance was reached.

The women under study had their mean BMI analysed according to the type of UI. The T-test statistical test was carried out to assess whether there exists any statistical significance between the prevalence of either type of UI in women with a BMI of ≥ 30 kg/m^2 and those with a BMI <30 kg/m^2. In this study, no statistically significant relationship was found between UI of any type and BMI.

The relationship between various metabolic factors and the mean cystometric capacity was analysed. Women with hyperlipidaemia were found to have a significantly lower mean cystometric capacity than those with normal serum HDL cholesterol and/or serum triglyceride levels (mean difference −76.484; 95% confidence interval −134.473 to −18.495). No significant associations were found in the mean cystometric capacity in hypertensive, diabetic, or menopausal women.

The women with a history of a previous normal vaginal delivery were analysed to see whether there was any relationship to the type of UI they were experiencing. Fisher's exact test was carried out to analyse the data. In this study, a statistically significant association was found between women who had a previous history of a normal vaginal delivery and USI. The participants were then analysed to check whether a history of previous instrumental delivery was associated with any type of UI. Statistical analysis using Mann-Whitney U test revealed no statistical significance between any type of UI and a history of instrumental delivery.

The different types of UI and the corresponding ICIQ-UI Short Form scores were analysed to check for any statistically different score between the different types of UI. No statistical significance was observed between the different types of UI and the ICIQ-UI Short Form scores.

Multiple linear regression models were applied to check for any confounding variables with respect to SUI against DM and menopause. In this study, DM and the menopause were found to be independent risk factors for the development of SUI. Moreover, the odds of women with DM to develop SUI was found to be approximately 6.5 (OR 6.603, 95% CI 2.037–21.404), whilst the odds of menopausal women to develop SUI was approximately 3.5 (OR 3.448; 95% CI 1.305–9.109).

1.4 Discussion

The aims of this study were to analyse the biological risk factors that are affecting women being referred to the urodynamic clinic at the antenatal and gynaecology outpatients' department at Mater Dei Hospital as well as to shed light on the severity of UI experienced by women being referred for urodynamics.

1.4.1 Urinary Incontinence and Body Mass Index

According to the European Health Interview Survey, carried out by the EUROSTAT between 2013 and 2015, in 2014, 55.2% of Maltese women aged ≥18 were overweight (BMI ≥25–<30 kg/m^2) [65]. The same survey showed that the proportion of obese (BMI ≥30 kg/m^2) women stood at 23.9%, the highest amongst the 28 member states of the EU [65]. In 2014, the standardised death rates (per 100,000 inhabitants) for circulatory diseases, heart disease, and cancer of the uterus in Malta were higher than the average in the 28 member states of the EU [65]. Circulatory diseases, heart disease, and cancer of the uterus all share common risk factors. The risk factors which are common to these diseases include obesity and diabetes, which are the core risk factors for the development of the MetS. In this study, over a 6-month period, 65.7% of women who were referred for urodynamics were considered obese. Multiple studies have associated a high BMI, particularly central adiposity, with UI, with a predilection for MUI and SUI. In this study, however, no statistical significance was reached when analysing the mean BMI to the different types of UI.

1.4.2 Urinary Incontinence and Metabolic Factors

Data retrieved from the latest Atlas of the IDF revealed that in 2013, the estimated national prevalence of DM in Malta stood at 13.9%, with a range of between 7.9 and 17.1% [66]. Further to this, the report issued by Foundation of European Nurses in Diabetes (FEND) group in 2014 stated that this prevalence rate in Malta is envisaged to rise to a total of 36,810 individuals by 2035 [67]. Univariate analysis in this study has shown a statistically significant association between DM and the presence of SUI (0.000, $p = <0.000$) and OAB syndrome (0.005, $p = 0.004$). Multiple linear regression models in this study have shown that DM is an independent risk factor for SUI (OR 6.603; $p = 0.002$; 95% confidence interval: 2.037–21.404). Multiple studies have outlined this association. Gorbachinsky et al. [17] postulated that UUI is caused by increased vesical contractions with subsequent increased urgency. A reduction in vesical capacity was also postulated, resulting in frequency [17]. Diabetes is thought to increase the expression of muscarinic receptor with subsequent increase in sensitivity. This increased sensitivity results in OAB syndrome [17]. Meng et al. [68] pointed out three possible underlying factors for the development of OAB: factors related to intrinsic detrusor factors; neural factors; as well as urothelial factors. Amarenco et al. [69] postulated that chronic hyperglycaemia may have an effect of the pelvic parasympathetic ganglia with subsequent storage LUTS. In an animal model, Lee et al. [70] postulated the association between DM and vesical sensory dysfunction. Lee et al., in a study involving fructose-fed mice ($n = 120$), found that these mice exhibited increased provoked vesical contractions, as well as a significant decrease in mean vesical capacity, compared to controls ($n = 50$). An increase in vesical urothelial proteins, such as transient receptor potential vanilloid 1 and P2X3, and decrease in endothelial nitric oxide synthase were observed in fructose-fed mice. This imbalance resulted in bladder dysfunction. In relation to the study by Lee et al., the current study also found a significant decrease in the mean cystometric capacity in relation to the MetS, specifically to hyperlipidaemia. This finding can be explained in relation to the pro-inflammatory state that is present in patients with the MetS [17]. Gorbachinsky et al. pointed out that pelvic ischaemia promotes detrusor hypertrophy which in turn results in OAB. In two separate animal studies, Liu et al. [4] and Yoshida et al. [3] pointed out the association between chronic hyperlipidaemia and detrusor overactivity. In a randomised controlled study by Liu et al. involving 30 rabbits, hyperlipidaemic rabbits were shown to exhibit increased detrusor contractions on urodynamics, compared to control. Moreover, microscopic examination of the internal iliac arteries showed mild fibrosis, a thickened intima, as well as distortion of the endothelium. Analogous to the findings in the study by Lee et al., the expression of detrusor muscarinic receptors was found to be higher in the hyperlipidaemic group. In a similar randomised controlled study by Yoshida et al., hyperlipidaemic rabbits were found to exhibit LUTS similar to the OAB syndrome. In this study, cystometric studies on hyperlipidaemic rabbits showed low voiding pressures, a decrease in the micturition time, as well as a decrease in voiding urinary volumes. Analogous to the study by Liu et al., atherosclerosis and intima-wall thickening were found on microscopy. Further to this, histological examination of the detrusor muscle revealed a thin urothelium and a decrease in detrusor muscle area.

1.4.3 Urinary Incontinence and Parturition

This study pointed out the significant relationship between vaginal birth and SUI. Women who had a vaginal delivery, but not instrumental, were found to suffer from USI significantly more than nulliparous women or women who had had a caesarean section (0.050; $p = 0.028$). Vaginal birth, particularly if prolonged or involves instrumentation, is known to increase the risk of SUI secondary to damage to the pelvic floor musculature and innervation to varying degrees. This, in turn, results in a greater risk of pelvic-organ prolapse, particularly descent of the bladder with resultant change in the vesico-urethral angle. Intrinsic sphincteric deficiency, which is failure of the sphincter urethrae to adequately maintain a high resistance against the expulsion of urine, is another underlying cause of SUI. Risk factors for this condition include age; menopausal status; congenital disorders, such as central nervous system lesions; as well as vaginal birth [71].

1.4.4 Urinary Incontinence and Menopause

In this study, menopausal women were found to suffer significantly more from MUI (0.041, $p = 0.022$). Moreover, the hypo-oestrogenic state in women in this study has also been found to be an independent risk factor for SUI (OR 3.448; $p = 0.013$; 95% confidence interval 1.305–9.109). The menopause is a known risk factor for UI. This is thought to be secondary to ageing of the pelvic floor with subsequent laxity of the pelvic floor musculature. In an animal study conducted by Rizk et al. [72], ovariectomised rats were administered with oestradiol and ghrelin (growth hormone). Immunohistochemical analysis showed reversal of age-associated pelvic floor changes. In a recently published study analysing the relationship between SUI and hypo-oestrogenic states, Bodner-Adler et al. [73] found that women with SUI had significantly lower serum oestradiol and androstenedione levels than controls, postulating that a hypo-oestrogenic state results in LUTS with resultant SUI.

1.4.5 Urinary Incontinence and Quality of Life

In this study, 20.6% of participants reported slight (score of 1–5) UI severity on the ICIQ-UI Short Form scale. However, 67.7% of participants reported moderate (score of 6–12) or severe (score 13–18) subjective rating of UI, thus leading to a higher impact on QoL. Univariate analysis showed no significant association between the ICIQ-UI Short Form score and the type of UI. Multiple studies have shown that UI results in an inferior QoL with multiple medical, as well as psychosocial, sequelae, such as anxiety and depression [74].

1.4.6 Clinical Diagnosis Versus Urodynamic Diagnosis

Urodynamic investigation is an invaluable tool when used in the correct context. Objective information of the storage and voiding properties of the bladder can be achieved by the use of urodynamic studies [75, 76]. In this study, the level of agreement between the clinical and urodynamic diagnosis was measured using Kappa coefficient. This statistical measure is used specifically to measure the degree to subjective agreement between two or more observers [77]. Fair, moderate, and good agreements were reached in this study with respect to SUI, OAB, and MUI, respectively (0.329 vs. 0.430 vs. 0.960). With its first applications in clinical settings taking place in the late 1950s, urodynamics have long been referred to as the 'gold standard' to objectively diagnose UI, making it pivotal to formulate a diagnosis back then [78–80]. Several studies have analysed the correlation between the clinical and urodynamic diagnosis [80–83]. In 1983, Bolla et al. [80] studied the relationship between clinical and urodynamic diagnosis in a cohort of patients in a hospital in Birmingham, UK. The results of their study favoured the use of urodynamics to achieve clinical diagnosis on the basis that clinical history alone was insufficient and that treatment plans for patients had to be changed following an invasive urodynamic study. Contrary to these findings, Katz et al. [82] found major disagreements between the clinical and urodynamic diagnoses of patients with different lower urinary tract complaints. In a study conducted by Leitner et al. [84] involving healthy subjects with no lower urinary tract complaints, 70% of the subjects under study had an abnormal urodynamic finding.

In recent years, many clinicians and researchers have asked the role urodynamics play in clinical practice and as to when they ought to be performed. Guidelines published by various urological societies have emphasised that urodynamics ought to be carried out only when invasive treatments are being considered [19, 85, 86]. Invasive urodynamic studies should not be carried out on a routine basis, particularly when implementing conservative therapy [75, 87]. Careful considerations must be taken when the clinical history and the urodynamic diagnosis do not correlate, especially in the geriatric population [88]. Judicious use of invasive urodynamics is of utmost importance.

1.5 Conclusion

UI is a common complaint in women of all ages. Multiple risk factors have been attributed to the aetiology of this condition. The metabolic factors which constitute the MetS play a major role in the aetiology of UI. From a local perspective, women being referred to the urodynamics clinic at Mater Dei Hospital share common risk factors attributed to the MetS. In this research study, DM and the menopause have been shown to be independent risk factors for Maltese women with UI. Moreover, the menopause has been shown to be significantly associated with the development of MUI and SUI. Hyperlipidaemia in these women has been shown to decrease the mean cystometric capacity. Vaginal deliveries have been associated with USI. The majority of women being referred to the urodynamic clinic have rated their severity of UI as moderate and severe, thus impeding their QoL. The correlation between the clinical diagnosis of UI and the urodynamic profile has been shown to vary from fair to good, thus indicating an overall good quality of urodynamic interpretation by resident specialists and trainees in the department.

References

1. Irwin DE, Kopp ZS, Agatep B, Milsom I, Abrams P. Worldwide prevalence estimates of lower urinary tract symptoms, overactive bladder, urinary incontinence and bladder outlet obstruction. BJU Int. 2011;108(7):1132–8. https://doi.org/10.1111/j.1464-410X.2010.09993.x.
2. He Q, Babcook MA, Shukla S, Shankar E, Wang Z, Liu G, et al. Obesity-initiated metabolic syndrome promotes urinary voiding dysfunction in a mouse model. Prostate. 2016;76(11):964–76. https://doi.org/10.1002/pros.23185.
3. Yoshida M, Masunaga K, Nagata T, Satoji Y, Shiomi M. The effects of chronic hyperlipidemia on bladder function in myocardial infarction-prone Watanabe heritable hyperlipidemic (WHHLMI) rabbits. Neurourol Urodyn. 2010;29(7):1350–4. https://doi.org/10.1002/nau.20843.
4. Liu XG, Tang Y, Yu W, Wu SL, Jin J. [Effects of diabetic hyperlipidemia on bladder function and its possible mechanisms in a male rabbit model]. Zhonghua Yi Xue Za Zhi. 2013;93(42):3338–42.
5. Gharaee-Kermani M, Rodriguez-Nieves JA, Mehra R, Vezina CA, Sarma AV, Macoska JA. Obesity-induced diabetes and lower urinary tract fibrosis promote urinary voiding dysfunction in a mouse model. Prostate. 2013;73(10):1123–33. https://doi.org/10.1002/pros.22662.
6. Bump RC, Sugerman HJ, Fantl JA, McClish DK. Obesity and lower urinary tract function in women: effect of surgically induced weight loss. Am J Obstet Gynecol. 1992;167(2):392–7; discussion 7–9.
7. Suskind AM, Cawthon PM, Nakagawa S, Subak LL, Reinders I, Satterfield S, et al. Urinary incontinence in older women: the role of body composition and muscle strength: from the health, aging, and body composition study. J Am Geriatr Soc. 2017;65(1):42–50. https://doi.org/10.1111/jgs.14545.
8. Nambiar AK, Bosch R, Cruz F, Lemack GE, Thiruchelvam N, Tubaro A, et al. EAU Guidelines on Assessment and Nonsurgical Management of Urinary Incontinence. Eur Urol. 2018;73(4):596–609. https://doi.org/10.1016/j.eururo.2017.12.031.
9. Elia G, Dye TD, Scariati PD. Body mass index and urinary symptoms in women. Int Urogynecol J Pelvic Floor Dysfunct. 2001;12(6):366–9.
10. Schmitt AC, Cardoso MR, Lopes H, Pereira WM, Pereira EC, de Rezende DA, et al. Prevalence of metabolic syndrome and associated factors in women aged 35 to 65 years who were enrolled in a family health program in Brazil. Menopause. 2013;20(4):470–6. https://doi.org/10.1097/gme.0b013e318272c938.
11. Lean ME. Obesity: burdens of illness and strategies for prevention or management. Drugs Today (Barc). 2000;36(11):773–84.
12. Rubenstein AH. Obesity: a modern epidemic. Trans Am Clin Climatol Assoc. 2005;116:103–11; discussion 12–3.
13. Uzun H, Zorba OU. Metabolic syndrome in female patients with overactive bladder. Urology. 2012;79(1):72–5. https://doi.org/10.1016/j.urology.2011.08.050.
14. Eckel RH, Grundy SM, Zimmet PZ. The metabolic syndrome. Lancet. 2005;365(9468):1415–28. https://doi.org/10.1016/S0140-6736(05)66378-7.
15. Grundy SM, Brewer HB Jr, Cleeman JI, Smith SC Jr, Lenfant C, National Heart L, et al. Definition of metabolic syndrome: report of the National Heart, Lung, and Blood Institute/American Heart Association conference on scientific issues related to definition. Arterioscler Thromb Vasc Biol. 2004;24(2):e13–8. https://doi.org/10.1161/01.ATV.0000111245.75752.C6.
16. Chung HJ, Lin AT, Lin CC, Chen TJ, Chen KK. Patients with urinary incontinence appear more likely to develop upper urinary tract stones: a nationwide, population-based study with 8-year follow-up. PLoS One. 2016;11(8):e0161223. https://doi.org/10.1371/journal.pone.0161223.
17. Gorbachinsky I, Akpinar H, Assimos DG. Metabolic syndrome and urologic diseases. Rev Urol. 2010;12(4):e157–80.

18. Chu KF, Rotker K, Ellsworth P. The impact of obesity on benign and malignant urologic conditions. Postgrad Med. 2013;125(4):53–69. https://doi.org/10.3810/pgm.2013.07.2679.
19. Thuroff JW, Abrams P, Andersson KE, Artibani W, Chapple CR, Drake MJ, et al. EAU guidelines on urinary incontinence. Eur Urol. 2011;59(3):387–400. https://doi.org/10.1016/j.eururo.2010.11.021.
20. Teleman PM, Lidfeldt J, Nerbrand C, Samsioe G, Mattiasson A, WHILA Study Group. Overactive bladder: prevalence, risk factors and relation to stress incontinence in middle-aged women. BJOG. 2004;111(6):600–4. https://doi.org/10.1111/j.1471-0528.2004.00137.x.
21. Alberti KG, Zimmet P, Shaw J. Metabolic syndrome—a new world-wide definition. A Consensus Statement from the International Diabetes Federation. Diabet Med. 2006;23(5):469–80. https://doi.org/10.1111/j.1464-5491.2006.01858.x.
22. Irwin DE, Milsom I, Hunskaar S, Reilly K, Kopp Z, Herschorn S, et al. Population-based survey of urinary incontinence, overactive bladder, and other lower urinary tract symptoms in five countries: results of the EPIC study. Eur Urol. 2006;50(6):1306–14; discussion 14–5. https://doi.org/10.1016/j.eururo.2006.09.019.
23. ICS. In: ICS. https://www.ics.org/glossary. Accessed 11 Feb 2022.
24. Phelan S, Kanaya AM, Subak LL, Hogan PE, Espeland MA, Wing RR, et al. Prevalence and risk factors for urinary incontinence in overweight and obese diabetic women: action for health in diabetes (look ahead) study. Diabetes Care. 2009;32(8):1391–7. https://doi.org/10.2337/dc09-0516.
25. Demir O, Sen V, Irer B, Bozkurt O, Esen A. Prevalence and possible risk factors for urinary incontinence: a cohort study in the City of Izmir. Urol Int. 2017;99(1):84–90. https://doi.org/10.1159/000466705.
26. Mommsen S, Foldspang A. Body mass index and adult female urinary incontinence. World J Urol. 1994;12(6):319–22.
27. Hannestad YS, Rortveit G, Daltveit AK, Hunskaar S. Are smoking and other lifestyle factors associated with female urinary incontinence? The Norwegian EPINCONT Study. BJOG. 2003;110(3):247–54.
28. Nitti VW. Pressure flow urodynamic studies: the gold standard for diagnosing bladder outlet obstruction. Rev Urol. 2005;7(Suppl 6):S14–21.
29. Townsend MK, Danforth KN, Rosner B, Curhan GC, Resnick NM, Grodstein F. Body mass index, weight gain, and incident urinary incontinence in middle-aged women. Obstet Gynecol. 2007;110(2 Pt 1):346–53. https://doi.org/10.1097/01.AOG.0000270121.15510.57.
30. Townsend MK, Curhan GC, Resnick NM, Grodstein F. BMI, waist circumference, and incident urinary incontinence in older women. Obesity. 2008;16(4):881–6. https://doi.org/10.1038/oby.2008.14.
31. Peyrat L, Haillot O, Bruyere F, Boutin JM, Bertrand P, Lanson Y. Prevalence and risk factors of urinary incontinence in young and middle-aged women. BJU Int. 2002;89(1):61–6.
32. Danforth KN, Townsend MK, Curhan GC, Resnick NM, Grodstein F. Type 2 diabetes mellitus and risk of stress, urge and mixed urinary incontinence. J Urol. 2009;181(1):193–7. https://doi.org/10.1016/j.juro.2008.09.007.
33. Izci Y, Topsever P, Filiz TM, Cinar ND, Uludag C, Lagro-Janssen T. The association between diabetes mellitus and urinary incontinence in adult women. Int Urogynecol J Pelvic Floor Dysfunct. 2009;20(8):947–52. https://doi.org/10.1007/s00192-009-0888-8.
34. Park HM, Lee SS, Park CM, Park SM, Park JW, Yi SW, et al. An analysis of the risk factors for metabolic syndrome affecting stress urinary incontinence in Korean middle-aged and older women. Korean J Obstet Gynecol. 2008;51(2):212–9.
35. Otunctemur A, Dursun M, Ozbek E, Sahin S, Besiroglu H, Koklu I, et al. Impact of metabolic syndrome on stress urinary incontinence in pre- and postmenopausal women. Int Urol Nephrol. 2014;46(8):1501–5. https://doi.org/10.1007/s11255-014-0680-7.
36. Ho CH, Tai HC, Yu HJ. Urodynamic findings in female diabetic patients with and without overactive bladder symptoms. Neurourol Urodyn. 2010;29(3):424–7. https://doi.org/10.1002/nau.20727.
37. Karoli R, Bhat S, Fatima J, Priya S. A study of bladder dysfunction in women with type 2 diabetes mellitus. Indian J Endocrinol Metab. 2014;18(4):552–7. https://doi.org/10.4103/2230-8210.137518.
38. Tai HC, Chung SD, Ho CH, Tai TY, Yang WS, Tseng CH, et al. Metabolic syndrome components worsen lower urinary tract symptoms in women with type 2 diabetes. J Clin Endocrinol Metab. 2010;95(3):1143–50. https://doi.org/10.1210/jc.2009-1492.
39. Pathiraja R, Prathapan S, Goonawardena S. Urinary incontinence of women in a nationwide study in Sri Lanka: prevalence and risk factors. Urol J. 2017;14(3):3075–80.
40. Jackson SL, Scholes D, Boyko EJ, Abraham L, Fihn SD. Urinary incontinence and diabetes in postmenopausal women. Diabetes Care. 2005;28(7):1730–8.
41. Hong GS, Shim BS, Chung WS, Yoon H. Correlation between metabolic syndrome and lower urinary tract symptoms of males and females in the aspect of gender-specific medicine: a single institutional study. Korean J Urol. 2010;51(9):631–5. https://doi.org/10.4111/kju.2010.51.9.631.
42. Schreiber Pedersen L, Lose G, Hoybye MT, Elsner S, Waldmann A, Rudnicki M. Prevalence of urinary incontinence among women and analysis of potential risk factors in Germany and Denmark. Acta Obstet Gynecol Scand. 2017;96(8):939–48. https://doi.org/10.1111/aogs.13149.
43. Losada L, Amundsen CL, Ashton-Miller J, Chai T, Close C, Damaser M, et al. Expert panel recommendations on lower urinary tract health of women across

their life span. J Womens Health. 2016;25(11):1086–96. https://doi.org/10.1089/jwh.2016.5895.
44. Brown JS, Grady D, Ouslander JG, Herzog AR, Varner RE, Posner SF. Prevalence of urinary incontinence and associated risk factors in postmenopausal women. Heart & Estrogen/Progestin Replacement Study (HERS) Research Group. Obstet Gynecol. 1999;94(1):66–70.
45. Jackson RA, Vittinghoff E, Kanaya AM, Miles TP, Resnick HE, Kritchevsky SB, et al. Urinary incontinence in elderly women: findings from the Health, Aging, and Body Composition Study. Obstet Gynecol. 2004;104(2):301–7. https://doi.org/10.1097/01.AOG.0000133482.20685.d1.
46. Leroy Lda S, Lopes MH. Urinary incontinence in the puerperium and its impact on the health-related quality of life. Rev Lat Am Enfermagem. 2012;20(2):346–53.
47. Oliveira C, Seleme M, Cansi PF, Consentino RF, Kumakura FY, Moreira GA, et al. Urinary incontinence in pregnant women and its relation with socio-demographic variables and quality of life. Rev Assoc Med Bras. 2013;59(5):460–6. https://doi.org/10.1016/j.ramb.2013.08.002.
48. Abrams P, Avery K, Gardener N, Donovan J, Board IA. The international consultation on incontinence modular questionnaire: www.iciq.net. J Urol. 2006;175(3 Pt 1):1063–6; discussion 6. https://doi.org/10.1016/S0022-5347(05)00348-4.
49. In: Iciq.net. https://iciq.net/wp-content/uploads/2019/08/Sample-ICIQ-UI-Short-Form.pdf. Accessed 11 Feb 2022.
50. Hajebrahimi S, Corcos J, Lemieux MC. International consultation on incontinence questionnaire short form: comparison of physician versus patient completion and immediate and delayed self-administration. Urology. 2004;63(6):1076–8. https://doi.org/10.1016/j.urology.2004.01.005.
51. Avery K, Donovan J, Peters TJ, Shaw C, Gotoh M, Abrams P. ICIQ: a brief and robust measure for evaluating the symptoms and impact of urinary incontinence. Neurourol Urodyn. 2004;23(4):322–30. https://doi.org/10.1002/nau.20041.
52. Espuna Pons M, Castro Diaz D, Carbonell C, Dilla T. [Comparison between the "ICIQ-UI Short Form" Questionnaire and the "King's Health Questionnaire" as assessment tools of urinary incontinence among women]. Actas Urol Esp. 2007;31(5):502–10.
53. Ito H, Hagiwara M, Furuuchi T, Kanai K, Kodaira K, Ninomiya A, et al. [Assessments of quality of life in women with urinary incontinence using: King's Health Questionnaire and International Consultation on Incontinence Questionnaire-Short Form]. Hinyokika Kiyo. 2010;56(5):255–9.
54. Klovning A, Avery K, Sandvik H, Hunskaar S. Comparison of two questionnaires for assessing the severity of urinary incontinence: the ICIQ-UI SF versus the incontinence severity index. Neurourol Urodyn. 2009;28(5):411–5. https://doi.org/10.1002/nau.20674.
55. Seckiner I, Yesilli C, Mungan NA, Aykanat A, Akduman B. Correlations between the ICIQ-SF score and urodynamic findings. Neurourol Urodyn. 2007;26(4):492–4. https://doi.org/10.1002/nau.20389.
56. Karantanis E, Fynes M, Moore KH, Stanton SL. Comparison of the ICIQ-SF and 24-hour pad test with other measures for evaluating the severity of urodynamic stress incontinence. Int Urogynecol J Pelvic Floor Dysfunct. 2004;15(2):111–6; discussion 6. https://doi.org/10.1007/s00192-004-1123-2.
57. Simsek A, Ozgor F, Yuksel B, Kucuktopcu O, Kirecci SL, Toptas M, et al. Female sexual function after transobturator tape in women with urodynamic stress urinary incontinence. Springerplus. 2014;3:570. https://doi.org/10.1186/2193-1801-3-570.
58. Meschia M, Rossi G, Bertini S, Sommacal A, Foina S, Sandretti F, et al. Single incision mid-urethral slings: impact of obesity on outcomes. Eur J Obstet Gynecol Reprod Biol. 2013;170(2):571–4. https://doi.org/10.1016/j.ejogrb.2013.08.007.
59. Diez-Itza I, Espuna-Pons M, Grupo de Investigacion de Disfunciones de Suelo Pelvico en Mujer—GISPEM. Evaluating the results of stress urinary incontinence surgery with objective and subjective outcome measures. Eur J Obstet Gynecol Reprod Biol. 2014;180:68–71. https://doi.org/10.1016/j.ejogrb.2014.06.020.
60. Abrams P, Smith AP, Cotterill N. The impact of urinary incontinence on health-related quality of life (HRQoL) in a real-world population of women aged 45-60 years: results from a survey in France, Germany, the UK and the USA. BJU Int. 2015;115(1):143–52. https://doi.org/10.1111/bju.12852.
61. Martinez Franco E, Pares D, Lorente Colome N, Mendez Paredes JR, Amat Tardiu L. Urinary incontinence during pregnancy. Is there a difference between first and third trimester? Eur J Obstet Gynecol Reprod Biol. 2014;182:86–90. https://doi.org/10.1016/j.ejogrb.2014.08.035.
62. Nystrom E, Sjostrom M, Stenlund H, Samuelsson E. ICIQ symptom and quality of life instruments measure clinically relevant improvements in women with stress urinary incontinence. Neurourol Urodyn. 2015;34(8):747–51. https://doi.org/10.1002/nau.22657.
63. Timmermans L, Falez F, Melot C, Wespes E. Validation of use of the International Consultation on Incontinence Questionnaire-Urinary Incontinence-Short Form (ICIQ-UI-SF) for impairment rating: a transversal retrospective study of 120 patients. Neurourol Urodyn. 2013;32(7):974–9. https://doi.org/10.1002/nau.22363.
64. European Association for Cardiovascular Prevention and Rehabilitation, Reiner Z, Catapano AL, De Backer G, Graham I, et al. ESC/EAS Guidelines for the management of dyslipidaemias: the Task Force for the management of dyslipidaemias of the European Society of Cardiology (ESC) and the European Atherosclerosis Society (EAS). Eur Heart

J. 2011;32(14):1769–818. https://doi.org/10.1093/eurheartj/ehr158.
65. Eurostat: overweight and obesity—BMI statistics [Internet]. 2017. http://ec.europa.eu/eurostat/statistics-explained/index.php/Overweight_and_obesity_-_BMI_statistics#Body_mass_index. Accessed 1 May 2017.
66. IDF diabetes atlas. In: Diabetesatlas.org. https://diabetesatlas.org/. Accessed 11 Feb 2022.
67. In: Fend.org. https://www.fend.org/wp-content/uploads/2021/04/Policy-Puzzle-PP4finalweb.pdf. Accessed 11 Feb 2022.
68. Meng E, Lin WY, Lee WC, Chuang YC. Pathophysiology of overactive bladder. Low Urin Tract Symptoms. 2012;4(Suppl 1):48–55. https://doi.org/10.1111/j.1757-5672.2011.00122.x.
69. Amarenco G, Serikoff A, Chartier-Kastler E, Grise P, Fatton B, Bruyere F, et al. [Metabolic syndrome and urinary disorders]. Prog Urol. 2012;22(4):207–13. https://doi.org/10.1016/j.purol.2012.01.005.
70. Lee WC, Chiang PH, Tain YL, Wu CC, Chuang YC. Sensory dysfunction of bladder mucosa and bladder oversensitivity in a rat model of metabolic syndrome. PLoS One. 2012;7(9):e45578. https://doi.org/10.1371/journal.pone.0045578.
71. Cundiff GW. The pathophysiology of stress urinary incontinence: a historical perspective. Rev Urol. 2004;6(Suppl 3):S10–8.
72. Rizk DE, Hassan HA, Al-Marzouqi AH, Shafiullah M, Fahim MA. Combined estrogen and ghrelin administration decreases expression of p27(kip1) and proportion of isomyosin type I in the striated urethral and anal sphincters and levator ani of old ovariectomized rats. Int Urogynecol J Pelvic Floor Dysfunct. 2008;19(10):1363–9. https://doi.org/10.1007/s00192-008-0638-3.
73. Bodner-Adler B, Bodner K, Kimberger O, Halpern K, Rieken M, Koelbl H, et al. Role of serum steroid hormones in women with stress urinary incontinence: a case-control study. BJU Int. 2017;120(3):416–21. https://doi.org/10.1111/bju.13902.
74. Lai HH, Rawal A, Shen B, Vetter J. The relationship between anxiety and overactive bladder or urinary incontinence symptoms in the clinical population. Urology. 2016;98:50–7. https://doi.org/10.1016/j.urology.2016.07.013.
75. Bross S. [Indication for urodynamic testing]. Urologe A. 2015;54(3):325–9. https://doi.org/10.1007/s00120-014-3681-3.
76. Chapple CR, Macdiarmid SA, Patel A. Urodynamics made easy. Edinburgh: Churchill Livingstone; 2012.
77. Viera AJ, Garrett JM. Understanding interobserver agreement: the kappa statistic. Fam Med. 2005;37(5):360–3.
78. Rosier PF. The evidence for urodynamic investigation of patients with symptoms of urinary incontinence. F1000Prime Rep. 2013;5:8. https://doi.org/10.12703/P5-8.
79. Maes D, Wyndaele JJ. Correlation between history and urodynamics in neurologically normal incontinent women. Eur Urol. 1988;14(5):377–80.
80. de Bolla AR, Arkell DG. Urodynamic investigation in a district general hospital. Ann R Coll Surg Engl. 1983;65(3):173–5.
81. Summitt RL Jr, Stovall TG, Bent AE, Ostergard DR. Urinary incontinence: correlation of history and brief office evaluation with multichannel urodynamic testing. Am J Obstet Gynecol. 1992;166(6 Pt 1):1835–40; discussion 40–4.
82. Katz GP, Blaivas JG. A diagnostic dilemma: when urodynamic findings differ from the clinical impression. J Urol. 1983;129(6):1170–4.
83. Borges JB, Guarisi T, Camargo AC, Borges PC. Correlation between urodynamic tests, history and clinical findings in treatment of women with urinary incontinence. Einstein. 2010;8(4):437–43. https://doi.org/10.1590/S1679-45082010AO1611.
84. Leitner L, Walter M, Sammer U, Knupfer SC, Mehnert U, Kessler TM. Urodynamic investigation: a valid tool to define normal lower urinary tract function? PLoS One. 2016;11(10):e0163847. https://doi.org/10.1371/journal.pone.0163847.
85. Nambiar AK, Lemack GE, Chapple CR, Burkhard FC, European Association of Urology. The role of urodynamics in the evaluation of urinary incontinence: the European Association of Urology recommendations in 2016. Eur Urol. 2017;71(4):501–3. https://doi.org/10.1016/j.eururo.2016.09.045.
86. Winters JC, Dmochowski RR, Goldman HB, Herndon CD, Kobashi KC, Kraus SR, et al. Urodynamic studies in adults: AUA/SUFU guideline. J Urol. 2012;188(6 Suppl):2464–72. https://doi.org/10.1016/j.juro.2012.09.081.
87. Urinary incontinence and pelvic organ prolapse in women: management NICE guideline. In: Org. uk. 2019. https://www.nice.org.uk/guidance/ng123/resources/urinary-incontinence-and-pelvic-organ-prolapse-in-women-management-pdf-66141657205189. Accessed 11 Feb 2022.
88. Homma Y, Imajo C, Takahashi S, Kawabe K, Aso Y. Urinary symptoms and urodynamics in a normal elderly population. Scand J Urol Nephrol Suppl. 1994;157:27–30.

2 Invasive and Noninvasive Uroflowmetry

Şerife Esra Çetinkaya, Mehmet Murat Seval, Bulut Varlı, Merve Toy, and Fulya Dökmeci

2.1 Introduction

Urodynamics is the term used for all measurements assessing the function and dysfunction of the lower urinary tract by any appropriate method. It is described as noninvasive or invasive according to the insertion of catheters or any other transducers into the bladder and/or other body cavities during the tests [1]. Uroflowmetry is the urodynamic test involving the measurement of urine flow and may be accomplished both noninvasively (i.e., free uroflowmetry) and invasively (i.e., pressure-flow study).

Free uroflowmetry is the most widely used noninvasive urodynamic examination. It is easy to perform at low cost. Here, the voided volume and flow rate are measured over time during voiding and are displayed graphically while patients void into a flowmeter in a completely private room. It is recommended as a first step test for patients with lower urinary tract symptoms (LUTS) and especially for those with voiding dysfunction [2]. The maximum flow rate (Q_{max}), the volume voided and post-void residual (PVR) are reported at minimal; average flow rate (Q_{ave}), time to Q_{max}, voiding time and the characteristic shape of the curve may also be provided as outputs of uroflowmetry [2].

The pressure-flow study involves the simultaneous recording of pressures and flow together during micturition. It offers more detailed information about bladder outlet dynamics and dysfunctional voiding. The procedure is generally performed at the end of filling cystometry when the patient feels a full bladder with a standard flowmeter and monitoring of intravesical, abdominal, detrusor pressures and flow parameters. It begins immediately after permission to void and ends when the detrusor pressure has returned to the baseline value and/or when the flow rate returns to zero and/or when the patient considers the micturition complete [3]. In addition to the parameters obtained from free uroflowmetry, data regarding pressure measurements, such as pre-micturition pressure, opening time, opening pressure, maximum pressure, pressure at maximum flow, closing pressure, contraction pressure at maximum flow, and flow delay, are provided by pressure-flow studies [4]. Thus, the pressure-flow study enables to determine whether a slow urine stream is due to bladder outlet obstruction, detrusor underactivity, or both. It is also helpful in diagnosing detrusor-sphincter dyssynergia.

It should be emphasized that a detailed urogynecological evaluation, including a detailed history, assessment of symptoms, voiding diaries,

Ş. E. Çetinkaya (✉)
Department of Obstetrics and Gynecology, Ankara University School of Medicine, Cebeci Hospital, Ankara, Turkey

M. M. Seval · B. Varlı · M. Toy · F. Dökmeci
Department of Obstetrics and Gynecology, Ankara University School of Medicine, Ankara, Turkey
e-mail: seval@ankara.edu.tr

F. Dökmeci, D. E. E. Rizk (eds.), *Insights Into Incontinence and the Pelvic Floor*,
https://doi.org/10.1007/978-3-030-94174-1_2

laboratory tests, and a physical examination, should precede both free uroflowmetry and the pressure-flow study. Both tests should be conducted in a place ensuring patient privacy, with adequate draping, and in the most comfortable position for the patients [1]. Antibiotic prophylaxis is not necessary before the procedures even if catheterization is to be performed. However, any urinary infection should be excluded. It would be helpful to ask the patient to arrive with an empty bowel, preferably without having used laxatives prior to the procedure as they may cause excessive bowel movements. Generally, 6-8F catheters are used for pressure-flow studies with adequate fixation of catheters being mandatory to eliminate any artifacts and test failures [5]. Post-void residual urine volume should be measured either via ultrasound or via catheters at the end of the procedure.

Voiding dysfunction, defined as abnormally slow and/or incomplete micturition [4], is the main indication for both tests; identifying or eliminating voiding dysfunction is crucial for patients who are considered as candidates for surgical or medical treatment for urinary incontinence [6]. Whether performed with a noninvasive or invasive approach, both procedures evaluate the voiding pattern. However, several differences between the procedures, and especially the presence of catheters, seem to lead to discrepant results between these tests in the literature.

2.2 Literature Review

As mentioned previously, it is widely accepted that the pressure-flow study is the most detailed method in the assessment of voiding dysfunction. However, the mechanical effect of the catheters has been investigated in many studies in the last two decades as a confounding factor in the interpretation of the results and in establishing correct diagnoses.

Groutz et al. have evaluated the effect of a 7F transurethral catheter on urinary flow during pressure-flow studies, comparing data from a urodynamic database of 600 women who underwent both free uroflowmetry and pressure-flow studies. It was found that the presence of 7F transurethral catheters in pressure-flow studies may adversely affect the maximum flow rate and flow time. The maximum flow rate was found to be significantly less and the flow time significantly longer on pressure versus free uroflowmetry studies. Moreover, an intermittent flow pattern was found to be more common on pressure than in free uroflowmetry measurements (43% vs. 9%, respectively) [7].

Baseman et al. have evaluated the effect of 6F transurethral catheters on urinary flow rates during pressure-flow studies compared to free uroflowmetry in 20 healthy female volunteers. A significant reduction in the maximal flow rate with the presence of a 6F urethral catheter was reported. It was stated that even though these differences may represent the possible obstructive effect of the catheter, a number of other possible factors such as dysfunctional voiding in the urodynamic setting may also be considered as a confounding effect [8].

Grazia et al. evaluated the effect of a 4F urethral catheter in 85 women referred for lower urinary tract symptoms. However, they could not demonstrate any significant differences in the flow parameters and curves of uroflowmetry and pressure-flow studies [9].

Scaldazza et al. compared three different sized (4.5F, 6F, and 7F) catheters in a randomized controlled study of 60 women with lower urinary tract symptoms. Women were randomized into two groups and underwent free uroflowmetry. In the first group, two consecutive pressure-flow studies were performed using a 4.5F catheter once and a 6F catheter once. In the second group, two consecutive pressure-flow studies were performed using a 4.5F catheter once and a 7F catheter once. In all women, the maximum and average flow rates were significantly lower, the flow time was significantly longer, and the PVR was significantly larger for pressure-flow studies when compared with the equivalent free uroflowmetry parameters. In the two groups comparing the different sized catheters, a statistically significant difference was found in all flow and detrusor parameters between 4.5F and 7F catheters, but not between 4.5F and 6F catheters [10].

In another study evaluating the potential contribution of a 6F double lumen transurethral catheter to bladder outlet obstruction, data from 120 women who underwent noninvasive free-flow and pressure-flow studies were reviewed. The authors reported that the use of a 6F catheter created an obstructive effect on uroflowmetry by lowering the maximum flow rate, especially in patients who voided more than 250 mL. It was concluded that in order to lower the possible over-diagnoses of bladder outlet obstruction, free uroflowmetry should be performed on all patients before any urethral manipulation [11].

In a retrospective review of the Urinary Incontinence Treatment Network (UITN) Trial of Mid-Urethral Slings (TOMUS), Mueller et al. compared the flow rates and voided volumes in uroflowmetry and pressure-flow studies in women with stress urinary incontinence. The authors similarly demonstrated significant differences in maximum flow rates between these studies, similarly with increasing voided volumes; with a voided volume of 200 mL, Q_{max} at free uroflow was 14% higher than the Q_{max} at the pressure-flow study, and this difference increased to 30% at 700 mL [12].

Valentini et al. assessed the potential effects of a urethral catheter on flow parameters with the VBN® mathematical micturition model, which was used to make simulations of various pathophysiological hypotheses in a retrospective study. This model was defined as a quantitative description of the mechanistic phenomena governing micturition, such as bladder contractility, elasticity, viscoelasticity, urethral elasticity, urethral compression by the sphincter, and turbulent incompressible fluid hydrodynamics. The authors also demonstrated significant differences in the flow parameters between uroflowmetry and pressure-flow studies, similarly to the other studies discussed above. However, simulations with this model showed that the geometrical obstruction due to the urethral catheter could not explain every difference in the flow parameters. They additionally mentioned a compression-like effect, possibly due to a urethral reflex induced by the catheter, and a fading effect of detrusor excitation [13].

Valentini et al. used the same model in another study to analyze the potential obstructive effect of a 7F transurethral catheter on the voiding process during a pressure-flow study in women and again demonstrated that the decrease in the maximum flow rate did not appear to result from the geometric effect of only the catheter. They suggested that the incomplete relaxation of the sphincter during voiding, due to the patient's anxiety or a urethral reflex induced by the catheter, should be considered as the potential mechanism of decreased flow [14].

In another interesting study, Susskind and Smith conducted a prospective clinical study in order to evaluate the effect of transient urethral catheterization on uroflow parameters by comparing pre- and post-urodynamic uroflowmetry. In this study, women underwent "uninstrumented" uroflowmetry twice, first prior to the filling cystometry (pre-urodynamic uroflow) and second at the end of the filling cystometry after the removal of the urodynamic catheters (post-urodynamic uroflow). With this study, the authors demonstrated a negative effect of "transient catheterization" on uroflow parameters, suggesting that catheterization may cause more than simply a passive obstructive effect [15].

2.3 Case Study: Comparison of Uroflowmetry Parameters Between Free Uroflowmetry and Ambulatory Urodynamic Monitoring in Women with Lower Urinary Tract Symptoms

(a) **Aim and Scope**

This study aimed to investigate the impact of intravesical catheterization on flow parameters by comparing free uroflowmetry and pressure-flow studies after ambulatory urodynamic monitoring (AUM) in women with LUTS.

(b) **Study Design and Material Methods**

In this retrospective cohort study, records of women with LUTS, attending the

Urogynaecology Unit at Ankara University School of Medicine, Department of Obstetrics and Gynaecology, were reviewed (n = 1659). Of these women, data of who underwent both free uroflowmetry and pressure-flow studies were selected for analysis (n = 512). Women presenting with clinically significant prolapse (stages III and IV) were excluded (n = 148), and the final analysis comprised 364 women.

AUM was performed on all patients with a standardized protocol, in line with the standards of the sub-committee of the International Continence Society (ICS) for AUM [16]. The steps of the investigation were as follows: The patients were asked to arrive to the hospital with a full bladder. After informed consent, they voided to a PC-based wireless uroflowmeter in the sitting position. After the completion of free uroflowmetry, patients were examined in the dorsal lithotomy position. Post-void residual urine volumes were measured with a Foley catheter and were recorded. A 7F double lumen air-charged single-sensor bladder catheter (T-DOC, Laborie™) and a 7F single lumen air-charged rectal catheter (T-DOC, Laborie™) were inserted to measure intravesical and intra-abdominal pressures, respectively. Then, they were connected to a microcomputer (LUNA, Medical Measurement Systems™) worn over the shoulder, allowing patients to move freely. Each transducer was set to zero atmospheric pressure before each investigation with the patient in standing position. A standardized fluid volume of 500 mL of water was provided for each patient. When the patients felt severe bladder fullness and were unable to delay voiding, monitoring was ended by a pressure-flow study, which was performed by a PC-based wireless uroflowmeter (Flowmaster, Medical Measurement Systems™) in a special section of the urodynamic room to preserve privacy and to avoid embarrassment. Once the urodynamic study was completed, all data were transferred from the LUNA to a PC with the database software (MMS database, Medical Measurement Systems™). After verifying the quality of traces recorded during both subtracted cystometry and pressure-flow study, a trained supervisor performed data analysis and interpretation before the patients left.

Kolmogorov-Smirnov/Shapiro-Wilk test was used to determine the distribution of the variables. Descriptive analyses were presented as means and standard deviations for normally distributed variables or medians and ranges for non-normally distributed variables. Students' paired t-test for normally distributed continuous data were used to compare the parameters. The Chi-square test or Fisher's exact test, where appropriate, were used to compare the proportions between groups. A P value of <0.05 was considered statistically significant.

(c) **Results of the Study**

The mean age and mean body mass index of the patients were 52 ± 11 years and 30 ± 6 kg/m^2, respectively, and 54% were post-menopausal. Data of AUM are presented in Table 2.1. The most common diagnosis at AUM was mixed urinary incontinence (n = 153, 42%). The comparison of free uroflowmetry and pressure-flow study parameters is presented in Table 2.2. Bladder capacity and voided volume were similar with both tests (434 ± 203 mL vs. 430 ± 218 mL, and 388 ± 196 mL vs. 379 ± 213 mL). Post-void residual urine volume was found to be significantly higher after pressure-flow studies (50 ± 29 mL vs. 46 ± 32 mL, p = 0.026). Voiding time was

Table 2.1 Ambulatory urodynamic monitoring data of women with LUTS

Cystometry findings	All patients (n = 364)
Duration (minute), mean ± SD	85 ± 24
Maximum cystometric capacity (mL), mean ± SD	431 ± 219
Detrusor over activity, n (%)	241 (66)
UUI, n (%)	59 (16)
SUI, n (%)	80 (22)
MUI, n (%)	153 (42)
No urodynamic UI, n (%)	72 (20)

Table 2.2 Comparison of free uroflowmetry with pressure-flow study at AUM ($n = 364$)

	Free uroflowmetry	Pressure-flow study	p^a
Bladder capacity (mL), mean ± SD	434 ± 203	430 ± 218	0.770
Voided volume (mL), mean ± SD	388 ± 196	379 ± 213	0.459
Post-void residual urine volume (mL), mean ± SD	46 ± 32	50 ± 29	0.026
Q_{max} (mL/s), mean ± SD	32 ± 15	29 ± 15	<0.001
c-Q_{max} (mL/s), mean ± SD	1.74 ± 0.68	1.61 ± 0.81	0.001
Voiding time (s), mean ± SD	25 ± 18	35 ± 31	<0.001

Q_{max} Maximal flow rate
c-Q_{max} corrected maximal flow rate
[a] Paired t-test

significantly shorter (25 ± 18 s vs. 35 ± 31 s, $p < 0.001$), and Q_{max} and corrected Q_{max} (c-Q_{max}) were significantly higher at uroflowmetry (32 ± 15 mL/s vs. 29 ± 15 mL/s, $p < 0.001$, and 1.74 ± 0.68 vs. 1.61 ± 0.81, $p = 0.001$).

2.4 Discussion

Considering all the studies discussed above together with the case study, the catheterization in pressure-flow studies appears to have a significant influence on the flow parameters in women, such as Q_{max} (both corrected and not corrected with voided volume), voiding time, and PVR. With the exception of one study indicating no differences in the flow parameters with 4F catheters, all these data suggest a certain degree of difficulty in voiding with invasive uroflowmetry regardless of the size of the catheter.

Catheterization, even transient patient characteristics, and the setting of the tests may all influence the findings of the pressure-flow studies. Although the obstructive effect of catheterization has been shown to be the main reason for the difference between invasive and non-invasive uroflowmetry parameters, other factors due to non-physiological test conditions, such as the urethral reflex, incomplete sphincter relaxation induced by the catheter, or anxiety of the patients, have also been suggested to contribute. The increases in voided volumes were also shown to increase these differences. We demonstrated a similar obstructive effect with a 7F catheter on the flow parameters and PVR even though we used AUM, which offers a more physiological setting than conventional urodynamics.

The differences in the flow characteristics between invasive and noninvasive uroflowmetry may be clinically insignificant for patients with rather normal flowmetry findings; however, it may be important for those who have borderline flowmetry findings. Therefore, results of both tests should be evaluated together.

2.5 Conclusion

Both noninvasive and invasive uroflowmetry are essential tools for the assessment of patients with LUTS, which provide valuable information regarding the dynamics of voiding. However, it should be emphasized that one cannot replace the other, and the results of both should be interpreted for a more correct diagnosis.

References

1. Rosier PFWM, Schaefer W, Lose G, Goldman HB, Guralnick M, Eustice S, et al. International Continence Society Good Urodynamic Practices and Terms 2016: urodynamics, uroflowmetry, cystometry, and pressure-flow study. Neurourol Urodyn. 2017;36(5):1243–60.
2. Rosier PFWM, Kuo H-C, Agro EF, Gennaro MD, Gammie A, Kakizaki H, et al. Urodynamic testing. In: Abrams P, Cardozo L, Wagg A, Wein A, editors. Incontinence. 6th ed; 2017. p. 602–70.
3. Drake MJ, Doumouchtsis SK, Hashim H, Gammie A. Fundamentals of urodynamic practice, based on International Continence Society good urodynamic practices recommendations. Neurourol Urodyn. 2018;37(S6):S50–60.

4. Haylen BT, de Ridder D, Freeman RM, Swift SE, Berghmans B, Lee J, et al. An International Urogynecological Association (IUGA)/International Continence Society (ICS) joint report on the terminology for female pelvic floor dysfunction. Neurourol Urodyn. 2010;29(1):4–20.
5. Rosier PFWM, Kirschner-Hermanns R, Svihra J, Homma Y, Wein AJ. ICS teaching module: analysis of voiding, pressure flow analysis (basic module). Neurourol Urodyn. 2016;35(1):36–8.
6. Haylen BT. Voiding difficulty in women. Int Urogynecol J. 2000;11(1):1–3.
7. Groutz A, Blaivas JG, Sassone AM. Detrusor pressure uroflowmetry studies in women: effect of a 7fr transurethral catheter. J Urol. 2000;164(1):109–14.
8. Baseman AG, Baseman JG, Zimmern PE, Lemack GE. Effect of 6F urethral catheterization on urinary flow rates during repeated pressure-flow studies in healthy female volunteers. Urology. 2002;59(6):843–6.
9. Grazia ED, Bartolotta S, Nicolosi F, Nicolosi D. Detrusor pressure uroflowmetry studies in women: effect of 4 Fr transurethral. Arch Ital Urol Androl. 2002;74(3):134–7.
10. Scaldazza CV, Morosetti C. Effect of different sized transurethral catheters on pressure-flow studies in women with lower urinary tract symptoms. Urol Int. 2005;75(1):21–5.
11. Richard P, Ordonez N, Tu L. The effect of a 6 Fr catheter in women: are they obstructive? Can Urol Assoc J. 2013;7(5–6):185–8.
12. Mueller ER, Litman H, Rickey LR, Sirls L, Norton P, Wilson T, et al. Comparison of flowrates and voided volumes during non-instrumented uroflowmetry and pressure-flow studies in women with stress incontinence. Neurourol Urodyn. 2015;34(6):549–53.
13. Valentini F, Marti B, Robain G, Nelson P. Differences between the data from free flow and intubated flow in women with urinary incontinence. What do they mean? Neurourol Urodyn. 2008;27(4):297–300.
14. Valentini FA, Robain G, Hennebelle DS, Nelson PP. Decreased maximum flow rate during intubated flow is not only due to urethral catheter in situ. Int Urogynecol J. 2013;24(3):461–7.
15. Susskind AM, Smith PP. Evidence of a functional effect of transient transurethral catheterization on micturition in women. Int Urogynecol J. 2012;23(9):1245–8.
16. van Waalwijk van Doorn E, Anders K, Khullar V, Kulseng-Hanssen S, Pesce F, Robertson A, et al. Standardisation of ambulatory urodynamic monitoring: report of the Standardisation Sub-Committee of the International Continence Society for Ambulatory Urodynamic Studies. Neurourol Urodyn. 2000;19(2):113–25.

3 Single-Incision Slings

Berna Haliloglu Peker, Ali Gursoy, Erdin Ilter, Aygen Celik, Erdal Yucel, Serpil Bozkurt, Umit Ozekici, and Hakan Peker

3.1 Introduction

Stress urinary incontinence (SUI) is defined as the complaint of any involuntary loss of urine on effort or physical exertion) or on sneezing or coughing by the International Continence Society (ICS) [1]. Urinary incontinence is common among middle-aged women, affecting 40%, and increasing to 50% among older-aged women [2]. With the integral theory proposed by Petros and Ulmsten, it was accepted that urethral closure was not in the bladder neck but in the mid-urethra [3]. Acceptance of this theory paved the way for "tension-free vaginal tape" (TVT) operations for stress urinary incontinence [4]. According to long-term studies, TVT was regarded as the "gold standard" treatment [5]. To avoid severe intestinal and vascular complications of TVT, transobturator sling technique was started to be preferred to place the end of the tape. However, this approach brought specific complications as postoperative groin pain due to neural injury [6]. Finally, the third-generation minimally invasive slings also called single-incision slings (SIMs) were developed to decrease the groin pain and to avoid blind passing trocars through obturator canal and Retzius space using shorter length of mesh [7].

3.2 Literature Review

SIM meshes are 8–16 cm in length and have a mechanism at both ends that provide fixation to the obturator membrane. There are many SIMs on the market with different fixation mechanisms. Because of TVT-Secur (Gynecare, Bridgewater, NJ, USA), first introduced at 2006, is inferior to standard mid-urethral slings (MUS) for the treatment of women with SUI, it has already been withdrawn from clinical use. Then, various SIMs with stronger fixation have been developed. However, many SIM studies in the literature are performed with TVT-Secur; many reviews and meta-analyses have found that SIMs are less effective than MUS operations [8]. In recent studies, SIMs appear to have a similar efficacy to standard MUS procedures [9]. However, there is not enough evidence found for SIMs compared with standard MUS to allow reliable

B. Haliloglu Peker (✉) · A. Gursoy · E. Ilter
A. Celik · U. Ozekici
Department of Obstetrics and Gynecology, Maltepe University Faculty of Medicine, Istanbul, Turkey
e-mail: umit.ozekici@maltepe.edu.tr

E. Yucel
Department of Obstetrics and Gynecology, Zeynep Kamil Women and Children Diseases Training and Research Hospital, Istanbul, Turkey

S. Bozkurt
Private Clinic, Istanbul, Turkey

H. Peker
Nisantasi Vocational School, Nisantasi University, Istanbul, Turkey

F. Dökmeci, D. E. E. Rizk (eds.), *Insights Into Incontinence and the Pelvic Floor*,
https://doi.org/10.1007/978-3-030-94174-1_3

comparisons. In Cochrane review, no difference has been reported in clinical outcomes between SIMs and transobturator technique, but SIMs may be more cost-effective than transobturator approach based on 1-year follow-up [10].

3.3 Case Study: Long-Term Results of Contasure-Needleless Technique Versus TVT-O for the Treatment of Stress Urinary Incontinence (Video)

(a) **Aim and Scope**

We aim to compare prospectively the long-term results and complications of transobturator tension-free vaginal tape (TVT-O, Gynecare) with a single-incision tape procedure (Contasure-Needleless, Neomedic Int.) (Fig. 3.1).

(b) **Study Design and Material Methods**

Sixteen women who underwent TVT-O and 21 women who underwent Needleless were compared. The complications, preoperative and postoperative QoL scores, objective cure rates, subjective cure rates, and recommendation rate of procedure to others were assessed.

(c) **Results of the Study**

There was no significant difference regarding age, gravida, parity, smoking, diabetes, and delivery type between two groups. The mean follow-up period was 30.3 ± 19.3 and 43.3 ± 22.9 months in TVT-O group and Needleless group, respectively. The complication rates including mesh erosion and groin pain were not found to be statistically significant between the two groups. De novo urge incontinence rates were significantly higher in TVT-O group compared with Needleless group (62.5% vs 28.6%, respectively, $p = 0.042$). The objective cure rates were 62.5% in TVT-O group whereas 71.4% in Needleless group ($p = 0.411$). The subjective cure rates were 62.5% and 90.5% in TVT-O and Needleless groups, respectively ($p = 0.05$). The recommendation rate of Needleless procedure was significantly higher in Needleless group compared with TVT-O group (90.5% vs 62.5%, respectively, $p = 0.05$).

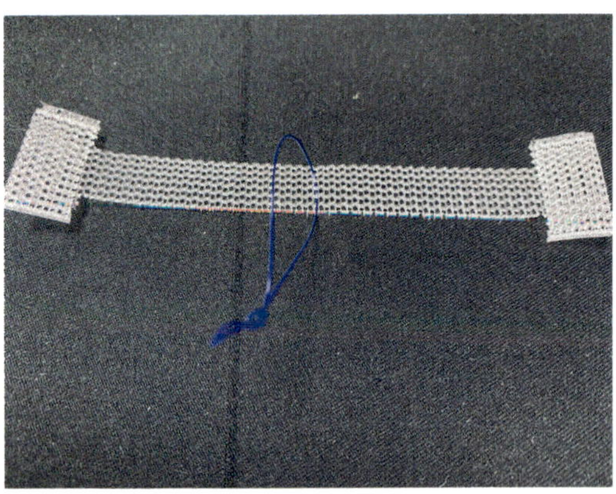

Fig. 3.1 The Contasure-Needleless System (with permission from Neomedic International SL)

3.4 Discussion

Although some studies show that SIMs are successful as transobturator approach [11–13], a meta-analysis showed higher reoperation rates and lower objective and subjective cure rates in SIMs [14]. Recently, SIMs were reported to have similar effectiveness compared with conventional MUS in short term [15]. There are several studies investigating the long-term cure rates of SIMs. Martinez-Franco et al. reported outcome of Needleless procedure at least 3 years after surgery [16]. In their study, objective and subjective cure rates were 84.7% and 90.7% respectively. They also showed that 8.4% of patients experienced de novo urgency and 0.8% experienced voiding difficulty. Lo et al. reported outcome of MiniArc (American Medical Systems, Minnetonka, MN, USA), another type of SIM, in a follow-up period of 74.1 ± 15.1 months [17]. They found that overall subjective cure rate was 80% and objective cure 84.7%. A meta-analysis determined that the MiniArc has similarly high cure rates when compared to transobturator approach. In addition, shorter operation time, less blood loss, faster recovery time, lower postoperative pain scores, less postoperative groin pain, and less urinary retention were observed in MiniArc slings [18].

3.5 Conclusion

Despite the equal effectiveness of TVT-O and Needleless technique in the long-term period, rate of de novo urgency seems to be less in Needleless procedure. This finding may be the reason of higher rates of subjective cure and recommendation of procedure to another patient in Needleless procedure.

In the future, well-designed, prospective randomized controlled trials comparing different SIMs and standard MUS procedures are needed.

Acknowledgment None.

References

1. Haylen BT, et al. An international Urogynecological Association (IUGA)/International Continence Society (ICS) joint report on the terminology for female pelvic floor dysfunction. Neurourol Urodyn. 2010;29:4–20.
2. Nitti VW. The prevalence of urinary incontinence. Rev Urol. 2001;3(Suppl 1):S2–6.
3. Petros PE, Ulmsten UI. An integral theory and its method for the diagnosis and management of female urinary incontinence. Scand J Urol Nephrol. 1993;153(Suppl):1–93.
4. Ulmsten U, Falconer C, Johnson P, Jomaa M, Lannér L, Nilsson CG, et al. A multicenter study of tension-free vaginal tape (TVT) for surgical treatment of stress urinary incontinence. Int Urogynecol J Pelvic Floor Dysfunct. 1998;9:210–3.
5. Lin L, Huang MC, Su TH, Lau HH. Comparison between tension-free vaginal tape and transobturator tape in treating stress urinary incontinence after vaginal mesh surgery. Taiwan J Obstet Gynecol. 2018;57:528–31.
6. Gambini-Ricapa J, García-Oms J, Barea M, Estrada A, Iturri A, Gambini-Buchon J, Gilabert-Estelles J. Endopelvic free anchor minisling technique for stress urinary incontinence treatment: 10 years of experience. Int Urogynecol J. 2016;27:1265–72.
7. Molden SM, Lucente VR. New minimally invasive slings: TVT Secur. Curr Urol Rep. 2008;9:358–61.
8. Linder BJ, Elliott DS. Synthetic midurethral slings: roles, outcomes, and complications. Urol Clin North Am. 2019;46:17–30.
9. Mostafa A, Lim CP, Hopper L, Madhuvrata P, Abdel-Fattah M. Single-incision mini-slings versus standard midurethral slings in surgical management of female stress urinary incontinence: an updated systematic review and meta-analysis of effectiveness and complications. Eur Urol. 2014;65:402–27.
10. Nambiar A, Cody JD, Jeffery ST, Aluko P. Single-incision sling operations for urinary incontinence in women. Cochrane Database Syst Rev. 2017;(7):CD008709.
11. Kennelly MJ, Moore R, Nguyen JN, Lukban JC, Siegel S. Prospective evaluation of a single incision sling for stress urinary incontinence. J Urol. 2010;184:604–9.
12. De Ridder D, Berkers J, Deprest J, Verguts J, Ost D, Hamid D, et al. Single incision mini-sling versus a transobutaror sling: a comparative study on MiniArc and Monarc slings. Int Urogynecol J. 2010;21:773–8.
13. Lee JK, Rosamilia A, Dwyer PL, Lim YN, Muller R. Randomized trial of a single incision versus an outside-in transobturator midurethral sling in women with stress urinary incontinence: 12 month results. Am J Obstet Gynecol. 2015;213:351–9.
14. Neuman M, Sosnovski V, Kais M, Ophir E, Bornstein J. Transobturator vs single-incision suburethral mini-slings for treatment of female stress urinary incontinence: early postoperative pain and 3-year follow-up. J Minim Invasive Gynecol. 2011;18:769–73.
15. Palmieri S, Frigerio M, Spelzini F, Manodoro S, Milani R. Risk factors for stress urinary incontinence recurrence after single-incision sling. Neurourol Urodyn. 2018;37:1711–6.
16. Martinez-Franco E, Amat Tardiu L. Contasure-Needleless® single-incision sling compared with transobturator TVT-O® for the treatment of stress urinary incontinence: long-term results. Int Urogynecol J. 2015;26:213–8.
17. Lo TS, Chua S, Kao CC, Uy-Patrimonio MC, Ibrahim R, Tan YL. Five-year outcome of mini-arc single-incision sling used in the treatment of primary urodynamic stress incontinence. J Minim Invasive Gynecol. 2018;25:116–23.
18. Jiao B, Lai S, Xu X, Zhang M, Diao T, Zhang G. A systematic review and meta-analysis of single-incision mini-slings (MiniArc) versus transobturator mid-urethral slings in surgical management of female stress urinary incontinence. Medicine (Baltimore). 2018;97:e0283.

4 Persistent Stress Urinary Incontinence

Fulya Dökmeci, Serife Esra Cetinkaya, and Ahkam Göksel Kanmaz

When we look at the history of anti-incontinence surgery in women, we see two techniques defined as the gold standard for the surgical treatment of female stress urinary incontinence (SUI): Burch colposuspension (BC) and mid-urethral slings (MUS) [1, 2]. However, with both gold standard techniques, short- and long-term surgical failures are reported in the literature with rates in a wide range [3–5]. The unresolved SUI complaints in women after anti-incontinence surgery have always been accepted as an indisputable surgical failure. Moreover, they have been defined as an "immediate failure" or as "persistent urinary incontinence". Authors usually attributed this condition to poor surgical technique, inaccurate pre-operative diagnoses or inadequate surgical indications [6]. However, there is still no standard definition for the situations that should be considered as recurrence or persistence, in other words, as surgical failure after anti-incontinence surgery.

Supplementary Information The online version contains supplementary material available at [https://doi.org/10.1007/978-3-030-94174-1_4].

F. Dökmeci (✉) · S. E. Cetinkaya
Department of Obstetrics and Gynecology, Ankara University School of Medicine, Ankara, Turkey

A. G. Kanmaz
Tepecik Education and Research Hospital, Obstetrics and Gynecology Clinic, İzmir, Turkey

Another controversial issue is the period to define the current situation as "recurrence". Some authors used the term "early recurrence" for incontinence in women who were very satisfied immediately after BC or other bladder neck surgeries but presented with the same complaint in a short time after surgery, while others interpreted the same condition in women who underwent MUS as "persistent urinary incontinence or surgical failure" and described an interval of 12 months. They reserved the term "recurrence" for cases in which SUI symptoms returned 12 months after MUS surgery.

It was assumed that the probable cause of the situation after a bladder neck operation was early return to physical activity and/or the patient's possible exposure to conditions increasing intra-abdominal pressure, damaging the patient's suspended tissues, so the authors defined it as "early postoperative recurrence", but not failure or persistence. However, the others chose the term "failure or persistence" for the recurrence of urinary leakage up to 12 months after MUS surgery, in which a permanent material was used. They also suggested that the term "recurrence" should be reserved for patients whose SUI symptoms returned after 12 months [6, 7]. Therefore, there is still no standard nomenclature covering all anti-incontinence surgical techniques in this context.

Whether early or postoperative recurrence, persistent/recurrent urinary incontinence is a

F. Dökmeci, D. E. E. Rizk (eds.), *Insights Into Incontinence and the Pelvic Floor*, https://doi.org/10.1007/978-3-030-94174-1_4

surgical failure from the patient's point of view. Therefore, evaluating the outcomes of anti-incontinence surgery from the patient's perspective and questioning whether the patient is satisfied with the surgery have gained as much importance as the objective criteria in recent years.

A comprehensive understanding of the underlying causes leading to unsatisfactory surgical outcome is important. All potential reasons such as de novo urgency incontinence, inadequate or over-elevation of the bladder neck, misplacement of the mesh, fistula formation due to surgical complication, poor tissue quality and poor surgical technique should be considered.

A thorough investigation of all women with persistent/recurrent urinary incontinence is mandatory to know the pitfalls before attempting to manage those women with this debilitating condition.

4.1 Literature Review

The prevalence of persistent/recurrent SUI (rSUI) has been reported to range from 3 to 20% and is mostly based on re-operation rates of women with failed primary anti-incontinence surgeries [8, 9]. Ashok et al. reviewed the literature of 10 years from PubMed between 1999 and 2009. In this review, covering randomised control trials, meta-analyses and prospective and retrospective cohort studies, the failure rates of both open and laparoscopic Burch colposuspension were between 6.3 and 43% in the long-term follow-up, and the retro-pubic MUS objective failure rates were between 10 and 19%. They also reported the surgical results of women with only stress urinary incontinence with the failure rates of 10–20% [9]. The authors concluded that menopause, advanced age, intrinsic sphincter deficiency, pre-operative detrusor overactivity and poor surgical technique were found to be the most related risk factors for surgical failure. A retrospective study of a case series includes 127 women who underwent open colposuspension who were followed up with a median of 12.4 years. A failure rate of 6.4% was reported with an emphasis that all failures were detected within the first year after BC [10].

Jelovsek et al. presented the anti-incontinence surgery outcomes after a median follow-up of 65 months and reported bothersome incontinence rates of 11 and 8% in the laparoscopic Burch and TVT groups, respectively [11]. However, the persistent urinary incontinence rate was found to be significantly higher (30%) after Burch colposuspension was performed concomitantly with the prolapse repair [12]. In a randomised controlled trial, 47 women with pelvic organ prolapse (POP) and SUI were grouped into two (abdominal POP repair with concomitant BC and abdominal POP repair alone) and were followed up to compare the surgical outcomes of different surgical approaches. Both mid-term and long-term follow-ups revealed that BC did not provide any additional benefit in women with SUI and apical prolapse, as the observed failure rates after abdominal POP repair (sacrocolpopexy and sacrohysteropexy) and concomitant BC were 54.2% at mid-term and 56.5% at long-term (5 years) follow-up. In other words, no increase was observed in the failure rate in the long-term. In the prolapse repair only group, 39.1 and 40.9% of women remained incontinent at mid-term and long-term follow-up, respectively. They also reported that four women underwent MUS due to persistent SUI at their mid-term follow-up and were found to be dry in the long-term [13, 14]. In the study performed by Cosson et al., the success rate of BC in cases with vault prolapse and SUI was found to be only 34%, when it was added concomitantly with sacrocolpopexy (SCP). The authors concluded that the long-term cure rate of isolated Burch procedure after 10–12 years (69%) decreases dramatically when it is performed concomitantly with abdominal prolapse repair [15]. The increase in the failure rate of concomitant BC with SCP is defined in the literature as possible consequences of inappropriate changes at the urethra-vesical angle and/or over-elevation of the bladder neck and, probably, by the accompanied elevation of the vaginal axis [12, 15].

Therefore, with this case study, the importance of the thorough evaluation of women with persistent urinary incontinence was summarised step by step to verify the underlying pathogenesis, in order to manage this devastating condition in a targeted manner.

4.2 Case Study: Worsening Urinary Incontinence After Abdominal Sacrocolpopexy and Concomitant Burch Colposuspension: Cystoscopy for Diagnosis of the Distorted Bladder Neck and for Guiding Management (Video Presentation)

A 61-year-old woman was admitted to the urogynaecology unit of the Ankara University School of Medicine Department of Obstetrics and Gynaecology with the chief complaint of worsening urinary incontinence initiated 1 year previously after her vaginal prolapse surgery.

Detailed history taking and examination of the past medical report revealed that she had also new-onset coital incontinence disabling her sexual function after the surgery, which was performed at another institute 1 year previously for her vaginal prolapse and mild SUI. From her medical reports, it was understood that the patient underwent both abdominal sacrocolpopexy and Burch colposuspension for her vault prolapse and mild SUI. She did not define any additional lower urinary tract symptoms suggestive of voiding dysfunction and/or an overactive bladder. She had seven full-term vaginal deliveries and two missed abortions, and she did not define any systemic disease and medication. Her past surgical history revealed that she underwent a total abdominal hysterectomy and bilateral salpingo-oophorectomy 15 years previously due to benign gynaecologic conditions.

Assessment of the severity of this patient's symptoms with the impact on her quality of life was performed with Turkish validated questionnaires, such as UDI-6 and IIQ-7. She has a total UDI-6 score of 18/24, and scores of the irritative, stress and obstructive sub-scales were found to be 8/8, 8/8, and 2/8, respectively. The IIQ-7 total and sub-scale scores indicated that quality of life was affected significantly, as indicated by a total IIQ-7 score of 21/21 with physical, travel, social and emotional sub-scale scores of 6/6, 6/6, 3/3 and 6/6, respectively.

In a thorough examination of the patient, no pelvic organ prolapse was recorded in the POPQ examination. The cough stress test and supine empty stress test were positive. Moreover, significant urinary leakage was observed with digital compression on the posterior vaginal wall (Video 4.1). Vaginal mucosa was examined carefully for any mesh extrusion as the complication of abdominal sacrocolpopexy; however, no mesh extrusion was recorded on examination of the vagina.

The post-void residual urine (PVR) was <50 mL. In order to evaluate urethral mobility, which is accepted as an essential part of the examination to assess urethral support in women with SUI and rSUI, a Q-tip test was performed and a result of <30° was found. Other recommended methods that can also be used to evaluate urethral mobility include imaging methods. Ultrasound may also offer valuable information in women with rSUI after MUS surgery to define both the in vivo time-related structural changes and position of the surgical tapes regarding urethral length and lumen [7].

Cystoscopy is recommended for all women suffering from persistent/recurrent urinary incontinence after anti-incontinence surgery. In this case, cystoscopy revealed urethral funnelling in which a pouch was created at the bladder neck interfering with adequate closure of the urethra. Additionally, Prolene sutures underneath the mucosa on the left side of the bladder wall were seen. Due to a distorted bladder cavity, the urethral orifices and ejection of urine were barely determined. No mesh erosion or fistula formation were observed on cystoscopy (Video 4.1).

Ambulatory urodynamic monitoring (AUM) during a single voiding cycle using the LUNA ambulatory monitoring recorder (MMS™) was performed. AUM has the advantage of allowing patients to perform activities or manoeuvre freely to be provocative for their urinary symptoms, such as listening to running water, hand washing, coughing, sitting, picking up an object from the floor, standing, walking or jumping. As AUM provides free movement for patients during cystometry, in cases of conventional urodynamics, it is worth emphasising that filling cystometry should also include an assessment in an erect position. During the single voiding cycle, no detrusor over-activity was recorded. Stress urinary incontinence, however, was confirmed. A pressure-flow study did not reveal any voiding dysfunction.

Surgery was performed to explore the space of Retzius and for mobilisation of the bladder neck. The observed Prolene sutures, passing through the bladder wall underneath the mucosa, were cut and extracted. The dense fibrotic tissues were dissected until the traction on the bladder neck resolved. In order to maintain continence, a retropubic tension-free vaginal tape was performed under direct vision of the space of Retzius. Preoperative urinary leakage during the compression on the posterior vaginal wall was no longer observed post-operatively. Control cystoscopy revealed an improvement of the bladder distortion, and appropriate closure of the urethra was visualised (Video 4.2).

Three months after the lysis of the adhesions at the Retzius space with the concomitant retropubic MUS, the patient defined no coital incontinence and a significant improvement in other lower urinary tract symptoms. Moreover, significant improvements in the UDI-6 and IIQ-7 total scores of 8/24 and 8/21, respectively, were also observed. The cough stress test was negative at a bladder volume of 500 mL with a post-void residue of 30 mL.

4.3 Discussion

All women suffering from persistent/recurrent SUI or new-onset symptoms of voiding dysfunction or an overactive bladder and pain or recurrent urinary tract infection after anti-incontinence surgery should be evaluated thoroughly. An individualised assessment should be performed, and treatment should be selected considering the primary failed surgery type. Additionally, while deciding on the surgical re-treatment and preferred surgical type, the existing status of urethral support should be evaluated according to the consensus report of ICI RS [7].

As poor surgical technique is one of the main reasons for the persistence of SUI, it is worth being reminded hitherto of all the surgical tips of the two gold standard anti-incontinence techniques that were reported on the grounds of pooled surgical experience. It was observed that every preventative measure against persistent/recurrent SUI regarding both BC and MUS mostly focused on the types of materials (sutures, tapes) being used and their placement technique in terms of route and/or tension. Permanent suture materials for BC, with two sutures on each side, and polypropylene macro-porous meshes with adequate tensile strength with retro-pubic and trans-obturator routes for mid-urethral tapes are recommended. Both routes are defined with different advantages in select women. Tensions on the sutures and on the tapes are not recommended in either technique. The authors emphasised a free space with various definitions in both techniques, between suture knots and iliopectineal ligaments in BC and between the urethra and the mesh in MUS. The placement of sutures on the endopelvic fascia at the level of the bladder neck and no higher in BC and the placement of tapes underneath the urethra at the level of the mid-urethra in MUS were considered as the mainstay of the surgical success for both techniques [4–6].

In the study of Zimmern et al., a secondary analysis of the selected participants from the SISTER and TOMUS trials was conducted to estimate the rate of recurrent SUI and to analyse the preferred re-treatment options. Additionally, the re-treatment free intervals after BC and autologous fascial and synthetic sling surgeries were examined. A surgical re-treatment rate of 6% with the mostly preferred options of injection of bulking agents or fascial slings was reported within 5 years after primary surgeries. Surgical or non-surgical treatment-free intervals of 5 years were found to be 87% for BC, 96% for autologous fascial slings, 97% for trans-obturator and 99% for retro-pubic MUS [16]. Due to a lack of evidence from high-quality studies, none of the currently available surgical options was found to be superior to be recommended as the most effective alternative for the treatment of persistent/recurrent SUI after failed anti-incontinence procedures [6, 17].

In light of the current literature reporting a wide range of MUS failure rates (8–57%) at 5 years of follow-up, it is apparent that a standardised terminology with clear definitions of surgical failure, "persistent and recurrent urinary incontinence" and "persistent and recurrent SUI" is needed [18].

A management strategy may consist of a single or combination therapy of the currently available retreatment options including both conservative and surgical alternatives, such as pelvic floor physiotherapy, incontinence pessary, vaginal or urethral mechanical devices, medical agents, periurethral injections of bulking agents, sling plication, repeat MUS with or without mesh removal, adjustable tapes, autologous fascial sling, Burch colposuspension and artificial urinary sphincters [7]. Although there is no consistent evidence supporting one surgical procedure over the other, the authors recommended retropubic sling operations as more effective options in women with previous failed incontinence surgery. They supported the use of autologous pubovaginal sling and retro-pubic mid-urethral tapes, as well as BC, trans-obturator tapes and urethral bulking agents with grade C recommendation [19]. However, repeat surgery choice is based on a number of factors, including surgeon and patient preferences, pathogenesis of the recurrence, risk factors of the patients and the type of previous failed surgery. Deciding on a strategic treatment plan should also include making a treatment contract with the patient according to their expected goals from the repeat surgery in order to achieve satisfactory patient-reported outcomes.

4.4 Conclusion

It is widely acknowledged that a detailed evaluation of women with persistent/recurrent urinary incontinence be mandatory to verify the underlying pathogenesis. The probable causes of surgical failure from all aspects should be borne in mind while investigating patients in order to perform an individualised management plan.

References

1. Burch JC. Cooper's ligament urethrovesical suspension for stress incontinence. Am J Obstet Gynecol. 1968;100:764–74.
2. Ford AA, Joseph VT, Veit-Rubin ON, Khullar V, Digesu A. Midurethral slings for treatment of stress urinary incontinence review. Neurourol Urodyn. 2019;38:70–5.
3. Lapitan MC, Cody JD. Open retropubic colposuspension for urinary incontinence in women. Cochrane Syst Rev. 2016;2:CD002912.
4. Dean N, Ellis G, Herbison GP, Wilson D, Mashayeki A. Laparoscopic colposuspension for urinary incontinence in women. Cochrane Syst Rev. 2017;7:CD002239.
5. Ford AA, Rogerson L, Cody JD, Aluko P, Ogah JA. Mid-urethral sling operations for stress urinary incontinence in women. Cochrane Database Syst Rev. 2017;7:CD006375.
6. Cardozo L, Hextall A, Bailey J, Boos K. Colposuspension after previous failed incontinence surgery: a prospective observational study. Br J Obstet Gynaecol. 1999;106:340–4.
7. Smith ARB, Artibani W, Drake MJ. Managing unsatisfactory outcome after mid-urethral tape insertion. Neurourol Urodyn. 2011;30:771–4.
8. Liapis A, Bakas P, Creatsas G. Long-term efficacy of tension-free vaginal tape in the management of stress urinary incontinence in women: efficacy at 5- and 7-year follow-up. Int Urogynecol J Pelvic Floor Dysfunct. 2008;19:1509–12.
9. Ashok K, Wang A. Recurrent urinary stress incontinence: an overview. J Obstet Gynaecol Res. 2010;36:467–73.
10. Langer R, Lipshitz Y, Halperin R, et al. Long-term (10-15 years) follow-up after Burch colposuspension for urinary stress incontinence. Int Urogynecol J. 2001;12:323–7.
11. Jelovsek JE, Barber MD, Karram MM, et al. Randomised trial of laparoscopic Burch colposuspension versus tension-free vaginal tape: long-term follow up. BJOG. 2008;115:219–25.
12. Lazarou G, Minis E, Grigorescu B. Outcomes of stress urinary incontinence in women undergoing

TOT versus Burch colposuspension with abdominal sacrocolpopexy. Int Urogynecol J. 2019;30:245–50.
13. Costantini E, Lazzeri M, Bini V, Zingaro DM, Zucchi A, Porena M. Burch colposuspension does not provide any additional benefit to pelvic organ prolapse repair in patients with urinary incontinence: a randomized surgical trial. J Urol. 2008;180:1007–12.
14. Costantini E, Lazzeri M, Bini V, Zingaro DM, Frumenzio E, Porena M. Pelvic organ prolapse repair with and without concomitant Burch colposuspension in incontinent women: a randomised controlled trial with at least 5-year follow up. Obstet Gynecol Int. 2012;1:1–6.
15. Cosson M, Boukerrou M, Narducci F, Occelli B, Querleu D, Crepin G. Long-term results of the Burch procedure combined with abdominal sacrocolpopexy for treatment of vault prolapse. Int Urogynecol J Pelvic Floor Dysfunct. 2003;14(2):104–7.
16. Zimmern EP, Gormley AE, Stoddard MA, Lukacz SE, Sirls L, Brubaker L, Norton P, Oliphant SS, Wilson T. Management of recurrent stress urinary incontinence after Burch and sling procedures. Neurourol Urodyn. 2016;35:344–34.
17. Bakali E, Johnson E, Buckley BS, Hilton P, Walker B, Tincello DG. Interventions for treating recurrent stress urinary incontinence after failed minimally invasive synthetic midurethral tape surgery in women. Cochrane Database Syst Rev. 2019;9:CD009407.
18. Kavanagh A, Sanaee M, Carlson VK, Bailly GG. Management of patients with stress urinary incontinence after failed midurethral sling. Can Urol Assoc J. 2017;11(6):143–6.
19. Medina AC, Costantini E, Petri E, Mourad S, Singla A, Colorado RS, Contreras OO, Doumouchtsis KS. Evaluation and surgery for stress urinary incontinence: a FIGO working group report. Neurourol Urodyn. 2017;36:518–28.

5 Vesicouterine Fistula

Ana Arrébola-Pajares, José Medina-Polo, Jose Manuel Duarte-Ojeda, Juan Justo-Quintas, Javier Gil-Moradillo, Raquel Sopeña-Sutil, and Alfredo Rodríguez-Antolín

5.1 Introduction

Genitourinary fistulas are one of the most devastating complications in the urogynecology setting. Vesicouterine fistula (VUF) is the rarest form of genitourinary fistulas, with an estimated prevalence of 1–4% for all genitourinary fistulas [1, 2]. In most cases, VUF is secondary to an iatrogenic injury during cesarean section (CS) or vaginal delivery after a previous CS [2, 3].

VUF was first described in the literature by Knipe [4] in 1908 but is known as Youssef's syndrome since its publication in 1957 [5]. Amenorrhea and menstrual bladder hemorrhage or menouria are the most common symptoms [1, 6].

Surgical treatment classically consists of an open surgical approach, with its associated significant morbidities in previously operated patients [1, 7]. Due to the advantages of laparoscopy, it has been proposed as a valid option for repairing VUF. However, there are few cases which report the feasibility of the laparoscopic repair of this entity [2].

A. Arrébola-Pajares (✉) · J. Medina-Polo
J. M. Duarte-Ojeda · J. Justo-Quintas
J. Gil-Moradillo · R. Sopeña-Sutil
A. Rodríguez-Antolín
Hospital Universitario 12 de Octubre, Urología, Madrid, Spain
e-mail: josemedinapolo@movistar.es

5.2 Literature Review

VUFs are rare in modern gynecological practice, with an estimated prevalence of 1–4% for all genitourinary fistulas [2]. A study by Rao et al. [6], which reported 12 patients with VUF, showed that 50% of fistulas occur following CS which were performed urgently. Naouar et al. [2], Unger et al. [8], and Bonillo et al. [9] reported that 83–93% of VUF were diagnosed after a CS.

Conservative therapeutic options, not including surgery, are only effective in 5% of the cases [10, 11]. Therefore, surgery should be considered the mainstay of treatment in the majority of patients. To date, most of the published literature consists of case reports and a case series with a small number of patients and short-term follow-up [2, 8, 10, 12–15]. A laparoscopic approach may be beneficial in terms of less invasive technique, faster recovery, and few anti-analgesic requirements in the postoperative period [8, 12]. However, few surgical reports are available demonstrating laparoscopic techniques repair for VUF. In 1999, Miklos et al. [16] reported the first successful laparoscopic repair of a VUF. The largest series of laparoscopic VUF repair has been reported by Abdel Karim et al. [1]. In the aforementioned study that included 14 patients with VUF, 8 of them were repaired using conventional laparoscopy. In contrast, the remaining 6 cases were repaired by laparoendoscopic single-site surgery (LESS). No complications and no

F. Dökmeci, D. E. E. Rizk (eds.), *Insights Into Incontinence and the Pelvic Floor*,
https://doi.org/10.1007/978-3-030-94174-1_5

conversion to open approach were reported. Purkait et al. [17] conducted the second-largest retrospective series of eight patients with VUF managed with a laparoscopy approach. They concluded that laparoscopic repair is safe, feasible, and effective with successful pregnancy rates in long-term follow-up. Several studies showed that the advantages of a laparoscopy approach are quicker patient recovery and decreased morbidity, shorter hospital stay, and higher patient satisfaction with better cosmetic results with similar success rates to open surgery [8, 12, 18].

Fertility after VUF repair is still a subject of considerable concern. However, it should be noted that reported pregnancy rates after VUF surgical repair range between 25 and 37% [17, 19]. Lotocki et al. [20] reported that, after a VUF repair, the overall pregnancy rate was 31% with full-term delivery at 25%. Bonillo et al. [9] reported two patients who maintain fertility and got pregnant 24 months after the surgery.

5.3 Case Study: Laparoscopic Repair of a Vesicouterine Fistula

(a) **Aim**

We aim to review the management of a VUF (Youssef's syndrome) with a laparoscopic approach.

(b) **Patient and Methods**

We presented a surgical technique with a laparoscopic approach for repairing a VUF using primary closure of the fistula and TachoSil® interposition.

A 40-year-old woman was referred to our department with urinary incontinence associated with menouria, 2 months following a late abortion at 22 weeks of pregnancy. The woman, otherwise healthy, had previously had six pregnancies, and her first child was born by caesarean section. After the birth of the fourth child, she presented vesicovaginal fistula that was satisfactorily managed with a bladder catheter.

At the clinic, vaginal examination showed normal vulva, vagina, and urethral meatus. Instillation of diluted methylene blue into bladder revealed vaginal leakage.

The cystoscopy (Fig. 5.1) confirmed the findings of a well-granulated fistulous tract at the posterior wall of the bladder. The computerized tomography (CT) showed the presence of VUF that connected the base of the bladder and the anterior uterine wall (Fig. 5.2).

A surgical management of the VUF was planned with a laparoscopic approach. The procedure was performed with general anesthesia, and the patient was placed in the lithotomy position. First of all, a cystoscopy

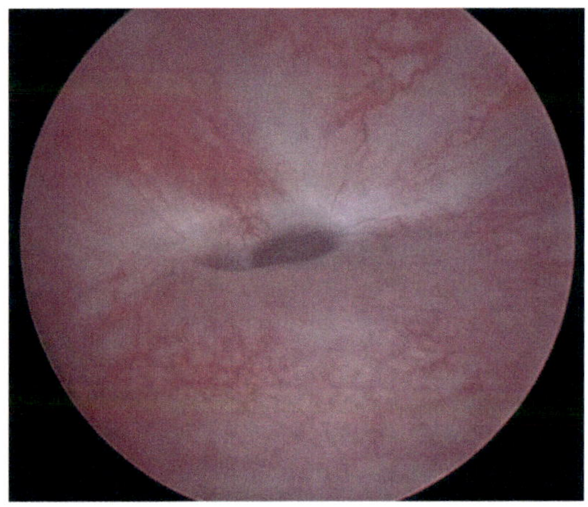

Fig. 5.1 Cystoscopy showed a hole smaller than 1 cm in the posterior bladder wall

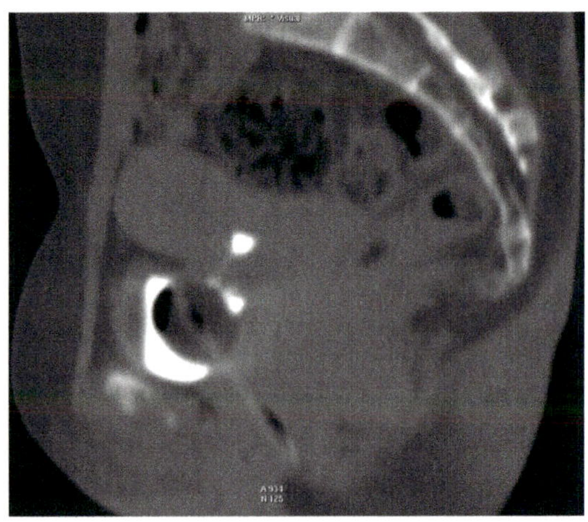

Fig. 5.2 CT showed the presence of VUF with a 1 cm filiform fistulous tract to the uterine cervix

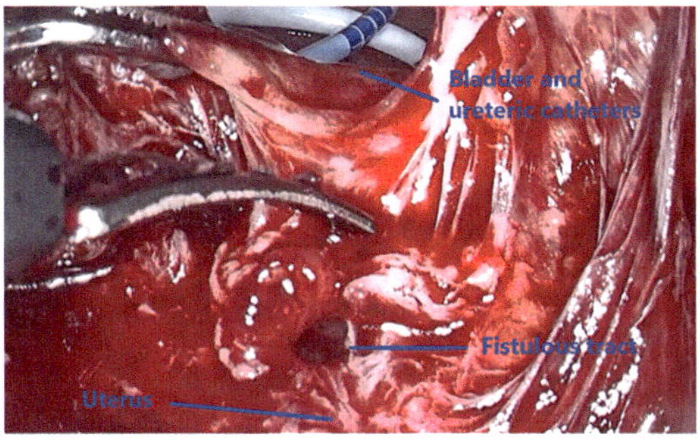

Fig. 5.3 Fistulous tract was excised

was performed with bilateral ureteric catheterization to help identify and protect the ureters. A catheter was also passed through the fistula to aid her identification, and then a urethral Foley catheter was inserted into the bladder. Thereafter, the patient was placed in a supine position with Trendelenburg. Pneumoperitoneum was created using open Hasson technique. One 10 mm and two 5 mm secondary ports were created in both right and left iliac fossae, under laparoscopic vision. As a surgical technique, in dissecting the plane between the uterus and the bladder, a malleable retractor was placed in the vagina to elevate the cervical stump and facilitate dissection of the bladder from the lower uterus. The dissection of the posterior bladder wall, near the fistula, was difficult due to the dense fibrous tissue. The fistulous tract was excised (Fig. 5.3), and the edges were removed by the endoscopic scissors in order to get better healing. The posterior wall of the bladder was completely mobilized. Bilateral ureteric catheters were removed before closing the bladder. The bladder was repaired with two V-locTM® running sutures, and the uterus defect was closed with three "figure eight" sutures of 2-0 polyglactin. Bladder integrity was checked with 250 mL of saline, with no leaks demonstrated. A fibrin sealant patch (TachoSil®) was interposed between the uterus and the bladder, over the sutures. Blood loss was minimal. The patient was discharged on day 2 with indwelling catheter drainage for 4 weeks.

No complications during surgery and postoperative period were reported.

(c) **Results of the Study**

The patients remained asymptomatic with the resumption of normal menses and no clinical evidence of fistula recurrence at 3 months follow-up (Fig. 5.4).

Despite the recommendations, 4 months after surgery, the patient got pregnant again. Due to the risk of fistula recurrence after VUF repair, delivery was performed by CS. At 37 weeks of pregnancy, a planned CS was underwent with no fistula recurrence at 22 months follow-up.

5.4 Discussion

VUF is an anomalous communication developing between the bladder and the uterus or cervix [2], a rare type of genitourinary fistula that accounts for 1–4% of all reported urogenital fistulas [1, 2, 21]. In development countries, VUF can occur following prolonged and obstructed labor. The most common etiology in developed countries is iatrogenic following gynecological surgery or CS [10, 15]. As lower uterine segment cesarean deliveries have increased in popularity, they have become the more common cause of VUF formation [8, 22], and the management of this entity becomes even more important. Other causes of VUF include uterine rupture (often in the context of a previous cesarean section), instrumental delivery, abnormal implantation of the placenta (previa or percreta), manual removal of the placenta, an intra-uterine device, inflammatory bowel disease, malignancy or radiotherapy [10, 15]. Congenital forms of ureterovesical fistula have also been described, but they are sporadic cases [23].

VUF can present with clinical symptoms varying from cyclic hematuria (menouria), amenorrhea, vaginal leakage, or urine infertility of first-trimester abortion [8, 10, 24, 25]. A classification of VUF based on the routes of menstrual flow has been proposed by Jozwik who divides VUF into three types. Type I (of menouria) is characterized by the triad of amenorrhea,

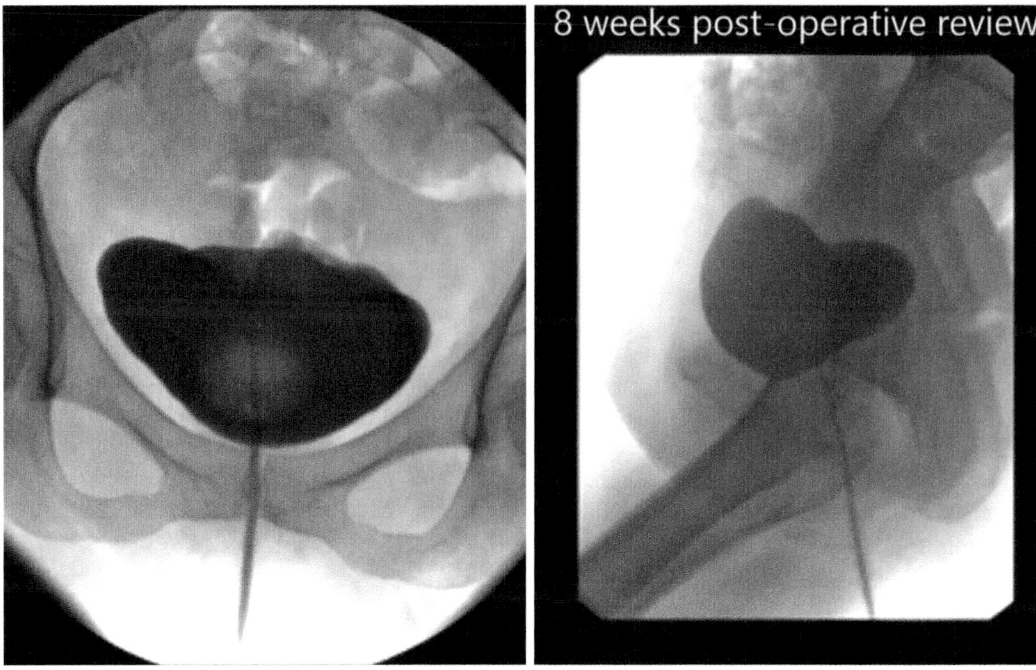

Fig. 5.4 Control cystography

menouria, and complete continence of urine. This triad has been known as Youssef's syndrome. Type II (double flow) is associated with the coexistence of menouria, vaginal menstruation, and constant or periodic urinary incontinence. Type III (vaginal menstruation) is characterized by lack of menouria, normal vaginal menstruation, and constant or periodic urinary incontinence [2, 3, 5].

Confirming the diagnosis of a VUF may be challenging. On pelvic examination, a fistula is usually not palpable. Hysteroscopy, cystoscopy, and cystography remain the "gold standard" in the diagnosis [2, 8]. The diagnosis can be confirmed by methylene blue instilled into the bladder. Additional modalities include CT and magnetic resonance imaging (MRI). MRI can delineate the fistula tract and its relation to the bladder and uterus [2, 10].

Treatment options depend upon fistula size, time of presentation, and symptoms. Conservative therapeutic options that have been proposed are bladder catheterization, hormonal therapy, and cystoscopic fulguration of the VUF. At least 3-week bladder catheterization is an option for patients who are in the early postpartum phase with a small fistula. Hormonal therapy consists of induction of artificial amenorrhea to prevent blood drainage through the fistula tract [2, 10, 21, 22]. However, conservative therapeutic options only show successful response in 5% of the cases [2, 10, 11]. In this way, surgery should be considered the mainstay of treatment in the majority of patients. Open surgical repair has been the traditional treatment with good results. As surgeons are becoming more proficient with minimally invasive techniques, it is now achievable to repair these fistulae laparoscopically. The basic surgical principles are release of the fistulous communication with a wide exposure and excision of scar tissues around the fistula, tension-free closure of the wound, and interposition of tissue to obliterate dead space and prevent hematoma formation. Absorbable sutures should be used to avoid necrosis. The repaired region must have a good blood supply [2, 17, 22]. All the steps of fistula repair that are usually performed in open surgery could be performed in laparoscopy surgery. We argue that this approach to surgery may be the most favorable by surgeons who are experienced in laparoscopy. Laparoscopic approach offer improvement in visualization resulting in excellent exposure to the vesicouterine pouch and retrovesical space, but intracorporeal suturing is the difficult part of the surgery [2, 21]. In our case, bilateral ureteric catheterization helps us to identify and protect the ureters during the surgery. The introduction of a malleable retractor into the vagina to elevate the cervical stump and the catheterization of the fistula were beneficial to localize the fistula tract, allowing meticulous dissection in the retrovesical space between the bladder and the uterus and resection of the fistula tract with minimal manipulation of the bladder. The interposition of a peritoneal or omental flap obliterates the dead space and prevents the formation of hematomas, avoiding the recurrence of the fistula. The first surgeon to introduce the concept of flap interposition was Martius in 1928 [26], who used a flap of adipose tissue obtained from the labia majora. In our case, rather than interpose a tissue flap, we used an absorbable fibrin sealant patch (TachoSil®), a collagen-rich spongy material covered with clotting factors, fibrinogen, and thrombin. Giusti et al. [27] reported successful laparoscopic repair of vesicovaginal fistulas in 16 patients with TachoSil® application as interposition tissue. They conclude that the use of TachoSil® can be considered a simple, quick, and atraumatic alternative that allows to simplify the procedure without impact on outcomes. Laparoscopy has proved advantages in terms of low morbidity, quicker convalescence, shorter hospital stay, and better cosmetic results while preserving the same success rates of the open surgical approaches [1, 2, 18]. Difficulties in the learning curve are the main obstacles in the practice of this minimally invasive approach [1, 12].

5.5 Conclusion

VUFs are a rare case in modern gynecological practice; most of these are the result of a previous cesarean section. Surgical repair is the standard treatment in most of the cases, and minimally invasive techniques started gaining ground as an alternative approach to traditional open surgical repair. Laparoscopic repair of a VUF is an effective and safe technique with successful outcome and low mobility, but the procedure is a technically challenging procedure that requires good laparoscopic skills.

References

1. Abdel-Karim A, Elmissiry M, Moussa A, Mahfouz W, Abulfotooh A, Dawood W, Elsalmy S. Laparoscopic repair of female genitourinary fistulae: 10-year single-center experience. Int Urogynecol J. 2020;31(7):1357–62.
2. Naouar S, Braiek S, El Kamel R. Laparoscopic repair of vesicouterine fistula: a case report and mini-review of the literature. J Curr Surg. 2016;6(3–4):75–7.
3. Garza Cortés R, Clavijo R, Sotelo R. Laparoscopic treatment of genitourinary fistulae. Arch Esp Urol. 2012;65(7):659–72.
4. Knipe WHW. Vesico-uterine fistula. Am J Obstet Gynecol. 1908;57:211–7.
5. Alonso M, Broseta E, y Jiménez, J. Cap 130: Fístulas urogenitales. In: Jiménez J, Rioja LA, editors. Tratado de Urología. 2nd ed. Barcelona: Prous SA; 2006. p. 2537–59.
6. Youssef AF. Menouria following lower segment cesarean section; a syndrome. Am J Obstet Gynecol. 1957;73(4):759–67.
7. Ghoniem GM, Warda HA. The management of genitourinary fistula in the third millennium. Arab J Urol. 2014;12(2):97–105.
8. Unger CA, Cohen SL, Einarsson JI, Morse AN. Laparoscopic repair of vesicouterine fistula. Female Pelvic Med Reconstr Surg. 2012;18(3):190–2.
9. Bonillo García MA, Pacheco Bru JJ, Palmero Martí JL, Alapont Alacreu JM, Alonso Gorrea M, Arlandis Guzmán S, Jiménez Cruz JF. Fístulas vesicouterinas. Nuestra experiencia tras 25 años [Vesicouterine fistula. Our experience of 25 years]. Actas Urol Esp. 2003;27(9):707–12.
10. Symeonidis EN, Sdralis E, Symeonidis A, Georgiadis C, Kalyvas V, Malioris A, Papathanasiou M. Vesicouterine Fistula (VUF) as a rare urogenital complication managed with delayed surgical repair: a case report and review of the literature. Case Rep Obstet Gynecol. 2018;2018:2394896.
11. Hadzi-Djokic JB, Pejcic TP, Colovic VC. Vesicouterine fistula: report of 14 cases. BJU Int. 2007;100(6):1361–3.
12. Chibber PJ, Shah HN, Jain P. Laparoscopic O'Conor's repair for vesico-vaginal and vesico-uterine fistulae. BJU Int. 2005;96(1):183–6.
13. Das Mahapatra P, Bhattacharyya P. Laparoscopic intraperitoneal repair of high-up urinary bladder fistula: a review of 12 cases. Int Urogynecol J Pelvic Floor Dysfunct. 2007;18(6):635–9.

14. Maioli RA, Macedo AR, Garcia AR, Almeida SH, Rodrigues MA. Laparoscopic repair for vesicouterine fistulae. Int Braz J Urol. 2015;41(5):1030–1.
15. Melon J, Chao F, Chan W, Rosamilia A. Video of the laparoscopic repair of a vesico-uterine fistula. Int Urogynecol J. 2018;29(4):599–600.
16. Miklos JR. Laparoscopic treatment of vesico-uterine fistula. J Am Assoc Gynecol Laparosc. 1999;6(3):339–41.
17. Purkait B, Mehrotra S, Sinha RJ, Bhaskar V, Singh V. Long-term outcome of laparoscopic vesicouterine fistula repair: experience from a tertiary referral centre. Turk J Urol. 2017;43(4):512–6.
18. Hemal AK, Kumar R, Nabi G. Post-cesarean cervicovesical fistula: technique of laparoscopic repair. J Urol. 2001;165(4):1167–8.
19. Rao MP, Dwivedi US, Datta B, Vyas N, Nandy PR, Trivedi S, et al. Post caesarean vesicouterine fistulae—Youssef syndrome: our experience and review of published work. ANZ J Surg. 2006;76(4):243–5.
20. Lotocki W, Jóźwik M, Jóźwik M. Prognosis of fertility after surgical closure of vesicouterine fistula. Eur J Obstet Gynecol Reprod Biol. 1996;64(1):87–90.
21. Singh V, Mandhani PA, Mehrotra S, Sinha RJ. Laparoscopic repair of vesicouterine fistula: a brief report with review of literature. Urol J. 2011;8(2):149–52.
22. Chang-Jackson SC, Acholonu UC Jr, Nezhat FR. Robotic-assisted laparoscopic repair of a vesicouterine fistula. JSLS. 2011;15(3):339–42.
23. Martinez Escoriza JC, Palacios Marques AM, Lopez Fernandez JA, Feliu Rey E, Martin Medina P, Herraiz Romero I, et al. Congenital vesicovaginal fistula with or without menouria: a literature review. Eur J Obstet Gynecol Reprod Biol. 2014;175:38–48.
24. Mercader VP, McGuckin JF Jr, Caroline DF, Chatwani A, Seidmon EJ. CT of vesicocorporeal fistula with menouria: a complication of uterine biopsy. J Comput Assist Tomogr. 1995;19(2):324–6.
25. Lenkovsky Z, Pode D, Shapiro A, Caine M. Vesicouterine fistula: a rare complication of cesarean section. J Urol. 1988;139(1):123–5.
26. Martius H. Die operative Wiederherstellung der vollkommen fehlenden Harnrohre und des Schiessmuskels derselbel. Zentralbl Gynakol. 1928;52:480–6.
27. Giusti G, Lucci Chiarissi M, Abate D, De Vita G, Angioni S, De Lisa A. Early repair of post-hysterectomy vesicovaginal fistulae through a laparoscopic transperitoneal extravesical approach. Experience of a single center. Urology. 2018;119:44–8.

Evaluation of Anal Sphincter Innervation

6

Diego Riva, E. Raimondi, A. Botter, Adolf Lukanović, Kristina Drusany Starič, Corrado Cescon, and Vita Zacesta

6.1 Introduction

Episiotomy is a surgical incision of the perineum with the aim to shorten the second stage of the delivery. Its rate in Europe ranges from 9% in Sweden to 58% in Italy [1]. It may have a significant impact on anal sphincter function, and therefore its relationship with muscular or neurological injuries is still discussed: several studies have demonstrated that midline episiotomy represents an independent risk factor for anal sphincter injuries [2–10]. Nevertheless, even the effect of mediolateral episiotomy is controversial, since some studies showed it to be an independent risk factor [11, 12], whereas other authors found it to be protective for fecal incontinence in primiparous women [13]. A mediolateral episiotomy should be at least 40° from the midline to avoid anal sphincter [4], but unfortunately in current practice it has been shown that no midwife and only 22% of doctors perform true mediolateral episiotomies [14]. However the decision to perform an episiotomy is a clinical judgment, and routine use of episiotomy is not advised anymore. Mediolateral episiotomy is recommended in association with instrumental-assisted deliveries, breech deliveries, and shoulder dystocia [15]. Moreover, when compared with a spontaneous tear, episiotomy may allow more accurate tissue apposition during primary repair with potential benefits in wound healing. The identification of anal sphincter injuries in the patients who had episiotomy is often difficult, and most of such lesions cannot be identified and therefore completely repaired.

The risk of pudendal nerve damage during physiological delivery or obstetric maneuvers represents a great point of interest too: it has been largely discussed in literature, but there is no general indication regarding the optimal location of episiotomy because of the large interindividual variability of EAS innervation [16, 17].

To investigate anal function after delivery, quantitative needle electromyography (EMG) has been used, but only a limited number of studies reached significative data [18, 19] because of

D. Riva (✉)
IRCCS Humanitas Research Hospital, Humanitas San Pio X, Milan, Italy

E. Raimondi
General Practitioner, Obstet Gynec Dept-Università, Varese, Italy

A. Botter
Laboratory for Engineering of the Neuromuscular System (Lisin), Department Electronics and Telecommunications-Politecnico, Torino, Italy

A. Lukanović · K. D. Starič
Gynec and Obst Dept Div., University of Ljubljana, Ljubljana, Slovenia

C. Cescon
Independent Researcher, Vacallo, Switzerland
e-mail: corrado.cescon@supsi.ch

V. Zacesta
Bellinzona and Valli Regional Hospital, Bellinzona, Switzerland

F. Dökmeci, D. E. E. Rizk (eds.), *Insights Into Incontinence and the Pelvic Floor*,
https://doi.org/10.1007/978-3-030-94174-1_6

the large variability of the results. The recruitment of the healthy subjects may be difficult because of the pain related to this invasive procedure. A study demonstrated that postpartum women affected by fecal incontinence show evidence of denervation/reinnervation of the EAS, when compared with asymptomatic women after their first vaginal delivery [19]. More significant data were recently reported by Zacesta and colleagues in 2018 [20] and by Cescon and colleagues [21] with mini-invasive EMG.

6.2 Literature Review

Fecal or anal incontinence is highly prevalent among adult women after delivery and has an important economic impact.

There are conflicting evidences from large studies, mostly observational, about the risk of FI and AI for women undergoing vaginal birth compared with cesarean delivery. A large recent Swedish national population-based study analyzed women who gave birth only by either vaginal or cesarean delivery between 1973 and 2015 and linked the delivery mode data to AI diagnoses between 2001 and 2015 [22]. They concluded that women who underwent only vaginal deliveries were 65% more likely to be diagnosed with AI compared with women who underwent only cesarean delivery. In contrast, a 2018 cohort study that recruited over 1500 women 5–10 years after their first delivery and followed them for up to 9 additional years did not support that cesarean delivery was associated with a reduced risk of AI, compared with women who had a spontaneous vaginal delivery [23].

Within the anorectum complex, normal continence is achieved, thanks to the interaction among the internal and external anal sphincter, puborectalis muscle, and sensory information that are under local, spinal, and central control [24]. The pudendal nerves innervate the external anal sphincter bilaterally. The development of incontinence may be caused by injuries to the levator ani muscle or changes in the anal sphincter muscle activation [25]. Recent advances in pelvic floor electromyography (EMG) allow the functional analysis of external anal sphincter with a minimally invasive rectal probe. If pudendal nerve or any of the continence mechanisms is altered during delivery, EMG signals should change at the postpartum investigation [26, 27].

Since 1996, when the World Health Organization recommended an episiotomy rate of approximately 10% (Birth. [28]), rates of episiotomy have generally been in decline. Sweden (6.6% in 2010), Iceland (7.3% in 2010), and Denmark (4.9% in 2010) are the only countries representing a very small overall episiotomy rate (Graham et al. [1]). Meanwhile Asian countries have very high overall episiotomy rates with the following leading countries: India (68% in 2008), China (85.5% in 2003), and Thailand (91.0% in 2005). Dynamic analysis made by Clesse in 2018 noted that 26 countries in Europe and North America showed a downward trend, often remaining below 30%; however these results correlate with an increased number of cesarean section [29].

6.3 Case Study: EMG Analysis of Anal Sphincter Innervation After Episiotomy

(a) **Aim and Scope**

The objective of this study was to evaluate the effect of episiotomy on the sphincter innervation, submitting patients to pre- and postpartum intra-anal, minimally invasive EMG. The knowledge before delivery of the individual location of the innervation zones (IZs) of the anal sphincter will suggest the best side to perform episiotomy, if necessary, reduce the likelihood of creating asymmetries, and, at the end, lead to a reduction of the consequences of this obstetric maneuver [27] on anal sphincter.

(b) **Study Design Materials and Methods**

Five hundred eleven primiparous women participated in the study. Nine clinical partners from five European countries (Germany, Italy, Latvia, Slovenia, Ukraine) were involved in the study. Each clinical partner obtained the approval from the local ethical committee. The inclusion criteria were nulliparous woman, cephalic presentation, no episodes of anal incontinence before pregnancy, no previous pelvic operations, no presence of neuropathies affecting pelvic innervation, no planned cesarean section, and no third-degree hemorrhoids. Each subject was informed about the study protocol and signed an informed consent form prior to the tests.

Questionnaires describing the clinical situation before, during, and after delivery were collected by questioning the subjects and analyzing medical records regarding the delivery.

Multichannel EMG is the summation of electrical contributions from individual motor units (MUs) detected with minimally invasive electrode arrays. Recent signal processing techniques provide tools to identify the location of the innervation zone (IZ) of individual motor units [30, 31]. The IZ is the region where the axonal terminal branches connect to muscle fibers through the neuromuscular junctions (NMJ). The muscle fiber action potentials start at the NMJ, propagate along each fiber, and extinguish at its ends.

Signals were detected using the probe shown in Fig. 6.1. The probe is a plastic support of 14 mm diameter holding a plastic circuit with 16 electrodes equally spaced along the circumference (Cescon and Merletti [32]). The depth for the anal insertion is marked on the probe. During the EMG measurements, each subject was laying on her back in a gynecologic chair with legs in stirrups while a trained doctor or midwife was holding the EMG probe in place. The probe was inserted for 15–20 mm in the anal canal in order to have the electrode array in correspondence of the anal verge. The orientation of the electrodes was always the same, with the midline between the 1st and the 16th electrode in ventral position (Fig. 6.1).

Each experimental session consisted of a series of EMG measurements performed as follows. The tip of the probe was lubricated with a drop of glycerol and inserted in the anal canal. After 2 min, when the EMG signals were stabilized, three acquisitions of 10 s were performed without the subject contracting the sphincter (rest), with 2-min pause in between, to test possible trends of muscle activity. The subjects were then asked to perform three maximal voluntary contractions (MVCs) for 10 s each of the EAS with 2-min pause in between. A total of six recordings were performed for each experimental session (three rest and three MVCs).

The MVCs were preceded and followed by increasing and decreasing force ramps of about 5 s in order to avoid movement artifacts due to sudden force changes.

The duration of the measurement protocol was approximately 12 min with 5–10 additional minutes for paper work, instructions, and positioning of the patient in the gynecologic chair.

Acquisition System

The 16 surface EMG signals were acquired in single differential derivation (Fig. 6.1) with an EMG-USB amplifier (LISiN and OT Bioelettronica, Torino, Italy, with gain variable from 100 to 10,000 in seven steps, 10,500 Hz 3 dB bandwidth, roll-off of 40 dB/decade, noise level lower than 1 μVRMS), sampled at 2048 Hz, and stored on a PC after 12bit A/D conversion. Slow signals produced by active smooth muscles (if any) were rejected because of the high-pass filter at 10 Hz.

Signal Processing

Signals were divided in epochs of 0.5 s. For each channel and epoch, average rectified value (ARV) of the EMG signals was computed after visual inspection of the raw signals for absence of artifacts and interferences. The ARV values were averaged along the 20 epochs in order to have one ARV value for each channel and extract the ARV distribution in the anal canal during rest and one during MVC.

Single MUAPs were identified from surface EMG signals by a decomposition method based on the Convolution Kernel Compensation (Holobar et al. [33]). The main limitation of the decomposition algo-

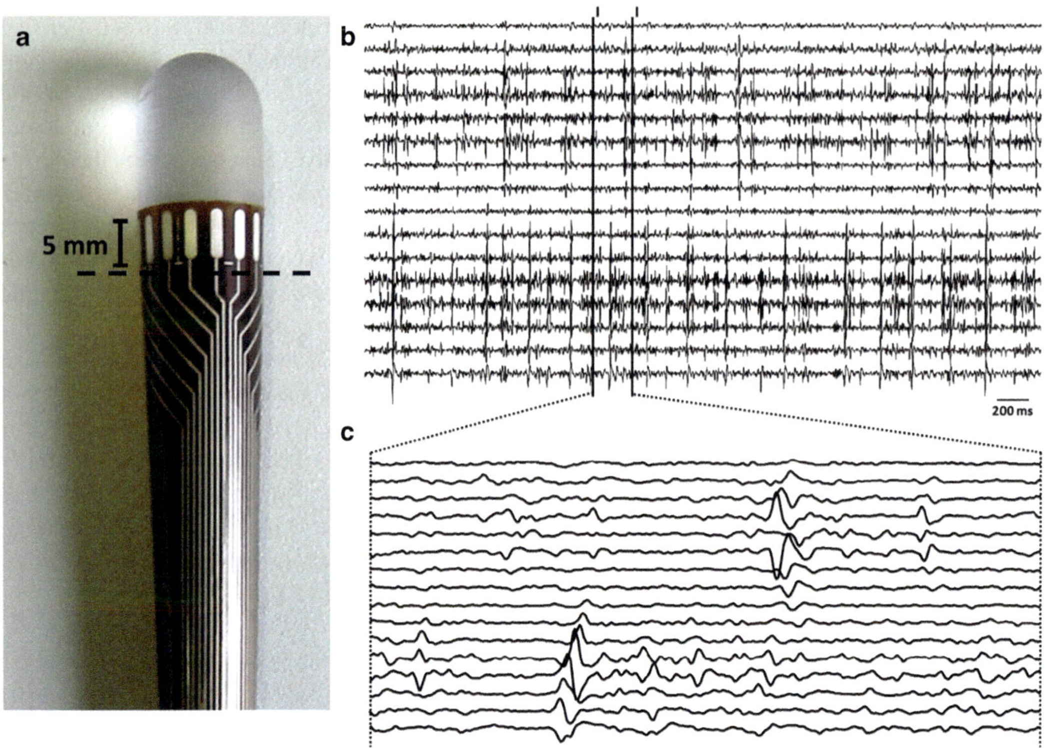

Fig. 6.1 (**a**) Picture of the disposable rectal probe. The probe is a plastic support of 14 mm in diameter holding an electric circuit printed on a thin plastic film with 16 equally spaced electrodes. (**b**) Example of sEMG signals detected from the external anal sphincter of a subject during rest. It is possible to observe action potentials of motor unit with different innervation zones. (**c**) Two large motor units with different innervation zones are visible in the zoomed EMG signal portion. (Reproduced with permission from Springer-Verlag, Italy [21])

rithm and of surface EMG in general is that the number of active and visible MUs is lower than the total number of active MUs, but it was already applied to EMG signals from EAS muscle and was proved to be robust to noise, allowing a complete reconstruction of up to ten concurrently active MUs (Holobar et al. [34]). The IZCorr2 algorithm (Cescon [30]) was applied to the MU templates to identify the innervation zone of each motor unit.

The study was conducted in a double blind fashion, meaning that the clinical partners did not receive any information regarding the IZs of the patients and that the signal analysis was performed without having information regarding the type of delivery. Two measurement sessions were performed for each subject: the first during pregnancy at the 28th to 34th week of gestation and the second at 6–8 weeks after the delivery (end of puerperium).

(c) **Results of the Study**

Among the 511 women recruited for this study, none of them had fourth-degree lacerations and in none of them forceps or vacuum extraction had been used. Only 331 patients returned for the second measurement after the delivery. The percentage of dropout patients was therefore 35%.

All C-section patients included in the analysis had their C-section performed during the first stage of labor.

The signals were visually inspected and classified in five different classes according to the overall signal quality. The quality was

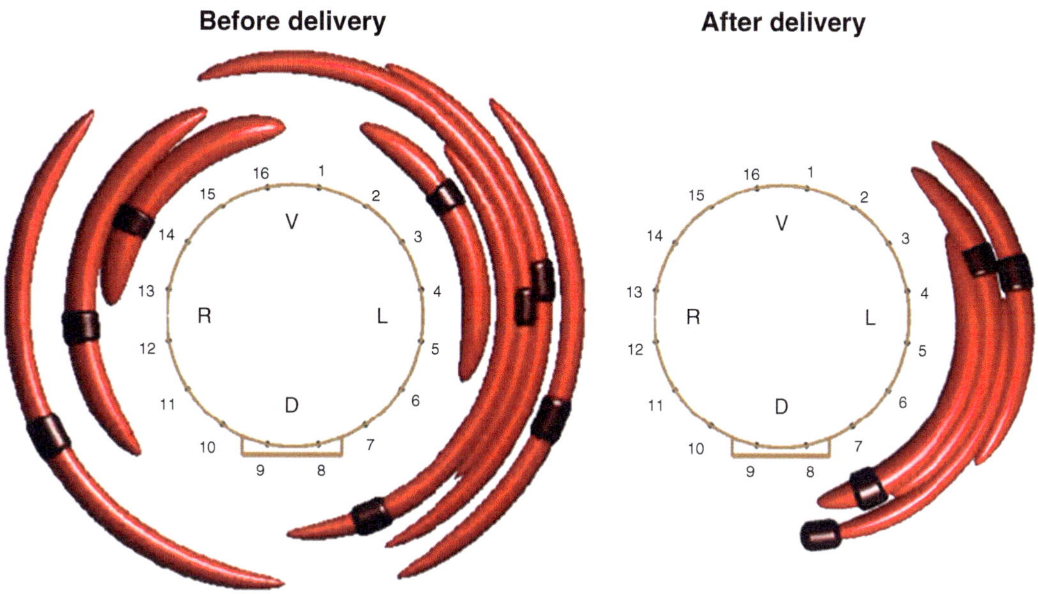

Fig. 6.2 Shows an example of distribution of innervation zones for a subject who had a vaginal delivery with right mediolateral episiotomy of more than 3 cm at approximately 30–40° from the midline. (Reproduced with permission from Springer-Verlag, Italy [21])

assessed on the basis of the absence of (a) artifacts due to contact problems and movement of the probe, (b) power line interference, (c) short circuits between electrodes, (d) saturation of the EMG channels, and (e) noise level. Therefore signals were classified from Q1 to Q5 on the basis of the quality of signals. The patients with signals of quality Q1 and Q2 (bad signals) in any of the two measurement sessions were discarded from the analysis: the final number of women included in the following analysis was 249 out of 331. The channel signals of quality Q3 and Q4 were reconstructed interpolating the adjacent good channels.

Subject Grouping

The 249 women with signal quality Q3-Q4-Q5 were divided in groups according to the type of delivery (vaginal or with cesarean section, n = 189 and 60 respectively), and in case of vaginal delivery they were divided in intact perineum (n = 32), spontaneous perineal tears/lacerations (n = 75), and mediolateral right episiotomy (n = 82). No statistically significant difference was observed as regards the subject weight and infant parameters between the four groups of subjects (one-way ANOVA).

A significant difference was observed in subject age (one-way ANOVA, $F = 6.09$; $p < 0.01$), with older patients receiving more frequently C-section or episiotomy with respect to younger subjects who had spontaneous lacerations or no damage.

The MUs on the right side of the sphincter can no longer be detected after delivery, suggesting neural or muscular damage on the right side (Fig. 6.2).

Estimates of the difference (pre-post) in the number of innervation zones in the four quadrants for two groups of subjects (cesarean section, episiotomy). Estimates and their 95% confidence intervals, in brackets, are reported. The only significant difference is for the right ventral (RV) quadrant of the women who had episiotomy ($p < 0.05$) (Fig. 6.3) Table 6.1.

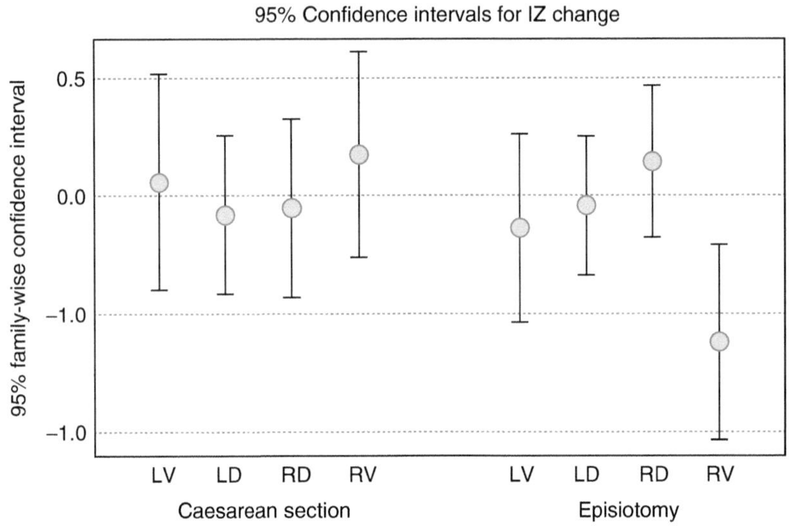

Fig. 6.3 Shows the confidence intervals for the change in the number of innervation zones in the four EAS quadrants and in the two groups of patients of interest (cesarean sections as control group and episiotomies as cases). Bars not cutting the zero line are significant at $p < 0.05$. The only difference was seen in the right ventral quadrant after episiotomy. (Reproduced with permission from Springer-Verlag, Italy [21])

Table 6.1 Estimates and their 95% confidence intervals, in brackets, are hetre reportedThe only significant difference is for the right ventral (RV) quadrant of the Estimates and their 95% confidence intervals, in brackets, are hetre reported. The only significant difference is for women who had episiotomy (p<0.05)

Quadrant delivery	Left ventral	Left dorsal	Right dorsal	Right ventral
C. section Mean [95%CI]	0.05 [−0.40 0.51]	−0.08 [−0.41 0.25]	−0.04 [−0.42 0.32]	0.17 [−0.25 0.60]
Episiotomy mean [95%CI]	−0.13 [−0.53 0.26]	−0.04 [−0.34 0.24]	0.14 [−0.17 0.46]	−0.62 [−1.03 −0.21]

6.4 Discussion

6.4.1 Limitations and Weaknesses of the Study

The first limitation in the analysis of the database is the high drop-off rate for the second measurement (postpartum). This phenomenon might be attributed to many reasons, including the limited availability of the subjects due to maternal duties and the lack of compliance for a second test of purely scientific relevance. However, as we were able to collect delivery data from 73 of the 180 women who did not return for the second measurements, it is reasonable to assume that the lack of data due to the non-returning women did not affect the results.

A second limitation of the study is the relatively high number of low-quality signals which is likely due to the lack of experience of the operators in using the lubricant, as well as to the limited time devoted for performing the tests.

The innervation of the sphincter is only a proxy for anal incontinence (the final clinical endpoint) which has not been assessed in this study. The proxy is valid if there is a causal connection between innervation and incontinence. This connection is suggested in the literature [35].

6.4.2 Strengths of the Study

This is the first observational study investigating innervation of the EAS pre- and postpartum. Although the focus was on episiotomy, a number of additional findings are now available. Some of these findings were predictable but have never been previously documented by an electrophysiological analysis of the EAS.

Cesarean section did not modify the number of innervation zones in any quadrant in a statistically significant way. The same results can be observed for the vaginal delivery with no evident perineal damage and for the spontaneous laceration group, fourth-degree lacerations being absent.

Although the obvious conclusion would be that episiotomy should be avoided in order to preserve EAS innervations, clinicians have to take into account the other risk factors related to C-section and the benefits of episiotomy during vaginal delivery.

A Cochrane review to determine the possible benefits and risks of the use of restrictive episiotomy versus routine episiotomy during delivery [36] found that the restrictive use of episiotomy shows a lower risk of clinically relevant morbidities including severe perineal trauma.

In addition, the guidelines from the Royal College of Obstetricians and Gynaecologists (RCOG) and from the British National Institute for Health and Clinical Excellence (NICE) indicate that routine episiotomy should not be carried out during spontaneous vaginal birth and that it should be performed only if there is a clinical need such as instrumental birth or suspected fetal compromise.

In our studies all episiotomies were performed because of suspect fetal compromise or threat of severe perineal tears, and no routine episiotomy was performed. In this case we cannot predict the degree of spontaneous lacerations that would have occurred if episiotomy had not been performed, but according to the literature [36], the lacerations would have likely been of third or fourth degree.

In our group of subjects, the spontaneous lacerations are mostly of first or second degree, and none is of fourth degree. These lacerations did not significantly affect the innervation of the EAS muscle. In addition, occult lacerations or sphincter injuries could have occurred also in the group of vaginal delivery without evident damage. For this reason the cases considered in the final analysis were only episiotomies (as cases) and C-sections (as controls).

The conclusion of this work is that episiotomy causes a loss of innervation on the side where it is performed. The operator should then choose the side which is less innervated in order to reduce possible damage due to the loss of innervation. Follow-up studies are necessary to evaluate the possible reinnervation of the EAS and to observe if anal incontinence will occur more likely in patient who had severe loss of innervation of this muscle.

We must underline that episiotomy is usually performed at the right side because the operators are right handed. The finding that a left mediolateral episiotomy is preferable when the dominant innervation is in the right side implies the development or adaptation of surgical instrumentation to perform left episiotomy with the right hand.

6.5 Conclusion

A rigorous statistical analysis (generalized mixed linear model) was applied to evaluate interactions between factors such as EAS quadrant, type of delivery, and time (before and after delivery) for the count variable "IZ number." The results of the analysis showed that there is a statistically significant decrease of the number of innervation zones (mean = 0.62, 95%CI [−1.03: −0.21]) in the right ventral quadrant of the EAS in women who have had mediolateral right episiotomy. Statistically significant changes of the number of innervation zones were not observed in the cases of cesarean section or vaginal delivery with spontaneous lacerations.

Knowledge of the pre-partum distribution of IZs allows gynecologists and obstetricians to evaluate the risk of episiotomy and to choose the side where to perform it in case it would be deemed necessary at the time of delivery. This knowledge, which can be obtained with a disposable probe and a minimally invasive surface EMG pre-partum test, is expected to reduce the consequences of episiotomy.

Acknowledgment The authors are grateful to Prof R Merletti for his studies and support to this publication and to project TASI that was financially supported by Compagnia di San Paolo, Torino, Italy.

References

1. Graham ID, Carroli G, Davies C, Medves JM. Episiotomy rates around the world: an update. Birth. 2005;32(3):219–23.
2. Andrews V, Sultan AH, Thakar R, Jones PW. Risk factors for obstetric anal sphincter injury: a prospective study. Birth. 2006;33(2):117–22.
3. Handa VL, Blomquist JL, McDermott KC, Friedman S, Muñoz A. Pelvic floor disorders after vaginal birth: effect of episiotomy, perineal laceration, and operative birth. Obstet Gynecol. 2012;119(2 Pt 1):233–9.
4. Dudding TC, Vaizey CJ, Kamm MA. Obstetric anal sphincter injury: incidence, risk factors, and management. Ann Surg. 2008;247(2):224–37.
5. Edwards NI, Jones D. The prevalence of fecal incontinence in older people living at home. Age Ageing. 2001;30:503–7.
6. Fitzgerald MP, Weber AM, Howden N, Cundiff GW, Brown MB. Risk factors for anal sphincter tear during vaginal delivery. Obstet Gynecol. 2007;109(1):29–34.
7. Kudish B, Blackwell S, Mc Neeley S, et al. Operative vaginal delivery and midline episiotomy: a bad combination for the perineum. Am J Obstet Gynecol. 2006;195:749–54.
8. McKinnie V, Swift SE, Wang W, et al. The effect of pregnancy and mode of delivery on the prevalence of urinary and fecal incontinence. Am J Obstet Gynecol. 2005;193:512–7.
9. Pirro N, Sastre B, Sielezneff IJ. What are the risk factors of anal incontinence after vaginal delivery? J Chir (Paris). 2007;144(3):197–202.
10. Pretlove SJ, Thompson PJ, Toozs-Hobson PM, Radley S, Khan KS. Does the mode of delivery predispose women to anal incontinence in the first year postpartum? A comparative systematic review. BJOG. 2008;115(4):421–34.
11. Sartore A, De Seta F, Maso G, et al. The effects of mediolateral episiotomy on pelvic floor function after vaginal delivery. Obstet Gynecol. 2004;103:669–73.
12. Wheeler TL, Richter HE. Delivery method, anal sphincter tears and fecal incontinence: new information on a persistent problem. Curr Opin Obstet Gynecol. 2007;19(5):474–9.
13. De Leeuw JW, Vierhout ME, Struijk PC, Hop WC, Wallenburg HC. Anal sphincter damage after vaginal delivery: functional outcome and risk factors for fecal incontinence. Acta Obstet Gynecol Scand. 2001;80(9):830–4.
14. Tincello DG, Williams A, Fowler GE, et al. Differences in episiotomy technique between midwives and doctors. BJOG. 2003;110:1041–4.
15. Začesta V, Rācene L, Cescon C, Plaudis H, Rezeberga D. Sphincter muscle activity before and after delivery. Does it depend on the type of birth? J Obstet Gynaecol Res. 2020;47:705–12.
16. Merletti R, Bottin A, Cescon C, Farina D, Mesin L, Gazzoni M, Martina S, Pozzo M, Rainoldi A, Enck P. Multichannel surface EMG for the non-invasive assessment of the anal sphincter muscle. Digestion. 2004;69:112–22.
17. Enck P, Franz H, Azpiroz F, Fernandez-Fraga X, Hinninghofen H, Kaske-Bretag K, Bottin A, Martina S, Merletti R. Innervation zones of the external anal sphincter in healthy male and female subjects. Digestion. 2004;69:123–30.
18. Podnar S, Lukanovic A, Vodusek DB. Anal sphincter electromyography after vaginal delivery: neuropathic insufficiency or normal wear and tear? Neurourol Urodyn. 2000;19(3):249–57.
19. Gregory WT, Lou JS, Simmons K, Clark AL. Quantitative anal sphincter electromyography in primiparous women with anal incontinence. Am J Obstet Gynecol. 2008;198(5):550.e1–6.
20. Začesta V, Rezeberga D, Plaudis H, Drusany-Staric K, Cescon C. Could the correct side of mediolateral episiotomy be determined according to anal sphincter EMG? Int Urogynecol J. 2018;29(10):1501–7.
21. Cescon C, Riva D, Začesta V, Drusany-Starič K, Martsidis K, Protsepko O, Baessler K, Merletti R. Effect of vaginal delivery on the external anal sphincter muscle innervation pattern evaluated by multichannel surface EMG: results of the multicentre study TASI-2. Int Urogynecol J. 2014;25(11):1491–9.
22. Larsson C, et al. Anal incontinence after caesarean and vaginal delivery in Sweden: a national population-based study. Lancet. 2019;393:1233–9.
23. Blomquist JL, Muñoz A, Carroll M, Handa VL. Association of delivery mode with pelvic floor disorders after childbirth. JAMA. 2018;320:2438.
24. Papaconstantinou HT. Evaluation of anal incontinence: minimal approach, maximal effectiveness. Clin Colon Rectal Surg. 2005;18:9–16.
25. Hallock JL, Handa VL. The epidemiology of pelvic floor disorders and childbirth: an update. Obstet Gynecol Clin North Am. 2016;43:1–13.
26. Drusany Staric K, Zacesta V, Cescon C, Vitagliano A, Bukovec P. Multichannel electromyography for the assessment of pelvic floor muscle function. Climacteric. 2018;21(6):617–8.
27. Drusany Staric K, Lukanovic A, Petrocnik P, Zacesta V, Cescon C, Lucovnik M. Impact of mediolateral episiotomy on incidence of obstetrical anal sphincter injury diagnosed by endoanal ultrasound. Midwifery. 2017;51:40–3.
28. Care in normal birth: a practical guide. Technical Working Group, World Health Organization. WHO recommendations: intrapartum care for a positive childbirth experience. Geneva: World Health Organization. Birth. 1997;24(2):121–3.
29. Clesse C, et al. Socio-historical evolution of the episiotomy practice: a literature review. Women Health. 2019;59(4):1–1.
30. Cescon C. Automatic location of muscle innervation zones from multi-channel surface EMG signals. In: Proceedings of the IEEE International Workshop on Medical Measurement and Applications (MeMeA2006), Benevento, Italy. 2006.

31. Ullah K, Afsharipour B, Cescon C, Merletti R. Automatic detection of motor unit innervation zones of the external anal sphincter by multichannel surface EMG. In: Proc of Int. Soc. Electromyog. and Kinesiol. 2014.
32. Cescon C, Merletti R. Conic disposable rectal probe. International Patent Nr. TO2009A000814. 2010.
33. Holobar A, Zazula D. Multichannel blind source separation using convolution kernel compensation. IEEE Trans Signal Process. 2007;55:4487–96.
34. Holobar A, Enck P, Hinninghofer H, Merletti R. Decomposition of surface EMG from external anal sphincter. In: XVII Congress of the International Society of Electrophysiology and Kinesiology, Niagara Falls, Ontario, Canada, June 18–21. 2008.
35. Wietek BM, Hinninghofen H, Jehle EC, Enck P, Franz HB. Asymmetric sphincter innervation is associated with fecal incontinence after anal sphincter trauma during childbirth. Neurourol Urodyn. 2007;26(1):134–9.
36. Carroli G, Belizan J, Stamp G. Episiotomy for vaginal birth. Cochrane Database Syst Rev. 1999;26(4):263. https://doi.org/10.1046/j.1523-536x.1999.00263.x. PMID: 10655834.

7 Impact of Delivery on the Anal Sphincter Innervation

Kristina Drusany Starič, Vita Zacesta, Adolf Lukanović, and Corrado Cescon

Several studies demonstrated that there is a significant correlation between external anal sphincter (EAS) damage during vaginal birth and subsequent development of anal incontinence [1]. The EAS is innervated by the somatic and autonomic nervous system, which is regulated from higher centres. Coordinated operation enables continence and excretion of faeces and flatus. The motor neurons that innervate the EAS muscles originate from the spinal segment from S2 to S4. Somatic nerves originate from the spinal cord and anterior and posterior roots, which merge into the spinal nerve. When it comes out of the intervertebral foramen, it splits into anterior and posterior branches [2]. The autonomic nervous system forms the pelvic plexus. Somatic nerves form the pudendal nerve. The pudendal nerve is most described as consisting of the anterior branches of the spinal nerves from S2 to S4. Research describes that innervation may occur from S1 rather than S4, meaning that the nerve is composed of anterior branches from S1 to S3 [3]. All the fibres form the main trunk—the pudendal nerve—which continues its way through the passage n. ischiadicus and then through the fossa ischiorectalis. Its branches innervate the EAS.

To date, pelvic floor nerve research has been invasive, based on intramuscular EMG. Intramuscular EMG is performed with needles, thus is a painful examination, so it is rarely performed, especially in healthy people. Therefore, relatively little is known about pelvic floor innervation in healthy people, about the asymmetric innervation of the EAS. There is ongoing discussion about the diversity between individuals, but little about the diversity between the left and right side in them [4]. Recently, advanced methods have been developed to try to answer the question whether the innervation of sphincters is symmetrical or asymmetrical. If the innervation is predominant on one side, a damage to the nervous system on the same side would lead to a complete damage of the sphincter function. If the innervation is symmetrical, a damage on one side would lead to a reduction of functionality to 50%. If the injury is on the opposite side, in case of asymmetric sphincter innervation, the damage would be negligible [5]. It is likely that despite the anatomical symmetry of innervation, nerve function is asymmetric in some individuals, as in some other organs, e.g., in the oesophagus [6].

The results of a recent research showed that approximately 20% of external anal sphincters

K. D. Starič (✉) · A. Lukanović
Univerzitetni Klinicni Center Ljubljana, Ginekološka Klinika, Ljubljana, University of Ljubljana, Medical Faculty, Ljubljana, Slovenia
e-mail: kristina.drusany@kclj.si

V. Zacesta
Riga Stradins University, Riga, Latvia

Dipartimento di Ginecologia e Ostetricia, Ente Ospedaliero Cantonale, Bellinzona, Switzerland

C. Cescon
Independent Researcher, Vacallo, Switzerland

F. Dökmeci, D. E. E. Rizk (eds.), *Insights Into Incontinence and the Pelvic Floor*,
https://doi.org/10.1007/978-3-030-94174-1_7

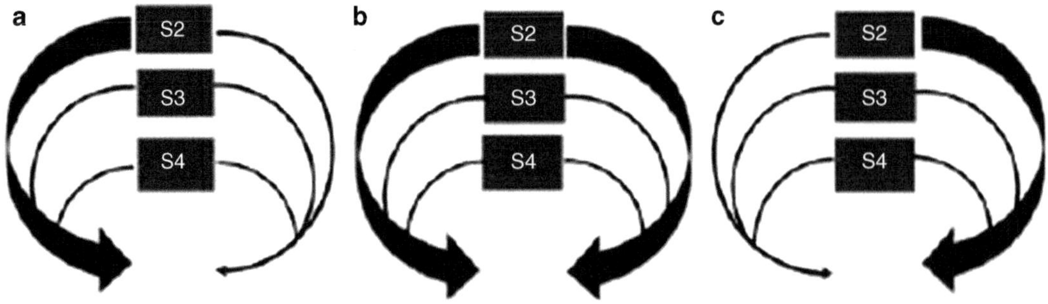

Fig. 7.1 The innervation of the anal sphincter is unique in every individual. On picture (**a**), the innervation is predominantly from the right, on picture (**b**) it is symmetrical and on picture (**c**) it is predominantly on the left site

are asymmetrically resuscitated and their function is symmetrical [5]; schematic examples of possible innervation are shown in the Fig. 7.1.

A new non-invasive method—surface electromyography (sEMG)—has been shown to be useful to detect the innervation pattern of EAS.

Surface EMG is, compared to needle, a minimally invasive method. The sEMG signal is the sum of electrical contributions from individual muscle motor units (MUs) of the muscle detected by minimally invasive electrodes located on the surface of the rectal probe. The most common arrangement for surface sensing EMG signals is a bipolar configuration that detects the difference between the signals of two electrodes placed on the same muscle at a certain distance, usually along the direction of the fibres. By summing the signals of electrical activity, we can obtain information on the location of the innervation zones (IZ) of motor units from multi-channel EMG signals [7]. This method of detection has been used in many studies to assess the function of the EAS using different probes and different electrode placements. Due to improvements in surface EMG technology and accuracy, variability in skeletal muscle innervation was found among subjects [5, 8]. Modern signal processing techniques enable the interpretation of information on the locations of IZ from multi-channel EMG systems [9].

Recognition of the distribution of IZ by the eye has been shown to be reproducible during measurements on different days [10]. Clinical electrophysiological studies can identify the IZ of the EAS [7, 8, 11]. They discovered exceptionally large variations between individuals. A standard pattern of EAS innervation was not found [10, 12].

The latest method, which automatically detects signals, was first tested on simulated signals, and then experimentally lives on 150 subjects. It has been found to be suitable for motor unit (MU) detection but has not been used in major studies to date [9].

During one measurement 5–15 active MUs that are on the surface and have the longest action potentials can be displayed. EMG cannot show in what order the IZ is distant from the probe; only their position with respect to the position of the electrodes can be recognised.

7.1 Case Study: Changes of External Anal Sphincter Innervation Pattern After Delivery

Kristina Drusany Starič, Vita Zacesta, Adolf Lukanović and Roberto Merletti

Univerzitetni Klinicni Center Ljubljana, Ginekološka Klinika, LjubljanaSlovenia
Riga Stradins University, RigaLatvia
Lisin, Politecnico Di Torino, TorinoItaly

Mediolateral episiotomy is the commonly used obstetrical intervention, usually performed on the right side with the aim to facilitate the delivery.

The aim of this study was to show variability of innervation among population and the impact of the episiotomy on the innervation of the anal sphincter.

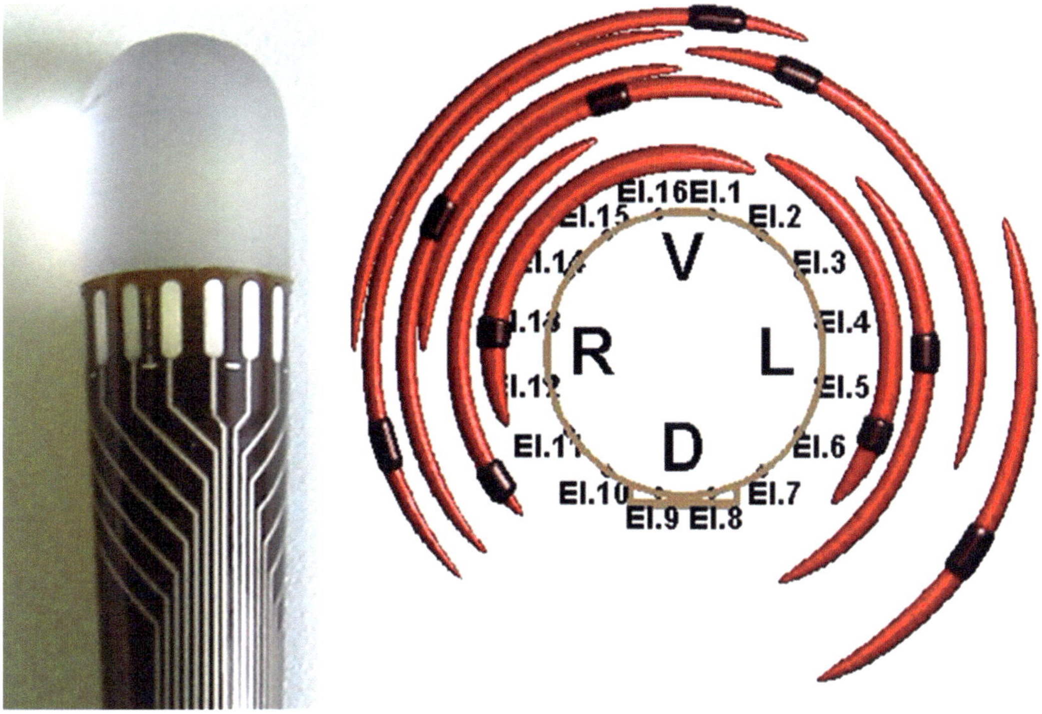

Fig. 7.2 On the left side, a probe with 16 electrodes for the detection of electromagnetic activity is shown. On the right site, the reconstructed motor units are shown. Innervation zones are shown as black dots as a part of motor units, and the propagation of the impulse is shown as a red half circle. The location of the motor unites is determined by the sequential number on the probe. *V* ventral, *D* dorsal, *L* left, *R* right

The signals were detected with a probe developed by the LISiN, Politecnico di Torino, which consists of a plastic support with an electric circuit including 16 silver electrodes equally spaced along the circumference of the probe (Fig. 7.2). With the probe the electrical activity of a small portion closer to the probe of the anal sphincter is measured. On Fig. 7.2 the reconstruction of the MU and IZ is shown. On Fig. 7.3 two examples of the reconstruction of IZ of the anal sphincter are shown. With this method the proximity of the IZ to the anal canal cannot be determined.

The study took place in University Medical Centre in Ljubljana, Slovenia, and Department of gynaecology and obstetrics, Division of Gynaecology and Stradins University in Riga, Latvia. The study was double blind, and it was approved by Republic of Slovenia National Medical Ethics Committee.

Data from the 33 primiparous women with subsequent right mediolateral episiotomy at labour were analysed. EMG measurements were performed with a disposable rectal probe at the 28th to 34th gestational week and 6–8 weeks after delivery. The IZs of single MU were identified by means of a recently developed signal processing technique [9]. Women were divided into three groups according to the distribution of IZ pre-partum: innervated predominantly left, symmetric or right.

Eighteen subjects were predominantly innervated left, 6 were symmetric and were predominantly right. The measurement of the IZs showed that in women with a prevalence of IZ on the right, a statistically significant reduction of the number of IZs was observed after delivery (Wilcoxon signed-rank test, $p = 0.0156$), while predominantly left or symmetric innervated women did not show any changes in their innervation pattern as is shown in Fig. 7.4.

sEMG measurement proved that the innervation pattern is individual and often asymmetric.

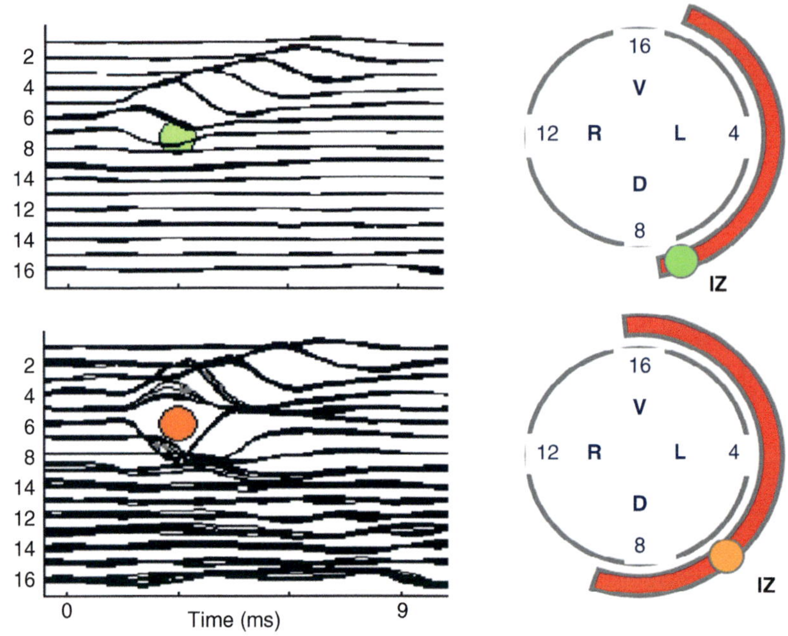

Fig. 7.3 The images on the left side show the EMG patterns. In the middle of the pattern, the green and orange dot show position of the innervation zone. The same innervation zones are shown on the right figures. The location of the motor unit is described by the sequential number of the electrode. *V* ventral, *D* dorsal, *L* left, *R* right

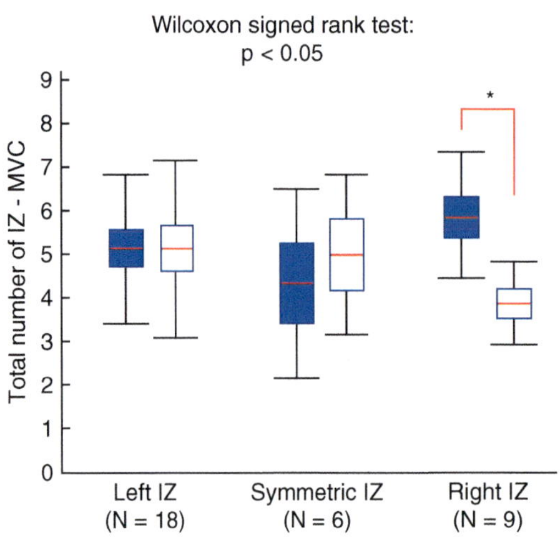

Fig. 7.4 Comparison of the three groups of patients; the total number of the IZ measured by the sEMG is presented with box-plots. The blue boxes show the IZ before the delivery and the white ones after the delivery. The median value is shown with the red stripe. Significant loss of IZ zones is shown with the asterix

Similar results were obtained also in other studies [5, 13–15]. It was not only proved that the difference of innervation exists between the subjects but also the innervation is different on the left and right side in the same subject. If the episiotomy was performed on the predominantly innervated side of the sphincter, it caused a significant damage to the innervation of the EAS as also shown on Fig. 7.5.

If innervation of EAS is from the side of episiotomy, it can be damaged by the procedure, which results in impaired function even if there is no anal sphincter injury (Fig. 7.6).

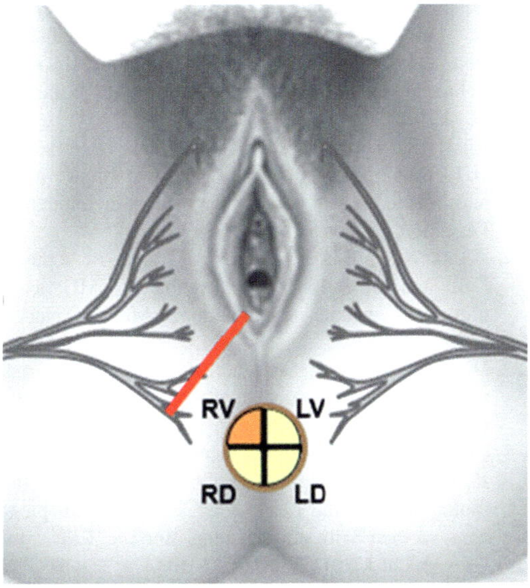

Fig. 7.5 The position of right mediolateral episiotomy in relation to anal sphincter. The quadrants are described as *RV* right ventral, *LV* left ventral, *RD* right dorsal, *LD* left dorsal

7.2 Conclusion

In this chapter, intra- and inter-subject diversity of external anal sphincter innervation was proved. The reduced innervation under the episiotomy has been proven by diminishing of IZ after the delivery. Obtaining the information about the innervation pattern before delivery could help the obstetricians to choose which side would be preferable for the episiotomy and presumably reduce the incidence of anal incontinence.

Acknowledgments We would like to thank Prof. Roberto Merletti for critical reading of the chapter and international project TASI-2 conducted by LISiN, Torino, that was the core project for our research. The authors would like to thank Ana Karolina Starič Drusany for the designs of Figs. 7.1 and 7.6.

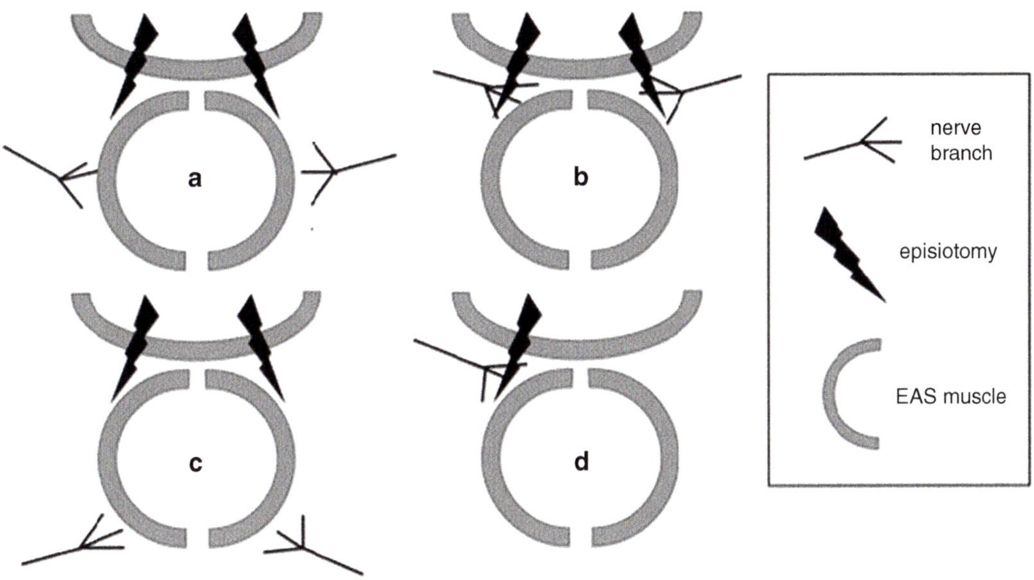

Fig. 7.6 The examples of innervation patterns of the anal sphincter are shown. In the patterns (**a**) and (**c**), episiotomy does not interfere with innervation. In the patterns (**b**) and (**d**), there is danger of nerve injury with episiotomy and subsequently reduced innervation of external anal sphincter

References

1. Haylen BT, de Ridder D, Freeman RM, et al. IUGA/ICS joint report on the terminology for female pelvic floor dysfunction, standardisation and terminology committees IUGA and ICS, joint IUGA/ICS working group on female terminology. Neurourol Urodyn. 2010;29(1):4–20.
2. Kobe V, Dekleva A, Lenart IF, Širca M, Velepič M. Anatomija. 1993;3:55.
3. Marani E, Pijl MEJ, Kraan MC, Lycklama à Nijeholt GA, Videleer AC. Interconnection of upper ventral rami of the human sacral plexus: a reappraisal for dorsal rhizotomy in neurostimulation operations. Neurourol Urodyn. 1993;12:585–98.
4. Vodušek D. Anatomy and neurocontrol of the pelvic floor. Digestion. 2004;69:87–92.
5. Enck P, Franz H, Azpiroz F, et al. Innervation zones of the external anal sphincter in healthy male and female subjects. Digestion. 2004;69:123–30.
6. Hamdy S, Aziz Q, Rothwell JC, Crone R, Hughes D, Tallis RC, Thompson DG. Explaining oropharyngeal dysphagia after unilateral hemispheric stroke. Lancet. 1997;350:686–92.
7. Cescon C. Automatic location of muscle innervation zones from multi-channel surface EMG signals. In: Proceedings of the IEEE International Workshop on Medical Measurement and Applications (MeMeA2006), Benevento (Italy), IEEE. 2006.
8. Merletti R, Bottin A, Cescon C. Multichannel surface EMG for the non-invasive assessment of the anal sphincter muscle. Digestion. 2004;69:112–3.
9. Ullah K, Cescon C, Afsharipour B, Merletti R. Automatic detection of motor unit innervation zones of the external anal sphincter by multichannel surface EMG. J Electromyogr Kinesiol. 2014;24(6):860–7.
10. Enck P, Hinninghofen H, Wietek B, Becker HD. Functional asymmetry of pelvic floor innervation and its role in the pathogenesis of fecal incontinence. Digestion. 2004;69(2):102–11.
11. Podnar S, Rodi Z, Lukanovic A, Trsinar B, Vodusek DB. Standardization of anal sphincter EMG: technique of needle examination. Muscle Nerve. 1999;22(3):400–3.
12. Dirro N, Sastre B, Sielezneff J. What are the risk factors of anal incontinence after vaginal delivery? J Chir. 2007;144:197–202.
13. Cescon C, Raimondi EE, Začesta V, Drusany-Starič K, Martsidis K, Merletti R. Characterization of the motor units of the external anal sphincter in pregnant women with multichannel surface EMG. Int Urogynecol J. 2014;25(8):1097–103.
14. Drusany Staric K, Zacesta V, Cescon C, Vitagliano A, Bukovec P. Multichannel electromyography for the assessment of pelvic floor muscle function. Climacteric. 2018;21(6):617–8. https://doi.org/10.1080/13697137.2018.1514007. Epub 2018 Oct 2. PubMed PMID: 30277095.
15. Začesta V, Rezeberga D, Plaudis H, Drusany-Staric K, Cescon C. Could the correct side of mediolateral episiotomy be determined according to anal sphincter EMG? Int Urogynecol J. 2018;29(10):1501–7. https://doi.org/10.1007/s00192-018-3560-3. PubMed PMID: 29480430.

Part II

Male Urinary Incontinence

8 Suburethral Slings

Javier Gil Moradillo, Jose Medina Polo, Ana Arrebola Pajares, Juan Justo Quintas, Esther García Rojo, Daniel Gonzalez Padilla, Manuel Alonso Isa, Borja Garcia Gomez, and Javier Romero Otero

Bulbourethral slings were designed to be an alternative to artificial sphincters in the treatment of PPI. Since their appearance, RTS have been widely used for the treatment of stress incontinence in men, with a majority use in cases, as previously mentioned, in mild-to-moderate PPI and no previous history of RT. However, most of the available evidence is a short, retrospective, one-center series, with important differences in the definition of "improvement" and "cure" [1, 2].

There is only one systematic review of the literature published in 2016 regarding PPI treatment [3] and few nonsystematic reviews of the surgical treatment of PPI [4–6]. This again demonstrates the lack of quality evidence regarding the use of these devices.

8.1 AdVance/AdVanceXP

The AdVance sling (Boston Scientific) was introduced in 2007. It is the most widely used retrourethral transobturator sling. It consists of a polypropylene mesh which is placed under the membranous urethra through a transection of the centrum tendineum by a transobturator approach.

J. G. Moradillo (✉) · J. M. Polo · A. A. Pajares · J. J. Quintas · E. G. Rojo · D. G. Padilla · M. A. Isa · B. G. Gomez · J. R. Otero
Urology Department, Hospital Universitario 12 De Octubre, Madrid, Spain
e-mail: josemedinapolo@movistar.es

The procedure was initially demonstrated in a cadaver series, which showed that the proximal urethra was repositioned into the pelvic outlet 3–4 cm with a retrograde leak point pressure (RLPP) greater than 60 cm H_2O following tensioning of the mesh. It was theorized that the AdVance sling action is multifactorial by relocating the posterior urethra as well as sphincter region into its original position, an increase of the venous sealing effect, and an increase of the functional urethral length [2].

In 2010, the second generation of the AdVance male sling (AdVanceXP) was introduced. It incorporated mesh barbs to limit sling slippage and loosening. This device is currently available in Europe and Australia but has not been approved for use in the United States by the Food and Drug Administration (FDA).

Follow-up for the AdVance sling is still short. Mid-term outcomes have shown durable results compared with initial reports. In their original study, Rehder and Gozzi reported a cure rate of 40% and an improved rate of 30% [2]. More extended follow-up has been described. In 2012, Rehder and colleagues reported 3-year outcomes following AdVance sling placement (mean: 40.1 months of follow-up) on 156 consecutive patients [7]. Patients were defined as having mild (1–2 pads/day), moderate (2–4 pads/day), or severe (5 pads/day) incontinence. Most patients (64.1%) had mild or moderate incontinence, whereas 35.3% had severe incontinence. Success

F. Dökmeci, D. E. E. Rizk (eds.), *Insights Into Incontinence and the Pelvic Floor*,
https://doi.org/10.1007/978-3-030-94174-1_8

was defined as cured (0–1 pad for security reasons only) or improved (1–2 pads per day, a 50% reduction in daily pad usage from baseline). The durable cure rates reported were 53.8% at 12 months and 53% at 36 months. Overall success rates were 76.9% and 76.8% at 12 and 36 months, respectively. Complications were common, but most of them are mild and transient, including perineal pain (50.0%), urinary retention (9.0%), and dysuria (4.5%).

The authors reported an extended outcome analysis on 102 patients followed for an average of 36.2 months with similar definitions for success [8]. Overall success at final follow-up was 62% (40% cured and 22% improved). These results did not confirm the durability reported by previous series.

There is a single-center prospective study which compares AdVance and AdVanceXP, with a total of 221 patients (121 in AdVance arm and 110 in AdVanceXP) [9]. The cure rate was higher in AdVanceXP arm (65.9% vs 46.2%), but median follow-up is shorter (12 months vs 25 months). Rate of improvement is similar in both arms of study (23.1 for AdVance vs 24.4 for AdVanceXP). It seems that new AdVanceXP is more effective than the first device from Boston Scientific, but a longer follow-up is needed.

Another single-center study compares, in 124 mild to moderate PPI patients, AUS and AdVance (48 and 76 patients, respectively) [10]. A cure rate (0–1 pad) of 88.2% for AdVance and 87.5% for AUS was achieved. There was an important difference in follow-up time, with a median of 24 months for AdVance and 43 months for AUS.

8.2 Virtue Male Sling

The Virtue male sling (Coloplast, Denmark) is a quadratic retrourethral transobturator male sling that has four sling arms. The first study reporting outcomes was in 2014 [11]. They compared an implantation with a fixed anchoring technique with initial trials using a technique without fixation. The authors found objective success rates (defined as >50% weight reduction in standardized pad testing) of 79.2% compared with 41.9% in the initial patient cohort. Similarly, median reduction in pad weight was 88.3% after a follow-up of 12 months compared with 51.1% in the initial cohort.

Recently, several studies addressed the outcome after Virtue male sling placement. McCall et al. [12] reported outcomes of 32 patients after a median follow-up of 55 months. A 22% of patients underwent sling excision due to chronic pain (7%) or continence failure. Notably, the authors found increased failure rates in previously irradiated patients. Due to an overall failure rate of 68%, the authors concluded that Virtue male sling implantation should not be recommended.

A more recent prospective 2-center study with 23 mild to moderate PPI patients showed an improvement of daily urine loss based on 24-h pad testing [13]. The authors stated that the positive results remained stable throughout the follow-up period of 36 months. The overall complication rate was 58.6% and, in all cases, has a Clavien I event.

8.3 I-STOP TOMS

I-STOP TOMS (CL Medical, Lyon, France), which consists in a four-arm transobturator male sling, is an adapted version of the two-arm TOMS. The classical implantation procedure consists of a perineal access incision followed by exposure of the bulbospongiosus muscle, without dissecting the central tendon. The bulbar urethra is not detached from the perineum, and urethral repositioning does not occur. The sling is placed over the muscle (which makes a difference from other slings) and compresses at the bulbous urethra by suspending through the transobturator foramen.

In a prospective, multicenter study of 103 patients with a follow-up for at least 12 months after the implementation of I-STOP TOMS, a 59.4% of the patients were cured (completely dry), while 87% showed improvement. No acute urinary retention or mesh erosion occurred; however, wound infection occurred in 2% of patients [14].

There is one long-term study of a median 59 months of follow-up for 100 patients after the implementation of the I-STOP TOMS with mild to moderate incontinence (24-h pad test <400 g). The cure (completely dry) rate after 1 year was 40% (77% "socially continent" which was up to 1 pad) in 1 year. This rate decreased to 15% (22% socially continent) of dry patients after 5 years of follow-up. So the long-term treatment effect does not appear to be good [15].

Recently, a new technique of placing the I-STOP TOMS sling on the superficial fascia was introduced. Of the 34 patients who could be followed up for 1 year, 52.9% were pad-free, while 73.5% showed improvement [16].

More data is necessary to determine the exact durability and success rates that can be expected by a general urologist performing this procedure with either version of the AdVance sling. It will be interesting to review 5- and 10-year outcomes following AdVance sling placement when they become available.

Of the transobturator retrourethral sling devices, most studies reported on the AdVance sling, which has relatively good outcomes. In particular, good results can be expected in patients who have good residual sphincter function, no previous treatment with RT, and mild to moderate PPI. Overall, relatively few complications occur and most of them are mild.

One disadvantage is that adjustment is impossible after surgery, and the success rate of the surgery may not be good in patients who previously had radiation treatment, those with severe PPI, or those who have a defect in the sphincter function [10]. However, there is evidence that re-treatment with a second sling is feasible and secure, and there is no need to remove the previous sling [17].

8.4 Case Study: Suburethral Sling for Male Urinary Incontinence—Our Experience and Results

Due to the lack of solid evidence on which is the best sling for patients with PPI, in our center we developed experience in the use of the AdVanceXP and the Virtue. Our intention was to review our functional results in the short and medium term (2, 12, and 24 months), as well as the safety profile, and thus adapt the treatment to the best practice in our environment.

A retrospective, single-center analysis of patients with mild to moderate stress urinary incontinence (less than 400 g in pad testing) undergoing suburethral sling (AdVanceXP or Virtue) between 2013 and 2017, at the Hospital Universitario 12 de Octubre, in Madrid (Spain). There is a total of 32 patients that completed follow-up (11 treated with AdVanceXP sling and 21 patients with Virtue sling). We made a descriptive analysis of rate of success (1 security pad/day) at 2, 12, and 24 months, as well as rate and severity (measured by Clavien-Dindo classification) of complications.

There were 32 patients with an average age of 69 years, checking the homogeneity between both groups for the demographic characteristics. 90.6% (n = 29) had stress urinary incontinence due to a prostate adenocarcinoma treated by radical prostatectomy, 6.25% (n = 2) secondary to endourological surgery of the BPH and 3.1% (n = 1) secondary to pelvic trauma (to remark all patients with both endourological surgery and trauma SUI were treated with Virtue sling). No patient had a previous history of radiotherapy. Two patients (6.25%) have a previous history of cervical sclerosis (previously treated by endoscopic urethrotomy), one being treated with Virtue and the other with AdVanceXP. The pad test prior to surgery was 236 cc (±135) combining both groups of study, 270 cc (±136) for the Virtue sling group, and 175 cc (±118) for the AdVanceXP sling group.

The continence rate (described as 0–1 security pad/day) at 2 months after surgery was 62.5%, 74% after 12 months, and 78.5% after 24 months of follow-up for the total of the RTS patients. In the AdVanceXP group, we observed an 81.8% rate of continence at 2 months, 91% after 12 months, and the same rate, 91%, at 24 months. In the Virtue sling group, we observed a 52.4% of continence at 2 months, a 66.6% after 12 months, and a 71.4% after 24 months of follow-up. There was one patient who was treated with a Virtue sling who underwent to the implantation of an AUS during follow-up. None of our patients was retreated with a second sling. Both patients with previous history of cervical sclerosis achieved continence.

If we focus in the complications rate, we observed that a 21.8% ($n = 7$) of the patients presented any postoperative complications. In the group of the AdVanceXP sling, there were complications in two patients (18.2%), one of them being classified as Clavien III (urinary outlet obstruction) that required surgical treatment (urethrolysis) and the other one, a mild complication, classified as Clavien I. In the Virtue sling group, a total of five patients (rate of 23.8%) presented complications, being all mild, with a Clavien I classification. One Virtue patient needed the implementation of an AUS due to lack of efficacy. The sling was not previously removed, and the patient achieved continency.

8.5 Discussion

Our results appear to be consistent with published evidence regarding their effectiveness in treating mild to moderate PPI. Although we have been guided by previous experiences when choosing the sling to be implanted and the patient profile, both study groups are similar in characteristics, so it seems that, despite the evident limitations of the study, they may be comparable groups. Due to previous results by other authors, we have not included patients previously submitted to radiotherapy [18]. However, two patients with urethrovesical anastomosis sclerosis were included, who subsequently had good continence results. In general, the main limitation of the studies is the lack of uniformity when defining the cure, since, although the objective must be that the patient is completely dry, it seems important to measure QoL of the patient after the procedure and to demonstrate an improvement, as many of the studies do not focus on QoL outcomes but in urine volume loss.

Regarding the results obtained, although in the literature about Virtue sling we see that there are studies that objectify acceptable rates of continence [11, 13], the rates of complications seem to be high, particularly in the study by McCall et al. [12], since a 22% of explant rate is remarkable. In our case, we did not need to perform any explants, nor have we reported any case of secondary chronic pelvic pain.

While it is true that we have had a more serious complication in the AdVanceXP group, the overall complication rate appears better than in the Virtue group. Furthermore, in the long term, the cure rate is excellent and is maintained over time (up to 24 months or follow-up).

In our center we have no experience with the I-STOP TOMS, but the results reported in the literature present a similar safety and effectiveness profile.

The indications for the use of RTS are being established little by little, being included in the clinical reference guidelines for patients with mild to moderate PPI who have not received radiotherapy [1, 19]. The challenge for the coming years will be to finish defining the patient population that can benefit from this surgical treatment for PPI, as well as to standardize the results reported to discern which sling is the best for our patient.

8.6 Conclusion

The suburethral transobturator sling is an established treatment of male urinary incontinence for selected patients (mild to moderate SUI). It has a good security profile and has a demonstrated effectiveness. Although more standardization in the studies is needed for acquiring better evidence in terms of effectiveness, it is a good therapeutic option for selected patients.

There are several different sling options available, and we have tested two of them in a single-center study. Although both the AdVanceXP sling and the Virtue sling have adequate functional results and an acceptable complication rate, it seems that more quality comparative studies and randomized clinical trials are needed between the different devices to determine which one to use in each single patient.

References

1. Burkhard FC. EAU guidelines on urinary incontinence in adults [Internet]. 2020. https://uroweb.org/guideline/urinary-incontinence/.
2. Rehder P, Gozzi C. Transobturator sling suspension for male urinary incontinence including post-radical prostatectomy. Eur Urol. 2007;52(3):860–6.
3. Kretschmer A, Hübner W, Sandhu JS, Bauer RM. Evaluation and management of postprostatectomy incontinence: a systematic review of current literature. Eur Urol Focus. 2016;2(3):245–59.
4. Kretschmer A, Nitti V. Surgical treatment of male postprostatectomy incontinence: current concepts. Eur Urol Focus. 2017;3(4–5):364–76.
5. Doudt AD, Zuckerman JM. Male slings for post-prostatectomy incontinence. Rev Urol. 2018;20(4):158–69.
6. Ko KJ, Kim SJ, Cho ST. Sling surgery for male urinary incontinence including post prostatectomy incontinence: a challenge to the urologist. Int Neurourol J. 2019;23(3):185–94.
7. Rehder P, Haab F, Cornu J-N, Gozzi C, Bauer RM. Treatment of postprostatectomy male urinary incontinence with the transobturator retroluminal repositioning sling suspension: 3-year follow-up. Eur Urol. 2012;62(1):140–5.
8. Zuckerman JM, Edwards B, Henderson K, Beydoun HA, McCammon KA. Extended outcomes in the treatment of male stress urinary incontinence with a transobturator sling. Urology. 2014;83(4):939–45.
9. Cornu J-N, Melot C, Haab F. A pragmatic approach to the characterization and effective treatment of male patients with postprostatectomy incontinence. Curr Opin Urol. 2014;24(6):566–70.
10. Hoy NY, Rourke KF. Stemming the tide of mild to moderate post-prostatectomy incontinence: a retrospective comparison of transobturator male slings and the artificial urinary sphincter. Can Urol Assoc J. 2014;8(7–8):273–7.
11. Comiter CV, Rhee EY, Tu L-M, Herschorn S, Nitti VW. The virtue sling—a new quadratic sling for post-prostatectomy incontinence—results of a multinational clinical trial. Urology. 2014;84(2):433–8.
12. McCall AN, Rivera ME, Elliott DS. Long-term follow-up of the virtue quadratic male sling. Urology. 2016;93:213–6.
13. Ferro M, Bottero D, D'Elia C, Matei DV, Cioffi A, Cozzi G, et al. Virtue male sling for post-prostatectomy stress incontinence: a prospective evaluation and mid-term outcomes. BJU Int. 2017;119(3):482–8.
14. Grise P, Vautherin R, Njinou-Ngninkeu B, Bochereau G, Lienhart J, Saussine C, et al. I-STOP TOMS transobturator male sling, a minimally invasive treatment for post-prostatectomy incontinence: continence improvement and tolerability. Urology. 2012;79(2):458–63.
15. Malval B, Rebibo J-D, Baron M, Nouhaud F-X, Pfister C, Cornu J-N, et al. Long-term outcomes of I-Stop TOMS™ male sling implantation for post-prostatectomy incontinence management. Prog Urol. 2017;27(17):1084–90.
16. Galiano M, Guillot-Tantay C, Sivaraman A, Slaoui H, Barret E, Rozet F, et al. Superficial implantation of the I-Stop TOMS transobturator sling in the treatment of postprostatectomy urinary incontinence: description of a novel technique and 1-year outcomes. Urology. 2016;90:195–8.
17. Soljanik I, Becker AJ, Stief CG, Gozzi C, Bauer RM. Repeat retrourethral transobturator sling in the management of recurrent postprostatectomy stress urinary incontinence after failed first male sling. Eur Urol. 2010;58(5):767–72.
18. Bauer RM, Soljanik I, Füllhase C, Buchner A, May F, Stief CG, et al. Results of the AdVance transobturator male sling after radical prostatectomy and adjuvant radiotherapy. Urology. 2011;77(2):474–9.
19. AUA Guidelines on Incontinence after prostate treatment [Internet]. 2020. https://www.auanet.org/guidelines/incontinence-after-prostate-treatment#x14393.

Adjustable Transobturator Male Systems

9

Enrico Ammirati, Paolo Geretto,
and Alessandro Giammò

Post-prostatectomy incontinence (PPI) is a common drawback of prostate surgery. In a large SEER cancer registry review, Kim et al. collected data on 16,348 men aged over 66 that had undergone radical prostatectomy; of them 1057 (6%) underwent at least 1 incontinence surgical procedure [1].

It has been hypothesized that the urethral sphincter complex and the supporting structures of the membranous urethra play a role in PPI. The urethral sphincter is made of two main components: an internal smooth muscle for passive continence and an external skeletal muscle for active continence. The finding of a positive coaptive test (a circumferential complete closure of the urethra on command at cystoscopy) usually implies the integrity of the muscle tissue with a good blood supply and innervation. Bladder neck sparing surgical techniques aim to reduce the damage to the internal sphincter muscle, maintaining a better passive continence and with a lower rate of PPI. The supporting structures of the membranous urethra comprehend an anterior compartment, a posterior compartment, and the pelvic floor. The anterior urethral support structures are the pubo-vesical ligament, the pubo-prostatic ligament, and the tendinous arch of the pelvic fascia; they keep the bladder neck and sphincter complex in position, close to the symphysis pubis. The posterior urethral support are Denonvilliers' fascia, the central perineal tendon, and the levator ani complex. Above this fascial plane, the pelvic floor, made up of the levator ani muscle with its surrounding fascia, represents the third urethral support. Many surgical procedures involve anterior, posterior, or total anatomical reconstruction of these structures to ameliorate continence results. With an analogy to the female population and the hammock theory, it has been hypnotized that after prostate surgery, a certain urethral hypermobility may arise due to the lack of anatomical supports of the bulbar urethra. The use of male slings was introduced after the studies of Burnett and Mostwin, demonstrating that the contraction of the external sphincter was associated with an upward movement of the sphincter complex [2, 3]. The first male sling was described by Kauffmann et al. in 1970, and many years thereafter Schaeffer et al. published their results of the implant of a bulbourethral sling for the treatment of PPI on 64 patients, with a 56% dry rate and a 27% revision rate [4, 5].

Even though the artificial urethral sphincter (AUS) represents the reference standard technique with a high continence rate up to 86%, the high costs, postoperative complications, and revision rates of the AUS favored the development of new devices in form of male slings and compressive devices [6]. New-generation slings can be distinguished between adjustable and fixed

E. Ammirati (✉) · P. Geretto · A. Giammò
Città Della Salute E Della Scienza Di Torino, Unità Spinale Unipolare-CTO-SC Neuro-Urologia, Torino, Italy

F. Dökmeci, D. E. E. Rizk (eds.), *Insights Into Incontinence and the Pelvic Floor*,
https://doi.org/10.1007/978-3-030-94174-1_9

suburethral transobturator slings. The main advantage of adjustable slings is the possibility of an easy post-implant tensioning to provide further urethral compression in case of persistent or recurrent PPI after sling implant. The mainly employed adjustable devices are Argus and Argus T (Promedon SA, Cordoba, Argentina), ATOMS (Adjustable Transobturator Male System, A.M.I. GmbH, Feldkirch, Austria), and ReMeEx (Readjustment Mechanical External, Neomedic International, Barcelona, Spain). Argus T and ATOMS are transobturator male slings, whereas Argus and ReMeEx are retropubic slings.

Argus and Argus T are both adjustable suburethral compressive male slings: the first is positioned with a retropubic approach and the second through the obturator foramen. The system is made of a central silicone foam pad that is positioned above the bulbouretralis muscle compressing the urethra and two silicone arms made of multiple small conical elements. A ring (washers) is fixed on each cone column to fix the device in place and with the right tensioning, usually up to a retrograde leak point pressure of 40–45 cmH_2O; the ring is placed against the rectus sheath for the Argus system and against the fibromuscular tissue of the obturator foramen for the Argus T system. The system can be progressively tensioned through a small skin incision under local anesthesia, and it can be de-tensioned thereafter, even if with a little difficulty.

Hübner et al. published the results of the implant of the retropubic Argus male sling on a cohort of 101 patients with a median follow-up of 2.2 years. The dry rate was 79.2% with a global reduction in 20 min pad test from a mean value of 30.9 g (1–117) to 2.2 g (0–90) ($p < 0.01$) and an increase in I-QoL score from the initial mean value of 28.8 (14.5 + 61.8) to 63.2 (16.4–115) ($p < 0.001$). Tensioning of the sling was required in 39 patients (38.6%); further second, third, and fourth tensioning were required in 6.9%, 3%, 1%, respectively. Complications included 14.9% transient perineal discomfort or moderate pain, 5% intraoperative bladder perforations, and one case of perineal infection treated conservatively; explant rate was 15.8% due to urethral erosion or infection [7]. Bochove-Overgaauw et al. described the results of a cohort of 100 patients subjected to Argus implantation with a median follow-up of 27 months (14–57), including 41 patients with severe incontinence, using 6–10 pads/day. The overall success rate at last follow-up was 72%, with a dry rate of 40%; dry rates in mild, moderate, and severe incontinence were 62%, 44%, and 28% respectively. A tightening revision procedure was required once in 24 patients, twice in 7, and thrice in 1. Complication rate was 55% with an explant rate of 11% due to infection (6%), bladder/urethral erosion (3%), sling rupture (1%), and pain (1%). Radio-treated patients had worse continence results and security profile, with a lower success rate (15% vs 79%) and a higher revision rate (67% vs 26%), sling explant rate (27% vs 8%), complication rate (60% vs 54%), and post-implant urethral strictures (20% vs 11%) [8].

The results of the retropubic Argus sling were compared with those of the transobturator Argus T by Loertzer et al. on a cohort of 106 patients (74 implanted with the classic Argus and 32 with Argus T) with a median follow-up of 44 months (24–64). Dry rate was 33.3% after Argus classic implant and 11.8% after Argus T ($p = 0.114$). The authors did not observe any statistically significant difference between Argus classic and Argus T in postoperative daily pad use (1.8 ± 1.6 vs 1.9 ± 0.9, $p = 0.336$) with a reduction of >50% in pad use in 76.9% and 64.7%, respectively. When observing the 24-h pad test, however, there was a significant better reduction after Argus classic implant (postoperative 24-h pad test 71 ± 162 g vs 160 ± 180 g, $p = 0.066$). Readjustments were required in 89.8% of the Argus classic subgroup and in 76.9% in the Argus T subgroup. Intraoperative complications were more frequent during Argus classic implant (23% vs 0%, $p < 0.01$), and postoperative complications were higher for Argus T implant (25.7% vs 60.6%, $p = 0.044$). Argus T implant showed a higher rate of inguinal pain (VAS 0.7 ± 0.9 vs 1.6 ± 1.8, $p = 0.033$), without statistical differences for perineal pain (1.1 ± 1.5 vs 1.7, p = 0.427), scrotal pain (0.6 ± 1.1 vs 2.1, p = 0.29), and pubic pain (0.5 ± 0.8 vs 1.0 ± 1.3, p = 0.125). Explantation rate was higher for Argus T (14% vs 23.3%, p = 0.371) [9]. Cunha Lima compared the results of the transobturator adjustable Argus T sling with the fixed transobturator Advance male sling in a randomized clinical trial. They implanted 11 Argus T slings and 11 Advance slings with 18 months follow-up. Social continence (0–1 pad/day and 24-h pad test <50 g) was reached in 45.5% in the Advance group and 77.8% in the Argus T group; only patients in the Argus T group had a statistically significant improvement in the 24-h pad test (Argus T from 674.44 ± 763.78 to 97 ± 218.6, p = 0.038; Advance from 620.91 ± 422.64 to 561.45 ± 890.09, p = 0.386). In accordance to continence results, patients in the Argus T group experienced a higher satisfaction degree (81.8% vs 36.4%) [10].

Chung et al. compared the personal patient choice between an adjustable and a fixed transobturator sling. Patients refusing an AUS implant were offered the choice to choose between an adjustable sling (Argus) and a fixed transobturator sling (Advance): 25 men (57%) underwent adjustable Argus implant and 19 (43%) a fixed Advance sling. The majority of patients asked for an adjustable sling because of the advantage of modulation in case of persistence of incontinence in the postoperative time with a simple procedure under local anesthesia. Patients choosing the fixed Advance sling preferred the single-incision design of the sling and the mechanism of action of the repositioning of the urethra (rather than a compressive effect) that may reduce the risk of retention and urethral complications. Continence results were comparable with social continence rates of 92% in the Argus group and 84% in the Advance group (p = 0.45) and a similar subjective satisfaction rate on a five-point scale (4.5 for Argus and 4.3 for Advance, p = 0.36) [11].

The ATOMS system is an adjustable transobturator compressive device in the form of a sling with a working mechanism similar to the AUS. The main differences are that the device does not compress the urethra circumferentially and that it is designed for postoperative adjustments. The device is made of a silicone cushion that is placed over the bulbouretralis muscle, compressing the urethra, anchored to two macroporous monofilament polypropylene mesh arms that are sutured to the device after the transobturator passage. The cushion is connected to a titanium port that is placed in the scrotum for the third-generation device, allowing intraoperative filling up to pressure equalization and postoperative adjustments with a percutaneous injection of saline solution until continence is reached.

In a retrospective series, Giammò et al. evaluated the results in terms of efficacy and safety on a cohort of 52 patients with a mean follow-up of 16.7 months (range: 2.7–35.6). This population had a high prevalence of previous incontinence surgery (57.7%; in 26 cases a ProACT device, in 1 case an artificial sphincter FlowSecure, in 2 cases both a ProACT device and an artificial sphincter AMS800, in 1 case both an intraurethral bulking therapy and subsequently a ProACT) and a relatively low rate of radio-treated patients (11.5%). At last follow-up dry rate was 30.8%, >50% improvement rate was 59.6%, and social continence rate was 73.1% (use of 0 or 1 security pad/day). Subgroup analysis evidenced that there is no statistically significant difference with regard to complete dryness and social continence between RT and non-RT patients (p = 0.99–p = 0.99) and between patients with and without previous urethral surgery (p = 0.56–p = 0.98); there is a statistically significant difference with regard to complete dryness (p = 0.04) but not to social continence (p = 0.49) between patients with and without previous incontinence surgery. Complication rate was 19% without episodes of device infection or device explantation (five cases of displacement of the scrotal port and surgical replacement, two cases of catheterization difficulties and difficulty to deflate the device, one case of epididymitis and concomitant superficial wound infection) [12].

9.1 Case Study: Implant of Atom System for the Treatment of Postoperative Male Stress Urinary Incontinence—An Italian Multicentric Study

Alessandro Giammò, Enrico Ammirati, Giuseppe Morgia, Sandro Sandri, Carlo Introini, Giorgio Canepa, Luca Timossi, Cristina Rossi, Cristina Mozzi and Roberto Carone

Città Della Salute E Della Scienza Di Torino, Unità Spinale Unipolare-CTO-SC Neuro-Urologia, Torino, Italy
Azienda Ospedaliera Universitaria Policlinico Vittorio Emanuele, Dipartimento Di Urologia, Catania, Italy
Asst Ovest Milanese, Ospedale Fornaroli Di Magenta, Magenta, Italy
Ente Ospedaliero Ospedali Galliera, Dipartimento Di Urologia, Genova, Italy
Ospedale Evangelico Internazionale, Dipartimento Di Urologia, Genova, Italy
ASL Alessandria, Ospedale San Giacomo Di Novi Ligure, Dipartimento Di Urologia, Novi Ligure, Italy

Giammò et al. extended the experience with ATOMS implant in a national multicentric study enrolling 98 patients with a median follow-up of 21.5 ± 18.38 months. This population had a higher incidence of adjuvant radiotherapy (14.3%) and a lower previous incontinence surgery rate (31.6%). The study population had prevalently a low to medium grade of incontinence (39.8% mild incontinence, 50% moderate incontinence, and 10.2% severe incontinence). Median surgical time was 47.00 ± 13.50. Median refilling number was 1 ± 3, and median total cushion filling volume was 10 ± 8. Dry rate was 47.96% and social continence rate was 79.59%, with a significant reduction in 24-h postoperative pad test (median 0 ± 100 g; $p < 0.01$) and 24-h postoperative pad count (median 1 ± 1; $p < 0.01$). Subjective benefit was demonstrated by a significant reduction in ICIQ-UI SF questionnaire from a median value of 16 ± 2 to a median value of 8 ± 4 ($p < 0.01$). A lower grade of incontinence was associated with a higher reduction in 24-h pad count and pad test ($p = 0.0019$, $p < 0.01$), whether a higher incontinence grade was associated with a lower dry rate ($p = 0, 0001$) and social continence rate ($p = 0.165$). Radiotherapy and previous incontinence surgery seemed to have a negative impact on continence rate, with patients without a history of RT having a higher dry rate ($p = 0.043$) and social continence rate ($p = 0.0244$) and patients without a history of previous incontinence surgery having a higher dry rate (<0.001) and social continence rate ($p = 0.0118$). Even previous urethral surgery (urethrotomy and bladder neck resection) has a negative impact on dry rate ($p = 0.0069$) and to social continence rate ($p = 0.0147$). Complication rate was 33.7% (10.2% scrotal and perineal pain and numbness persisting >4 weeks, 10.2% scrotal port displacement requiring surgical repositioning in six cases and removal of the entire device in four cases due to scrotal port erosion, 7.1% temporary scrotal edema, 6.1% transient dysuria treated with partial deflate of the device, 2% superficial wound infection, removal of the device in one case due to the persistence of scrotal/perineal pain) [13].

9.2 Discussion

Results are in line with a systematic review of literature of Esquinas et al. on 20 different studies (13 retrospective and 7 prospective, of which 3 multicentric) with 1393 patients. Mean dry rate was 67% (95%CI 0.61–0.72), and mean improvement rate was 90% (95% CI 0.86–0.94), with a significative reduction of the pad count (mean −4.14, 95%CI −4.52/−3.76) and 24-h pad test (mean −443 g, 95%CI −482.6/−403.5 g). Mean total refilling number was 2.4 (95%CI 1.82–2.9). Subjective satisfaction was declared by 87% of patients (95%CI 83–89.8). Studies with a high percentage of radio-treated patients showed a lower dry rate (59%, 95%CI 54–64% vs 76%, 95%CI 67–84, $p = 0.014$), but a similar improvement rate than the rest (89%, 95%CI 81–95 vs 92%, 95%CI 87–96, $p = 0.56$). After a median follow-up of 20.9 months, they reported a 35.6% rate of transient postoperative dysesthesia

(95%CI 86.5–93.1) and a 16.4% complication rate (95%CI 12.1–21.2), with major complications in 3% (95%CI 2.8–9.5) [14].

Angulo et al. compared the results of the ATOMS system with those of the ProACT in a systematic review. ProACT is an extra-urethral compressive device made of a silicone balloon that is positioned in a peri-urethral position under the bladder neck and that is connected to a titanium port for postoperative modulation. Forty-one studies were eligible for this systematic review, with populations equivalent for baseline continence severity (pad count 5.05, 95%CI 4.8–5.3 vs 4.6, 95%CI 3.9–5.3, $p = 0.27$) and proportion of patients with previous incontinence surgery (16.1%, 95%CI 9.7–23.5 vs 11%, 95%CI 5.05–18.6, $p = 0.29$). Dry rate was higher in ATOMS implants than ProACT (68%, 95%CI 62–73 vs 55%, 95%CI 47–63, $p = 0.01$) as well as the improvement rate (91%, 95%CI 87–94 vs 80%, 95%CI 72–87, $p = 0.007$); pad count was lower after ATOMS implant rather than after ProACT (1.1 pads/day, 95%CI 0.9–1.3 vs 2.1 pads/day, 95%CI 1.7–2.5, $p < 0.0001$) as well as mean differential pad test (−426 mL, 95%CI −462/−389 vs −211 mL, 95%CI −312/−111, $p < 0.0001$). On the other hand, the total number or refilling procedures was lower for the ATOMS system rather than for ProACT (2.4, 95%CI 1.9–2.9 vs 3.5, 95%CI 3–3.9, $p = 0.001$). Even though follow-up was lower for ATOMS implants (20.8 months, 95%CI 22.7–28.7 vs 20.8 vs 30.6 months, 95%CI 23–38.1, $p = 0.02$), ATOMS implants demonstrated a lower explant rate (5%, 95%CI 2–9, vs 25%, 95%CI 19–31, $p < 0.0001$) with a higher proportion of working devices during the first 3 years of follow-up. Global complication rate was lower after ATOMS implant, however without statistical significance (17%, 95% CI 13–22 vs 26%, 95%CI 18–34, $p = 0.067$), and severe complication rate was similar for the two devices (4.2%, 95%CI 1.7–7.7 vs 10.4%, 95%CI 3.15–20.7, $p = 0.15$) [15].

Ammirati et al. evaluated the ATOMS device also in neurogenic patients, in a retrospective cohort of eight male patients with neurogenic stress urinary incontinence and performing clean intermittent catheterization, four with myelomeningocele and four with cauda equine syndrome, with 12 months follow-up. A second refill of the device was required only in two cases with a low total filling volume (median 8 mL, IQR 6–8 mL). The device appeared to be effective even in such a fragile population, with all patients reaching dryness and a significant reduction in postoperative 24-h pad test (from a median of 225 g, IQR 180–275 to a median of 7.5 g, IQR 0–16.25, $p < 0.05$) and also in Qualiveen scores (from a median of 2.25, IQR 1.875–2.28 to a median of 1.625, IQR 1.5–1.65, $p < 0.05$). Even if the follow-up was limited to 12 months and the size of the cohort was small, there were no late postoperative complications in this pilot study. Any patient referred difficulty in performing clean intermittent catheterization, and there were no cases of device infection nor device removal [16].

The ReMeEx device is made of a monofilament polypropylene suburethral mesh with a monofilament traction threads on each side; the monofilament sutures are delivered in the retropubic space with a dedicated tunneler and are fixed to a mechanical regulator (varitensor) 2 cm above the pubis. The tension of the sling can be modulated postoperatively through a small skin incision under local anesthesia with a dedicated manipulator that allows to wrap the suture through the device.

In a multicentric European study involving seven centers, Sousa-Escandón et al. evaluated efficacy and safety of ReMeEx implant on a cohort of 51 patients. Regulations were required in 46 patients during the early postoperative time, a second regulation was required in 44 patients, and 17 patients required more than one delayed regulation during follow-up. With an average follow-up of 32 months (16–50), continence rate was 64.7%, with a 49% dry rate and a 15.7% social continence rate (one security pad/day). Complications included one case of urethral erosion of the mesh requiring removal, two infections of the varitensor that was removed tying together the extremities of the Prolene threads, five cases of intraoperative bladder perforation treated conservatively, and three mild perineal hematomas; most patients experienced transient pain or perineal discomfort, treated with oral drugs [17].

Angulo et al. evaluated the efficacy and safety of the ATOMS device compared to the ReMeEx implant in a systematic review including 29 studies with a mean follow-up of 24.5 months (95%CI 21.2–27.7). ATOMS and ReMeEx studies were homogeneous with regard to the population characteristics (radical prostatectomy in 87.1%, 95%CI 78.6–93.9 vs 95.6%, 95%CI 85.9–100, $p = 0.125$; previous radiotherapy in 23.1%, 95%CI 19.5–26.9, vs 23.9%, 95%CI 11.6–24.6, $p = 0.126$). Dry rate and overall improvement rate were higher after ATOMS implant than after ReMeEx implant (dry rates 69.3%, 95%CI 63.9–74.4, vs 53.4%, 95%CI 42.2–64.3, $p = 0.008$; improvement rates 90.8%, 95%CI 86.6–94.4 vs 80.2%, 95%CI 71.5–87.8, $p = 0.007$). The mean number of modulations was similar for ATOMS device and ReMeEx device (2.4, 95%CI 1.9–2.8 VS 2.7, 95%CI 1.5–3.8, $p = 0.656$). It is possible that the mechanical compression exerted by the sling could determine a reduced increase in intraurethral pressure, as the sling can apply a force only from one side. On the other hand, the peculiar compression of the bulbar urethra from the ATOMS device can determine a complex deformation of the urethral walls that can increase the intra-urethral pressure according to the Laplace law; this design difference may be, at least in part, responsible for the better functional outcomes after ATOMS implant. The safety profile appears to be slightly in favor of the ATOMS device with a lower complication rate (18.9%, 95%CI 14.1–24.1 vs 35.8%, 95%CI 15.9–58.3, $p = 0.096$) and a lower explant rate (5.4%, 95%CI 2.8–8.8 vs 13.9%, 95%CI 6.6–22.9, $p = 0.027$). It should be underlined that adjustments for the ATOMS system can be made with a simple percutaneous injection in the scrotal port, whereas the ReMeEx device requires a small skin incision for tensioning the threads [18].

Generally, it can be stated that the overall quality of the studies on adjustable male slings is poor, with mainly retrospective series including a limited number of patients and with the lack of long-term follow-up. Most studies describe mid-term results on a single device, and we lack randomized clinical trials comparing different devices that could help clinicians in deciding which is the best for a specific patient. According to the low quality of the studies regarding adjustable slings, functional outcomes are heterogeneous. Argus device is reported to give a dry rate ranging from 11.8 to 79.2%, while continence improvement (usually reported as "social continence" or >50% continence improvement) is higher and ranges from 64.7 to 92% [7, 8]. Transobturator approach (Argus T device) seemed to give lower functional results than retropubic approach (Argus classic) in a recent multicenter study [9]. Continence outcomes are generally satisfactory after ATOMS device implant as well. Literature reports dry rates ranging from 30.8 to 67%, while improvement rate exceeds 90% in most studies [12–15]. However, the lack of direct comparisons between ATOMS and Argus devices does not allow to state clearly which device gives the best functional results. Oppositely, a recent systematic review by Angulo et al. seems to clarify the functional superiority of ATOMS device over the ReMeEx sling, which is reported to result in a dry rate of 53.4% and an improvement rate of 80.2% [18].

Along with clinical effectiveness, safety and complication rates are other paramount aspects to be considered. Argus device is associated with a complication rate ranging from 20 to 60%. Most of the complications described in literature are mild and transient (such as temporary surgical site discomfort and pain or minor perineal hematoma). Explantation rate is about 15% in all studies, even though transobturator approach (Argus T) seems to be associated with a higher explantation rate than retropubic approach (Argus classic). Argus T is related to higher postoperative complications as well, despite lower intraoperative complications [7–9]. ATOMS device is associated with comparable complication rates (16–33%) although the explantation of the device seems less likely than after Argus device implantation (about 5% in most studies). Nevertheless, the lack of prospective comparative studies does not allow clear states about the superiority of one device over the other [12–15]. On the other hand, the study by Angulo et al. suggests a lower complication rate of the ATOMS device compared to the ReMeEx male sling [18]. The solid point about adjustable slings is that those devices are generally safe and can be proposed to patients without high risk of short- and long-term complications.

The major advantage of adjustable devices is the possibility to modulate the compressive tension on the urethra in the postoperative time with a simple procedure, giving a higher possibility to reach good continence results with time. In fact, the mean number of regulations needed to optimize the continence is 2–3, with no evident difference between devices. Therefore, when choosing a device, particular attention should be given to the facility of modulation of the compression over the urethra. Comparing the three aforementioned devices, ATOMS devices is the only one which allows to adjust the compression postoperatively without further surgical incisions.

9.3 Conclusion

Despite the slight differences among devices, adjustable slings appear to be safe and effective. AUS is still considered the gold standard for the treatment of stress urinary incontinence in males. Despite the very satisfactory continence outcomes of the AUS, the main drawbacks are high costs and high complication and explantation rates. According to the previous studies, adjustable slings could be considered as the first choice for selected patients, in particular with low to medium incontinence severity. Nevertheless, literature lacks prospective randomized studies indicating the differences of outcomes between AUS and adjustable slings. Therefore, it is still unclear what the ideal subject for adjustable sling implantation over AUS could be. Prospective randomized studies are strongly advocated in order to better define what patients could benefit the most from adjustable slings.

References

1. Kim PH, Pinheiro LC, Atoria CL, Eastham JA, Sandhu JS, Elkin EB. Trends in the use of incontinence procedures after radical prostatectomy: a population based analysis. J Urol. 2013;189(2):602–8.
2. Heesakkers J, Farag F, Bauer RM, Sandhu J, De Ridder D, Stenzl A. Pathophysiology and contributing factors in postprostatectomy incontinence: a review. Eur Urol. 2017;71(6):936–44.
3. Burnett AL, Mostwin JL. In situ anatomical study of the male urethral sphincteric complex: relevance to continence preservation following major pelvic surgery. J Urol. 1998;160(4):1301–6.
4. Kaufman JJ. A new operation for male incontinence. Surg Gynecol Obstet. 1970;131(2):295–9.
5. Schaeffer AJ, Clemens JQ, Ferrari M, Stamey TA. The male bulbourethral sling procedure for post-radical prostatectomy incontinence. J Urol. 1998;159(5):1510–5.
6. Van Der Aa F, Drake MJ, Kasyan GR, Petrolekas A, Cornu JN. The artificial urinary sphincter after a quarter of a century: a critical systematic review of its use in male non-neurogenic incontinence. Eur Urol. 2013;63:681–9.
7. Hübner WA, Gallistl H, Rutkowski M, Huber ER. Adjustable bulbourethral male sling: experience after 101 cases of moderate-to-severe male stress urinary incontinence. BJU Int. 2011;107(5):777–82.
8. Bochove-Overgaauw DM, Schrier BP. An adjustable sling for the treatment of all degrees of male stress urinary incontinence: retrospective evaluation of efficacy and complications after a minimal follow up of 14 months. J Urol. 2011;185(4):1363–8.
9. Loertzer H, Huesch T, Kirschner-Hermanns R, Anding R, Rose A, Brehmer B, Naumann CM, Queissert F, Nyarangi-Dix J, Homberg R, Grabbert M, Hofmann T, Pottek T, Hübner W, Haferkamp A, Bauer RM, Kretschmer A. Retropubic vs transobturator Argus adjustable male sling: results from a multicenter study. Neurourol Urodyn. 2020;39(3):987–93.
10. Lima JP, Pompeo AC, Bezerra CA. Argus T® versus Advance® Sling for postprostatectomy urinary incontinence: a randomized clinical trial. Int Braz J Urol. 2016;42(3):531–9.
11. Chung E, Smith P, Malone G, Cartmill R. Adjustable versus non-adjustable male sling for post-prostatectomy urinary incontinence: a prospective clinical trial comparing patient choice, clinical outcomes and satisfaction rate with a minimum follow up of 24 months. Neurourol Urodyn. 2016;35(4):482–6.
12. Giammò A, Ammirati E, Tullio A, Bodo G, Manassero A, Gontero P, Carone R. Implant of ATOMS® system for the treatment of postoperative male stress urinary incontinence: results of a single centre.Int Braz. J Urol. 2019;45(1):127–36.
13. Giammò A, Ammirati E, Tullio A, Morgia G, Sandri S, Introini C, Canepa G, Timossi L, Rossi C, Mozzi

C, Carone R. Implant of ATOMS® system for the treatment of postoperative male stress urinary incontinence: an Italian multicentric study. Minerva Urol Nefrol. 2020;72(6):770–7. https://doi.org/10.23736/S0393-2249.19.03457-X.
14. Esquinas C, Angulo JC. Effectiveness of Adjustable Transobturator Male System (ATOMS) to treat male stress incontinence: a systematic review and meta-analysis. Adv Ther. 2019;36(2):426–41.
15. Angulo JC, Giammò SSA, Abellán FJ, Arance I, Lora D. Systematic review and meta-analysis comparing Adjustable Transobturator Male System (ATOMS) and Adjustable Continence Therapy (ProACT) for male stress incontinence. PLoS One. 2019;14(12):e0225762.
16. Ammirati E, Manassero A, Mosiello G, Falcone M, Geretto P, Giammò A. First experience with ATOMS system implant in neurogenic stress urinary incontinence. Neurourol Urodyn. 2020;39(6):1837–41. https://doi.org/10.1002/nau.24433.
17. Sousa-Escandón A, Cabrera J, Mantovani F, Moretti M, Ioanidis E, Kondelidis N, Neymeyer J, Noguera R. Adjustable suburethral sling (male remeex system) in the treatment of male stress urinary incontinence: a multicentric European study. Eur Urol. 2007;52(5):1473–9.
18. Angulo JC, Ruiz S, Lozano M, Arance I, Virseda M, Lora D. Systematic review and meta-analysis comparing Adjustable Transobturator Male System (ATOMS) and male Readjustment Mechanical External (REMEEX) system for post-prostatectomy incontinence. World J Urol. 2021;39(4):1083–92. https://doi.org/10.1007/s00345-020-03300-1.

10 Quality of Life After Suburethral Slings

Barbara Padilla-Fernandez, Ana Teresa Roberto-Alcacer, Mónica Paola Coderque-Mejía, Cristina Salvatierra-Pérez, Alejandro Sousa-Escandón, Alejandro Sanz-Ruiz, María Begoña García-Cenador, José Antonio Mirón-Canelo, and María Fernanda Lorenzo-Gómez

10.1 Introduction

Prostate cancer is the second most commonly diagnosed cancer in men, with an estimated 1,276,106 diagnoses worldwide in 2018, accounting for 7.1% of all cancers diagnosed (including both sexes) [1]. Family history and racial/ethnic background are associated with an increased incidence suggesting a genetic predisposition, but less than 10% of men with prostate cancer have true hereditary disease [2]. A wide variety of exogenous/environmental factors have been discussed as being associated with the risk of developing the disease; however, currently there are no known effective preventative dietary or pharmacological interventions [2].

Watchful waiting and active surveillance have been adopted as treatment strategies in the last decades, but radical prostatectomy is still the preferred management option by most urologists. Although many patients will experience a return to urinary continence [3], temporary urinary incontinence is common early after surgery, reducing quality of life [2]. Urinary incontinence rates are not significantly different between open, laparoscopic, or robot-assisted radical prostatec-

B. Padilla-Fernandez
Departamento de Cirugía, Facultad de Medicina, Universidad de La Laguna, Tenerife, Spain

A. T. Roberto-Alcacer · M. B. García-Cenador
Department of Surgery, University of Salamanca, Salamanca, Spain

M. P. Coderque-Mejía
Department of Urology, Complejo Asistencial Universitario de Salamanca, Salamanca, Spain

C. Salvatierra-Pérez
Department of Urology, Hospital Universitario San Pedro, Logroño, Spain

A. Sousa-Escandón
Department of Urology, Hospital de Monforte de Lemos, Lugo, Spain

A. Sanz-Ruiz
Department of Urology, Complejo Asistencial Universitario de León, León, Spain

J. A. Mirón-Canelo
Department of Public Health, University of Salamanca, Salamanca, Spain

M. F. Lorenzo-Gómez (✉)
Department of Surgery, University of Salamanca, Salamanca, Spain

Department of Urology, Complejo Asistencial Universitario De Salamanca, Salamanca, Spain

F. Dökmeci, D. E. E. Rizk (eds.), *Insights Into Incontinence and the Pelvic Floor*, https://doi.org/10.1007/978-3-030-94174-1_10

tomy [4–6]. Patients with bothersome lower urinary tract symptoms after robot-assisted radical prostatectomy have higher baseline ICIQ-MLUTs scores and significant worsening of total scores at 6, 12, and 18 months after surgery compared with the baseline [7]. On the other hand, patients with a body mass index over 26 kg/m^2, higher prostate volumes (>70 mL), a low glomerular filtration rate (<60 mL/min), or a Charlson comorbidity index higher than 2 have a higher tendency to develop post-prostatectomy incontinence [8].

External beam radiation therapy (EBRT) and brachytherapy can also be considered in the treatment algorithm of prostate cancer. The Prostate Cancer Outcomes Study (PCOS) [9] reported that at 5 years of follow-up, men who underwent radical prostatectomy had a higher prevalence of urinary incontinence and erectile dysfunction, while men treated with radiation therapy had a higher prevalence of bowel dysfunction. However, there were no significant differences in the adjusted odds of urinary incontinence, bowel dysfunction, or erectile dysfunction between radical prostatectomy and radiation therapy at 15 years [2, 9]. It has been suggested that urinary incontinence after EBRT is significantly associated with dose distributions in the trigone [10]. Furthermore, radiation therapy is associated with several other complications, including urethral stenosis, radiation cystitis with hematuria, refractory storage lower urinary tract symptoms, genitourinary pain, and prostate necrosis/abscess [11].

Nevertheless, prostate cancer treatment is not the only source of male stress urinary incontinence (SUI). The rate of persistent SUI in patients undergoing open, laparoscopic, or endoscopic surgical management of benign prostatic hyperplasia ranges between 0 and 8.4% [6, 12], and evaluation of these patients should be similar to those who have undergone radical prostatectomy [6]. The gold standard for the surgical treatment of bladder outlet obstruction of prostatic origin is the transurethral resection of the prostate (TURP). A recent systematic review including 59 randomized controlled trials (RCTs) reports that bipolar TURP may carry similar risk of urinary incontinence at 12 months (relative risk 0.20, 95% confidence interval 0.01–4.06; participants = 751; RCTs = 4; low certainty of evidence [CoE]), compared to monopolar TURP [13]. TURP following brachytherapy or EBRT has been associated with incontinence rates of up to 70% [6, 14]. Although up to 43% of patients have some degree of urinary incontinence 1 month after holmium laser enucleation of the prostate (HoLEP) surgery, persistent incontinence is typically mild and has been shown to affect between 0.5 and 10% of the patients [15–17]. Several risk factors have been related with persistent incontinence, including larger-volume prostates, longer operating times, operative blood loss, diabetes mellitus [18], removal of larger volumes of the transition zone of the prostate, and larger enucleation ratios [19]. SUI has not been reported after prostatic arterial embolization [20].

Incontinence after prostate treatment causes emotional and financial distress by delaying patient's re-entry into society, inhibiting relationships, and carrying an economic burden [6]. The first device developed for its correction was the artificial urinary sphincter (AUS), and it is still considered the gold standard. In the last decades, other implants have been launched in the market which have changed the landscape of incontinence surgery over the past 10 years.

10.2 Literature Review

The AUS has the longest track record of success in the treatment of incontinence after prostate surgery, and its complications and their management are well known [21]. The choice of AUS will be based upon patient dexterity, economics, degree of incontinence, previous incontinence surgery, and expectations from surgery [21]. High satisfaction rates of 87–90% are consistently reported, even without total continence [21]. Revision and explantation rates due to mechanical failure, urethral atrophy, infection, and erosion vary considerably among studies with reports of 8–45% and 7–17% [22]. However, it is still the preferred option in patients with previous radiation therapy and/or severe urinary incontinence [23].

Transobturator slings were first implanted in male patients in 2007 after a feasibility cadaveric study [24]. The authors hypothesized that cranial and posterior elevation of the proximal bulbar urethra allowed for more effective membranous urethral coaptation rather than directly compressing it. Later, urodynamic studies provided more evidence that the male transobturator sling in fact does not cause compression of the urethra [25]. In a dynamic MRI study, transobturator slings seemed to elevate the vesicourethral anastomosis (the craniocaudal distance from vesicourethral anastomosis to urethra at pubococcygeal line became longer), so when compared to controls, the difference was no longer significantly different after sling placement both at rest (1.06 cm control vs 0.63 cm post-sling, $p = 0.07$) and at Valsalva (1.09 cm control vs 0.7 cm post-sling, $p = 0.07$) [26]. This study supports the concept that the male transobturator sling improves continence by increasing the membranous urethral length. Predictors of sling failure are [21] prior radiation therapy (probably due to urethral fibrosis and inadequate urethral coaptation), prior urethral stricture, prior incontinence surgery, short functional urethral length, low maximal urethral closure pressure and abdominal leak point pressure, negative repositioning test, and severe urine leakage (24-h pad test over 400 g). Complications have been described [27]: acute urinary retention, pain or discomfort, de novo overactive bladder, perineal hematoma, perineal abscess, and urethral perforation. Serious complications requiring sling explantation are rare and are generally reported as <1% [21].

Papers specifically reporting the management of incontinence after prostatectomy for benign disease are scarce. Hogewoning et al. published a systematic literature search showing that only 59 studies included patients with post-TURP incontinence undergoing sling surgery, and only six papers differentiated the results between patients with previous radical prostatectomy and patients post-TURP, including a combined total of 23 patients [28]. The adjustable transobturator male system (ATOMS®, A.M.I., Feldkirch, Austria) has also been described as treatment of SUI secondary to TURP with or without previous radiation therapy with good continence results and patient's satisfaction scores [29]. A retrospective multicenter study describes the outcomes of adjustable continence balloons (ProACT™, Uromedica Inc., Plymouth, MN) in the treatment of SUI after TURP in 29 patients, including men with severe incontinence, showing an improvement rate of 76% and a dry rate (no pad or one security pad) of 45% [30]. A recent case series has evaluated the role of suburethral fixed slings (AdVance®, Boston Scientific, Boston, MA) in the management of post-HoLEP persistent stress urinary incontinence with good results, although only three patients were operated [17].

Stratification of treatment based on the degree of stress incontinence is the current trend. Men with milder degrees of incontinence and normal bladder function are candidates for either artificial urinary sphincter placement or sling surgery, each with similar success rates [21]. Sling surgery appears to have a lower risk of surgical complications in this population, and patient preference may be for a sling vs a mechanical device in this group of patients [31]. On the other hand, with more severe incontinence, AUS surgery has a more predictable success profile than sling surgery [21]. However, there is a lack of well-designed RCT comparing the outcomes of the different devices [12]. A protocol for a RCT including men with urodynamic SUI after prostatectomy (both for benign and malignant conditions) and who will be randomized for sling procedures or artificial urinary sphincter implantation has been published (ISRCTN49212975) [32].

10.3 Case Study: Male Adjustable Sling ReMeEx: Variables Affecting Quality of Life After Surgery

(a) **Aim and Scope**

The aim of our study is to identify which pre- and/or postoperative variables may influence patient's quality of life (QoL) after surgical correction of male urinary incontinence with the male adjustable sling (MRS®) with suprapubic ReMeEx® device.

(b) **Study Design and Material and Methods**

A retrospective, multicenter study was developed including men with urinary incontinence after prostate surgery (both for benign prostatic enlargement and cancer) or other pelvic treatments (i.e., radiation therapy for prostate cancer or for other malignancies). These patients underwent surgical treatment with the male adjustable sling (MRS®, Neomedic© Int, Terrassa, Spain) with suprapubic ReMeEx® device (Neomedic© Int, Terrassa, Spain) between January 2006 and June 2016 in three different hospitals in Spain: Hospital General Santísima Trinidad (Salamanca), Complejo Asistencial Universitario de Salamanca, and Hospital de Monforte de Lemos (Lugo). Patients with less than a year of postoperative follow-up were excluded.

Urinary incontinence was evaluated using the International Consultation on Incontinence Questionnaire-Urinary Incontinence Short Form (ICIQ-SF), which is a self-administered questionnaire that has been validated in Spanish [33]. Its better feasibility makes this questionnaire more useful in clinical practice than the King's Health Questionnaire [34]. Although mostly used in women, the construct validity of ICIQ-SF in the assessment of treatment for male stress incontinence has also been validated [35], and it correlates with 24-h pad usage [36].

The Short Form-36 (SF-36) Health Survey is a self-reported measure of health that is often used as a measure of a person or population's quality of life (QoL) [37]. It comprises 36 questions which assess eight domains of health: (1) limitations in physical activities because of health problems, (2) limitations in social activities because of physical or emotional problems, (3) limitations in usual role activities because of physical health problems, (4) bodily pain, (5) general mental health (psychological distress and well-being), (6) limitations in usual role activities because of emotional problems, (7) vitality, and (8) general health perceptions. The survey has been validated in Spanish and has been used by multiple researchers in several diseases [38, 39].

One hundred and seventy-four patients were identified, but only 90 patients answered the SF-36 before and after MRS® implantation. The patients were grouped according to their improvement in the SF-36 survey's scores:

- Group A (GA): improvement in SF-36 survey's scores greater than 30
- Group B (GB): improvement in SF-36 survey's scores between 10 and 30
- Group C (GC): improvement in SF-36 survey's scores less than 10

An Excel work sheet including the following variables was developed: age, body mass index (BMI), secondary diagnoses, concomitant treatment, toxic habits, medical and surgical background, urinary incontinence's etiology, pTNM and Gleason score in patients treated of prostate cancer, urethral size (calculated by flowmetry, urethrocystoscopy, and/or urethrocystography), continence after the procedure, postoperative care, and adjuvant treatment. Scores of both questionnaires (ICIQ-SF and SF-36) were compared before surgery and 1, 6, and 12 months after implantation and yearly after.

Data were analyzed using the NCSS 2007/GESS 2007 statistical system (NCSS, LLC; Kaysville, Utah, USA). Descriptive statistics, ANOVA test, and Student's t-test were used. $p < 0.005$ was considered significant.

(c) **Results of the Study**

Ninety patients were included in the final analysis. Average age of the sample was 70.06 years (range 45–86 years). Mean follow-up was 28.17 months (SD, 23.63; range, 12–156). Sixty patients belong to Group A (66.67%), 20 patients to Group B (22.22%), and 10 patients to Group C (11.11%).

Investigating the etiology of urinary incontinence, 61 patients have had a radical prostatectomy (RP), 6 patients a transurethral resection of the prostate (TUR-P), 8 patients laser enucleation/vaporization, 22 patients RP with adjuvant EBRT, 8 patients EBRT for prostate cancer, and 4 patients EBRT for other pelvic malignancies. The remaining 3 patients were incontinent after an abdominoperineal resection of the rectum plus colostomy and EBRT.

Before implantation, 18 patients with previous radical prostatectomy underwent endoscopic urethrotomy due to urethrovesical anastomosis fibrosis, and resolution was confirmed with a preoperative cystoscopy. No differences between groups regarding BMI, pTNM, and Gleason score were found. Readjustment was done in 34 patients (38%).

Late complications were detected in four patients: two with infection at the location of the varitensor treated with antibiotics (Clavien-Dindo II) and two urethral extrusions requiring device explantation (Clavien-Dindo IIIb).

Regarding the need of concomitant therapies, more patients in Group B accepted to receive physical and pain therapies, with good responses at 2–4 months. There was a trend in patients in Group C to decline other therapies.

Patients in Group C were older, and they had a higher rate of radiation cystitis, low maximum bladder capacity, diabetes, depression/anxiety, allergies, and pretreatment chronic pelvic pain.

10.4 Discussion

ReMeEx® (from the Spanish *Regulador Mecánico Externo*) is a device manufactured in Spain that initially was designed for the correction of recurrent female stress urinary incontinence and that was introduced in 2003 as an alternative in male incontinence (MRS®) [40]. The system consists of a polypropylene suburethral mesh measuring 3 × 4 cm with two Prolene® threads attached to both sides that are inserted in a subcutaneous regulator (Varitensor) measuring 1 × 1 × 2.5 cm and that should be implanted over the rectus abdominis fascia in the suprapubic area. These pieces act like an active pressure transmission system. A baseplate was added to the original design in order to avoid both varitensor migration and thread medialization. Postoperative adjustments can be done connecting an external handler to the varitensor with local anesthesia [40, 41].

A multicentre study published in 2007, including 51 patients with a median follow-up of 32 months, reported a success rate of 64.7%, improvement rate of 19.6% and failure rate of 15.7% [42]. Other studies with similar follow-up but smaller samples report also success rates around 60% and improvement in all patients according to the Incontinence Impact Questionnaire—Short Form (IIQ-7) scores, requiring a mean of 2.4 adjustments (range 0–6) [41].

The possibility of performing postoperative adjustments is the main characteristic of this device, but it can also be a reason for patient's dissatisfaction. Jiménez Parra et al. described 92.8% of continent patients after the first tensioning; however, incontinence recurs progressively and several readjustments are required, making the patient withdraw from treatment and to device removal in some cases [43]. Nevertheless, a trend toward reducing the number of adjustments with the MRS®-II has been reported [44].

According to the results published, the safety profile is comparable to other implantable devices. The most frequent intraoperative complication is bladder perforation (4–28.5%) [43–46] that does not exclude device implantation, but adjustment in the immediate postoperative time should be avoided, and the urethral catheter should be left in place for 4–5 days [41, 42, 45]. Acute urinary retention is rare after adjustment (0–35.7%) [41, 42, 46] and can be resolved releasing the thread [45] and/or leaving an indwelling catheter for 1 week [46]. Mild perineal hematoma can be managed conservatively [42]. Infection at the location of the varitensor has also been described when adjustments are performed in the follow-up, and explantation only of this piece has been performed [44]. In our study, this complication was successfully managed with antibiotics. We also found that 2.22% developed urethral extrusion requiring device explantation, and this rare complication has also been reported by other authors [42].

Radiation therapy is usually considered a contraindication for sling insertion. However, other groups have also reported their experience including patients with previous history of pelvic radiation [42, 47]. In our experience, it is feasible to perform the surgery in this group of patients (especially if they have limited hand dexterity), but they should be informed beforehand of the lower rate of cure in comparison with non-radiated patients [42, 48].

The best results are achieved when bladder compliance and capacity are not affected, confirming the device's strong control of the urethra. Thus, it is important to diminish treatments' adverse events on the bladder (i.e., poor compliance due to radiation therapy) or bladder dysfunction due to other comorbidities (i.e., diabetes mellitus and neurogenic bladder). These results persisted in the long term.

10.5 Conclusion

Male adjustable sling ReMeEx® is a good option for the correction of UI. Pre-surgical bladder capacity, diabetes, and chronic pain may influence patient's QoL after treatment.

Acknowledgment (Only of Funding) None.

References

1. Prostate Cancer fact sheet—GLOBOCAN. 2019. https://gco.iarc.fr/today/data/factsheets/cancers/27-Prostate-fact-sheet.pdf. Accessed 09/01/2020.
2. Mottet N, Cornford P, van den Bergh RCN, et al. EAU—EANM—ESTRO—ESUR—SIOG guidelines on prostate cancer. 2020. https://uroweb.org/wp-content/uploads/EAU-EANM-ESTRO-ESUR-SIOG-Guidelines-on-Prostate-Cancer-2020v4.pdf. Accessed 09/01/2020.
3. De Nunzio C, Pastore AL, Lombardo R, et al. The EORTC quality of life questionnaire predicts early and long-term incontinence in patients treated with robotic assisted radical prostatectomy: analysis of a large single center cohort. Urol Oncol. 2019;37(12):1006–13.
4. Ilic D, Evans SM, Allan CA, Jung JH, Murphy D, Frydenberg M. Laparoscopic and robotic-assisted versus open radical prostatectomy for the treatment of localised prostate cancer. Cochrane Database Syst Rev. 2017;9(9):Cd009625.
5. Haglind E, Carlsson S, Stranne J, et al. Urinary incontinence and erectile dysfunction after robotic versus open radical prostatectomy: a prospective, controlled, nonrandomised trial. Eur Urol. 2015;68(2):216–25.
6. Sandhu JS, Breyer B, Comiter C, et al. Incontinence after prostate treatment: AUA/SUFU guideline. J Urol. 2019;202(2):369–78.
7. MacKenzie KR, Davis J, Harding C, Aning JJ. Patient-reported outcomes and urodynamic findings in men with persistent lower urinary tract symptoms following robot-assisted radical prostatectomy. Neurourol Urodyn. 2019;38(5):1353–62.
8. Haga N, Takinami R, Tanji R, et al. Comprehensive approach for post-prostatectomy incontinence in the era of robot-assisted radical prostatectomy. Fukushima J Med Sci. 2017;63(2):46–56.
9. Resnick MJ, Koyama T, Fan KH, et al. Long-term functional outcomes after treatment for localized prostate cancer. N Engl J Med. 2013;368(5):436–45.
10. Schaake W, van der Schaaf A, van Dijk LV, van den Bergh ACM, Langendijk JA. Development of a prediction model for late urinary incontinence, hematuria, pain and voiding frequency among irradiated prostate cancer patients. PLoS One. 2018;13(7):e0197757.
11. Doiron RC, Witten J, Rourke KF. The scope, presentation, and management of genitourinary complications in patients presenting with high-grade urethral complications after radiotherapy for prostate cancer. Can Urol Assoc J. 2021;15(1):E6–E10.
12. Silva LA, Andriolo RB, Atallah ÁN, da Silva EM. Surgery for stress urinary incontinence due to presumed sphincter deficiency after prostate surgery. Cochrane Database Syst Rev. 2014;2014(9):Cd008306.
13. Alexander CE, Scullion MMF, Omar MI, et al. Bipolar vs. monopolar transurethral resection of the prostate for lower urinary tract symptoms secondary to benign prostatic obstruction: a Cochrane review. Can Urol Assoc J. 2020;14(12):423–30.
14. Mock S, Leapman M, Stock RG, Hall SJ, Stone NN. Risk of urinary incontinence following post-brachytherapy transurethral resection of the prostate and correlation with clinical and treatment parameters. J Urol. 2013;190(5):1805–10.
15. Sapetti J, Sakat J, Saad E, et al. [Urinary incontinence after HoLEP: incidence, evolution and predictive factors]. Prog Urol. 2019;29(2):101–7.
16. Elmansy HM, Kotb A, Elhilali MM. Holmium laser enucleation of the prostate: long-term durability of clinical outcomes and complication rates during 10 years of follow up. J Urol. 2011;186(5):1972–6.
17. Kleinguetl C, Virani S, Bird ET, El Tayeb MM. Safety and efficacy of male urethral slings for management of persistent stress urinary incontinence after holmium laser enucleation of the prostate. Proc (Baylor Univ Med Cent). 2020;33(4):554–6.

18. Elmansy HM, Kotb A, Elhilali MM. Is there a way to predict stress urinary incontinence after holmium laser enucleation of the prostate? J Urol. 2011;186(5):1977–81.
19. Cho KJ, Koh JS, Choi JB, Kim JC. Factors associated with early recovery of stress urinary incontinence following holmium laser enucleation of the prostate in patients with benign prostatic enlargement. Int Neurourol J. 2018;22(3):200–5.
20. Petrillo M, Pesapane F, Fumarola EM, et al. State of the art of prostatic arterial embolization for benign prostatic hyperplasia. Gland Surg. 2018;7(2):188–99.
21. Goldman HB, Averbeck MA, Bruschini H, et al. Surgical treatment of urinary incontinence in men. In: Abrahms P, Cardozo L, Wagg A, Wein A, editors. Incontinence. 6th ed. ICUD—ICS; 2017. p. 1645–724.
22. Gousse AE, Madjar S, Lambert MM, Fishman IJ. Artificial urinary sphincter for post-radical prostatectomy urinary incontinence: long-term subjective results. J Urol. 2001;166(5):1755–8.
23. Rivera ME, Linder BJ, Ziegelmann MJ, Viers BR, Rangel LJ, Elliott DS. The impact of prior radiation therapy on artificial urinary sphincter device survival. J Urol. 2016;195(4 Pt 1):1033–7.
24. Rehder P, Gozzi C. Transobturator sling suspension for male urinary incontinence including post-radical prostatectomy. Eur Urol. 2007;52(3):860–6.
25. Davies TO, Bepple JL, McCammon KA. Urodynamic changes and initial results of the AdVance male sling. Urology. 2009;74(2):354–7.
26. Kahokehr AA, Selph JP, Belsante MJ, et al. Mechanism of action of the transobturator sling for post-radical prostatectomy incontinence: a multi-institutional prospective study using dynamic magnetic resonance imaging. Urology. 2018;116:185–92.
27. Ye H, Haab F, de Ridder D, et al. Effectiveness and complications of the AMS AdVance™ male sling system for the treatment of stress urinary incontinence: a prospective multicenter study. Urology. 2018;120:197–204.
28. Hogewoning CRC, Meij LAM, Pelger RCM, Putter H, Krouwel EM, Elzevier HW. Sling surgery for the treatment of urinary incontinence after transurethral resection of the prostate: new data on the virtue male sling and an evaluation of literature. Urology. 2017;100:187–92.
29. Angulo JC, Fonseca J, Esquinas C, et al. Adjustable transobturator male system (ATOMS(®)) as treatment of stress urinary incontinence secondary to transurethral resection of the prostate. Actas Urol Esp. 2018;42(9):567–73.
30. Noordhoff TC, Finazzi-Agrò E, Scheepe JR, Blok BFM. Outcome and complications of adjustable continence therapy (ProACT(TM)) in the treatment of urinary incontinence after transurethral resection of the prostate: a multicenter study. Neurourol Urodyn. 2019;38(4):1111–9.
31. Kumar A, Litt ER, Ballert KN, Nitti VW. Artificial urinary sphincter versus male sling for post-prostatectomy incontinence—what do patients choose? J Urol. 2009;181(3):1231–5.
32. Constable L, Cotterill N, Cooper D, et al. Male synthetic sling versus artificial urinary sphincter trial for men with urodynamic stress incontinence after prostate surgery (MASTER): study protocol for a randomised controlled trial. Trials. 2018;19(1):131.
33. Espuña Pons M, Rebollo Alvarez P, Puig Clota M. [Validation of the Spanish version of the International Consultation on Incontinence Questionnaire-Short Form. A questionnaire for assessing the urinary incontinence]. Med Clin. 2004;122(8):288–92.
34. Espuña Pons M, Castro Díaz D, Carbonell C, Dilla T. [Comparison between the "ICIQ-UI Short Form" Questionnaire and the "King's Health Questionnaire" as assessment tools of urinary incontinence among women]. Actas Urol Esp. 2007;31(5):502–10.
35. Twiss CO, Fischer MC, Nitti VW. Comparison between reduction in 24-hour pad weight, International Consultation on Incontinence-Short Form (ICIQ-SF) score, International Prostate Symptom Score (IPSS), and Post-Operative Patient Global Impression of Improvement (PGI-I) score in patient evaluation after male perineal sling. Neurourol Urodyn. 2007;26(1):8–13.
36. Tienza A, Graham PL, Robles JE, et al. Daily pad usage versus the international consultation on incontinence questionnaire short form for continence assessment following radical prostatectomy. Int Neurourol J. 2020;24(2):156–62.
37. Ware JE Jr, Sherbourne CD. The MOS 36-item short-form health survey (SF-36). I. Conceptual framework and item selection. Med Care. 1992;30(6):473–83.
38. Alonso J, Prieto L, Antó JM. [The Spanish version of the SF-36 Health Survey (the SF-36 health questionnaire): an instrument for measuring clinical results]. Med Clin. 1995;104(20):771–6.
39. Vilagut G, Ferrer M, Rajmil L, et al. [The Spanish version of the Short Form 36 Health Survey: a decade of experience and new developments]. Gac Sanit. 2005;19(2):135–50.
40. Sanz-Ruiz A. Factores que influyen en los resultados de la corrección quirúrgica de la incontinencia urinaria por tratamiento del cáncer de próstata. Salamanca. España.: Departamento de Cirugía., Universidad de Salamanca. Salamanca.; 2017.
41. Navalón P, Pallás Y, Ordoño F, et al. Our experience in the treatment of male stress urinary incontinence with the male remeex system. Arch Esp Urol. 2010;63(6):432–9.
42. Sousa-Escandón A, Cabrera J, Mantovanic F, et al. Adjustable suburethral sling (male Remeex system®) in the treatment of male stress urinary incontinence: a multicentric European study. Eur Urol. 2007;52(5):1473–80.
43. Jiménez Parra JD, Cebrián Lostal JL, Hualde Alfaro A, et al. [REMEEX® system for the treatment of male urinary stress incontinence: our experience]. Actas Urol Esp. 2010;34(9):802–5.

44. Navalón-Monllor V, Ordoño-Domínguez F, Pallás-Costa Y, et al. Long-term follow-up for the treatment of male urinary incontinence with the Remeex system. Actas Urol Esp. 2016;40(9):585–91.
45. Sousa-Escandon A, León J, Flores J, Sousa-González D. Adjustable male slings: REMEEX. In: Singla A, Comiter C, editors. Post-prostatectomy incontinence. Evaluation and management. Cham: Springer; 2017. p. 91–104.
46. El Kharroubi A, Dergamoun H, Droupy S, Wagner L. [Retrospective multicentric evaluation of the efficacy of four-arms and adjustable male slings in the management of mild and moderate urinary incontinence after radical prostatectomy]. Prog Urol. 2019;29(16):989–94.
47. Leizour B, Chevrot A, Wagner L, Droupy S, Costa P. [Adjustable retropubic suburethral sling Remeex(®) in the treatment of male stress urinary incontinence: one-year results]. Prog Urol. 2017;27(4):238–43.
48. Burkhard FC, Bosch JLHR, Cruz F, et al. European Association of Urology guidelines on urinary incontinence in adults. Arnhem: ©European-Association-of-Urology-2020; 2020.

Part III

Pelvic Organ Prolapse

11 Inheritance of Pelvic Organ Prolapse

Fulya Tekşen, Fulya Dökmeci, Tülin Özkan, Şerife Esra Çetinkaya, and Fuat Kaplan

11.1 Introduction

Pelvic organ prolapse (POP) is a common health problem affecting approximately 50% of women over 50, with a significant burden on health and quality of life. Genetic predisposition has been suggested as an important risk factor in the etiology of pelvic organ prolapse (POP) in addition to menopause, aging, multiparity, vaginal delivery, chronic constipation, chronic obstructive lung disease, and obesity [1, 2]. It has been reported that 40% of women are susceptible to POP due to genetic effects [3]. Hence, family history has been proposed as an important risk factor for the prediction of genetic susceptibility.

Epidemiologic studies have shed light on the hereditary role of prolapse. Observations of advanced stages of prolapse in nulliparous women without any other risk factor apart from positive family history, and no vaginal prolapse in significant numbers of multiparous women with a negative family history, have been explained in this context [4, 5]. The rate of familial genetic incidence of genital prolapse has been reported as 60%, and a five times higher risk of developing prolapse has been found among siblings of young women (under 55 years of age) with severe prolapse, when compared with the general population [6–8].

Ethnic and racial variations also may play role in female pelvic floor disorders. Asian, African, and Native American women seem to have less risk compared to women of European and Hispanic descent [9]. Dietz et al. showed that Caucasian ancestry women have significantly high pelvic organ mobility, both antepartum and postpartum, as opposed to Asian women [10].

Defining the etiology and risk factors of this highly prevalent condition is of paramount importance in determining individuals at risk in order to provide preventative strategies or in planning the most appropriate management option for affected individuals. Therefore, a comprehensive understanding about the disease on a genetic basis and with a hereditary point of view

This study was presented at the Mediterranean Incontinence and Pelvic Floor Society (MIPS) Fourth Annual Meeting in Malta on 1–3 December 2016 and was awarded the First Oral Presentation Prize.

F. Tekşen · T. Özkan
Department of Medical Biology, Ankara University School of Medicine, Ankara, Turkey
e-mail: tozkan@ankara.edu.tr

F. Dökmeci
Department of Obstetrics and Gynecology, Ankara University School of Medicine, Ankara, Turkey

Ş. E. Çetinkaya (✉)
Department of Obstetrics and Gynecology, Ankara University School of Medicine, Cebeci Hospital, Ankara, Turkey

F. Kaplan
WCHN Rudy Ruggles Biomedical Research Institute Danbury, Danbury, CT, USA

F. Dökmeci, D. E. E. Rizk (eds.), *Insights Into Incontinence and the Pelvic Floor*,
https://doi.org/10.1007/978-3-030-94174-1_11

will be helpful not only in the treatment but also in the planning of effective preventative strategies for women who are genetically predisposed to develop POP [6].

Numerous studies have been performed so far to reveal the genetic basis of POP. This chapter will focus on and summarize these investigations, including an example of a case study, which will be reported and discussed briefly.

11.2 Literature Review

In order to observe the genetic component of POP, several methods have been used, such as the gene mutation/mutations causing the defect, the possible loci of the mutant gene/genes, linkage analyses, polymorphism studies such as single nucleotide polymorphism (SNP), epigenetic factors, animal studies, twin studies, family studies, and pedigree analyses to show the mode of transmission.

Homeobox (HOX) genes are a group of genes, which encode transcription factors that are necessary in embryonic development and are considered to play a role in the development of POP [11]. Altered gene expressions or mutations in the defined 39 HOX genes lead to human diseases. These HOX genes are classified in A, B, C, and D clusters, which are especially involved in the reproductive system [12, 13].

Animal models, as well as in vitro and human studies, have shown significant findings regarding these genes in the reproductive system. It has been reported that HOXA11 is responsible for the synthesis of Collagen Type III, matrix metalloproteinase 2 (MMP2), and the development of the lower uterine segment, cervix, and uterosacral ligaments (USLs) [14, 15]. Similarly, the HOXA13 gene is involved in the development of the upper vagina and has been reported to regulate the ECM constituents [13, 16, 17].

In the study of Ma, Y. et al., it has been reported that the knockdown of the HOXA11 gene in the USLs of mice and in fibroblasts has confirmed that it has a vital role in the homeostasis of connective tissue support [14]. Similarly, Connel et al. reported that HOXA11-null mice had no noticeable uterosacral ligaments, demonstrating that HOXA11 is essential for organogenesis [15]. These investigators further analyzed expressions of HOXA11, Collagen Type I, Collagen Type III, MMP2, and MMP9 in USLs of women with and without POP and found approximately 75-fold and 17-fold lower expression levels of HOXA11 (142958) and Collagen Type III (COL3A1; 120180), respectively, in the USLs of 18 pre- and postmenopausal women with pelvic organ prolapse. Moreover, matrix metalloproteinase MMP2 (120360) gene expression level was increased twofold in patients compared to controls. In the same study, in vitro studies on murine embryonic fibroblasts showed that HOXA11 increased Collagen III expression and decreased MMP2 expression levels. They concluded that HOXA11 is an essential gene for the development of the USLs and suggested that women with POP might have weakened connective tissue due to changes in the signaling pathway involving HOXA11, Collagen Type III, and MMP2 [15]. In another study comparing mRNA expressions of the HOXA11 and MMP2 genes in women with and without POP, no difference in HOXA11 mRNA expression was reported in either group, but an increased MMP2 mRNA expression has been found in women with prolapse [18]. On the other hand, data regarding the role of HOXA 13 in women with prolapse is scarce. Connel, K.A. et al. have investigated the mRNA expression of the HOXA 13 gene in the anterior apical vaginal tissues of women with POP and have shown a significantly lower expression compared to women with normal vaginal wall support in both pre- and postmenopausal women [17].

The synthesis and degradation of collagen and elastin are crucial in the maintenance of pelvic floor integrity. Alterations in collagen metabolism and the quantity and composition of various collagen subtypes have been shown in women with POP. Of more than 20 subtypes of collagen, Types I and III have been studied widely in the etiopathogenesis of prolapse. While Collagen Type I is nonelastic and provides great resistance to tensile forces, Collagen Type III has elastic properties and is extensively found in more flexible tissues. Alterations in their ratios have been suggested to cause connective tissue disorders [6, 19]. In this context, genes and their polymorphisms related to the connective tissue, mainly Collagen Type 1 alpha 1 (COL1A1), Collagen Type 3 alpha 1 (COL3A1), laminin gamma-1 (LAMC1), MMP9, MMP1 and 3, lysyl oxidase-like 1 (LOXL1), and estrogen and progesterone receptors, have also been studied in women with prolapse and have been analyzed in two meta-analyses [20, 21]. In these two systematic reviews and meta-analyses, the COL3A1 rs1800255 genotype AA was shown to be associated with prolapse in Asian and Dutch women, whereas the rs1800012 polymorphism of the COL1A1 gene was found to be correlated in Brazilian, Italian, Polish, and Israeli women [20, 21]. In a very recent study including 826 post-menopausal Brazilian women with mixed ancestries, polymorphisms rs1800012 of the Collagen I (COL1A1) and rs1800255 of the Collagen III (COL3A1) genes and their association with pelvic organ prolapse (POP) have been investigated, and no associations have been found [22]. There was insufficient evidence or no association with prolapse for LAMC1, MMP1, MMP3, and MMP9 genes, and although individual studies have suggested some significant associations between estrogen and progesterone receptors with prolapse, these associations could not be confirmed in the aforementioned meta-analyses [20, 21]. COL4A2, COL5A1, COL14A1, COL18A1, ESR, ZFAT, MMP-3, MMP-9, MMP-10, and LOXL-4 are other potential polymorphic genes that have been evaluated recently in the etiology of POP [23–27].

In the study we have conducted, the mRNA gene expression profiles of Collagen Type I (COL1A), Collagen Type III (COL3A), HomeoboxA11 (HOXA11), HomeoboxA13 (HOXA13), and estrogen receptor genes (ESR1 and ESR2) of round ligament (RL) and uterosacral ligament (USL) in a cohort of post-menopausal Turkish women with and without uterine prolapse were studied. Low expression levels of HOXA13 and COL3A genes in the USLs and ESR2 genes in the RLs were demonstrated especially in advanced stages of prolapse, implicating a role in the development of uterine prolapse [28].

As the familial occurrence rate was found to be 30% among women with vaginal prolapse [29], family studies and pedigree analyses not only suggest the genetic susceptibility to POP and provide the basis for molecular investigations but also provide significant knowledge for clinical practice in terms of preventative strategies for prolapse. In a meta-analysis on 1107 POP patients and 1941 controls, the overall OR of prolapse in case of a positive family history has been reported as 2.58 (95% CI 2.12–3.15) [30]. Twin studies also support the genetic basis of POP. In a female twin study comparing 3376 monozygotic and 5067 dizygotic twin pairs, twin similarity and the relative proportions of phenotypic variance resulting from genetic and environmental factors regarding POP and stress urinary incontinence (SUI) have been investigated. Data has been extracted from the Swedish Twin Register and the Swedish Inpatient Registry; same-sex female pairs born from 1926 to 1958 with known zygosity were included, and hospital admissions, surgeries, and discharges were evaluated. Environmental factors have been classified as shared and non-shared. In this study, it has been reported that there was greater similarity among monozygotic twin pairs than the dizygotic ones in developing POP. Genetic and non-shared environmental factors equally contributed about 40%, and shared environmental factors contributed about 20% of the variation in liability for the two disorders [3].

Genetic susceptibility has been shown to be significantly more common in younger (46%, age 45 and over) affected women compared to older (8%, under 55) in family history studies of women with POP [31]. Nikolova et al. have reported six affected individuals presenting with early onset of prolapse in a single multigenerational family. A higher genetic risk has been shown for the family members of patients with advanced prolapse, and it similarly suggests a five times higher risk for patients under 55 with advanced POP [8].

The risk of prolapse has been related not only to affected first-degree family members but also suggests being affected by distant relatives, such as third-degree relatives [32]. A retrospective study including 453,522 females showed that 4628 females treated with POP had 15,530 first-degree relatives, 33,782 second-degree relatives, and 66,469 third-degree relatives. It was also indicated that having a family history of three or more affected third-degree relatives and no affected first- or second-degree relatives was similar in risk to having one affected first-degree relative [33]. Briefly defined, first-degree relatives are parents, children, and siblings. Second-degree relatives are grandparents, grandchildren, aunts, uncles, nieces, nephews, and half-siblings. Third-degree relatives are great grandparents, great grandchildren, grand nieces/nephews, grand aunts/uncles, and first cousins. The RR (relative risk) is defined as the ratio of observed treated POP patients to expected treated POP patients among the probands, as shown by the following formula [33]:

$$\text{Relative risk}\left(\text{RR}\right)=\frac{\text{Observed POP treated}}{\text{Expected POP treated among probands}}$$

In addition to prolapse, the importance of family history has also been observed in conditions suggestive of deficient connective tissue, such as hernia or hemorrhoids, supporting the hypothesis that certain women with connective tissue problems are genetically more predisposed to POP [34]. Male cases with connective tissue problems, such as inguinal and other forms of hernia, have been reported among family members of POP patients, and patients with POP have been reported to be at risk for other hernias in their bodies [35, 36]. In fact, McLennan, M.T. et al. reported that 47.3% of their patients had family histories of prolapse and/or hernia compared with the control group having a 28.9% rate of prolapse and suggested to take the histories of the both male and female members of the family [35]. Segev, Y. et al. reported that 32% of POP patients had hernias elsewhere in their bodies, while this rate was only 5% in the control group ($n = 60$) [36].

Autosomal dominant, multifactorial patterns and sporadic cases with spontaneous mutations have been reported as the inheritance patterns of POP in the literature [7, 37]. Jack, G.S. et al. have reported an autosomal dominant pattern in their study in ten young POP patients (average age, 37; range, 27–51 years), with both maternal and paternal transmissions and high penetrance [7].

Familial cases aid the linkage analyses, which are performed to identify the genes and alleles involved in prolapse. Nikolova, G. et al. evaluated one family, with POP presenting in nearly 11 female relatives of a three-generation pedigree, all having severe prolapse and progression at younger ages. They genotyped nine individuals from that family, of whom six had prolapse, and reported a possible association between POP and LAMC1 [8]. Another linkage analysis showing a predisposition for pelvic floor disorders on chromosome 9q21 involved 32 families and 70 affected women, mostly sister pairs [38].

11.3 Case Study: Inheritance of Pelvic Organ Prolapses

(a) **Aim and Scope**
The aim of this study was to analyze the pedigrees of women affected with prolapse in order to evaluate the inheritance of POP in a cohort of Turkish women. Cases, with family members who have vaginal prolapse, were evaluated to observe the familial transmission of the disease.

(b) **Study Design and Material Methods**
The family histories of women with POP, who attended the Department of Obstetrics and Gynaecology of Ankara University School of Medicine between 2012 and 2015, were evaluated. Women who underwent surgery for POP (study group, POPQ stage ≥ 2, $n = 38$) and for other gynecological problems (control patients, POPQ stage <2, $n = 21$) were included. The family members of proband that are affected by hernia, in addition

to POP, were also evaluated. Women with malignancies and connective tissue disorders were excluded. At least three successive generations were investigated by pedigree analysis. Fischer's exact test was used for the statistical analysis.

(c) **Results of the Study**
Fifteen women (39.5%) in the study group and none in the control group (0%) were found to have a family history of POP ($p < 0.05$). Women in the study group were significantly older ($p < 0.001$) than the women in the control group ($p < 0.05$).

The pedigree analysis showed autosomal dominant inheritance of POP in seven families (18.4%). The mode of inheritance could not be clarified in eight cases (21.1%). Twenty-three cases with a negative family history were evaluated as sporadic cases (60.5%). Thus, autosomal dominant, multifactorial inheritance and sporadic occurrence were suggested for the familial transmission of the disease.

Some examples of the pedigrees of the families are given below.

As observed in Table 11.1, in 11 families, there was one other family member affected with POP, and in three families of the study group, there was more than one POP case other than the proband.

To explain the families with more than one case of POP, in the first family (Family 11, Fig. 11.1), there were two sisters of the proband with POP. In the second family, (Family 13, Fig. 11.2), there were three cases (proband's mother and two aunts) with POP, and in the third family (Family 14), the proband's mother and aunt were both affected with POP.

In addition to POP, hernias were also observed in the family members of some of the probands. In Family 13, there were two cases (proband's father and uncle) with hernia (Fig. 11.2), and in Family 1, the proband's mother and daughter were both affected with hernias, showing three successive generations.

The families without any members with POP seem to be sporadic cases if we do not consider the possible insufficient knowledge about the family history.

11.4 Discussion

According to the literature and the case study presented above, inheritance and genetics seem to have a significant role in the etiopathogenesis of POP. Numerous investigations have been performed so far. However, there are still many controversial and conflicting results. The mostly proposed reasons for this situation include the

Table 11.1 Family members of proband who are also affected with POP and/or hernia

Family no.	Proband (patient affected with POP)	Mother	Aunt	Sister	Father	Uncle/brother	Daughter	Others
1	P1	X*					X*	
2	P2	X						
3	P3			X				
4	P4			X				
5	P5	X						
6	P6			X				
7	P7			X				
8	P8	X						
9	P9							X
10	P10							X
11	P11			X X				
12	P12							X
13	P13	X	X X		X*	X*		
14	P14	X	X					
15	P15	X						

x: POP, x*: hernia

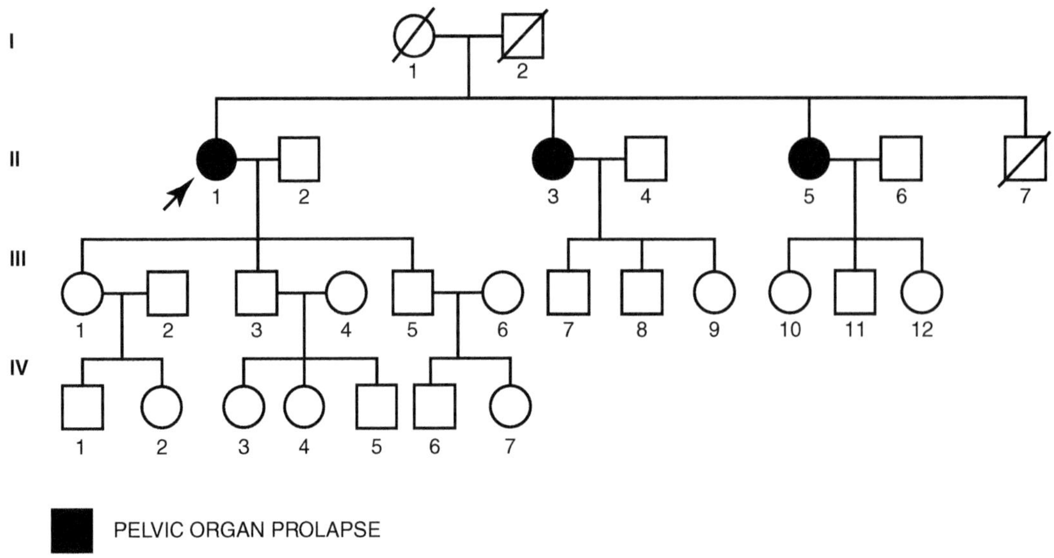

Fig. 11.1 Pedigree of Family 11

Fig. 11.2 Pedigree of Family 13

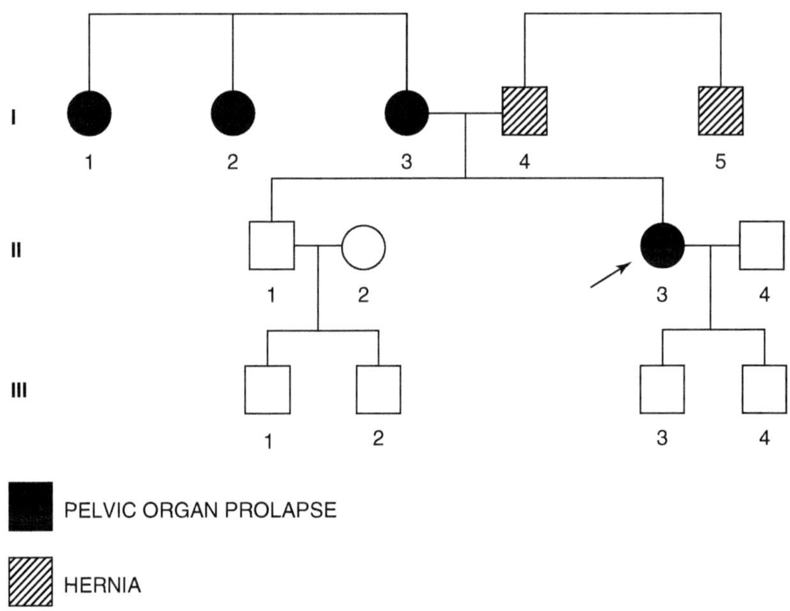

small sample sizes, the heterogeneous study populations that include women of different ethnicities, heterogeneous methodologies, various tissues sampled for analysis, their harvesting and extraction methods, the lack of longitudinal studies evaluating the natural history of POP with changes in the composition of pelvic tissues in a life span, and the multifactorial etiology of prolapse [6, 18, 19].

It is difficult to interpret the studies and predict the susceptibility and risk of prolapse due to its multifactorial nature. While inheritance has been reported to contribute significantly in the variance of POP, all non-genetic environmental factors (shared and non-shared) have also been shown to have a significant influence [3]. Shared and non-shared environmental effects, such as smoking habits, exercise, dietary and drinking habits, and socioeconomic status, are important in the expression of the genes that affect the phenotype. Thus, in these circumstances, it is not very easy to evaluate the factors separately in the families showing multifactorial inheritance.

In this context, genome-wide association studies may provide the knowledge regarding genotype-phenotype associations, testing genetic variants across the genomes of many individuals [39].

11.5 Conclusion

At present, in order to give appropriate genetic counseling to women who are predisposed to developing POP and to take preventative strategies in the management of the condition, larger population studies investigating the obstetrical, genetic, and environmental factors of women, and linkage analyses and genome-wide association studies are needed. Family studies and pedigree analyses shed light to the inheritance pattern of the disease and provide the basis for molecular studies.

References

1. Chow D, Rodríguez LV. Epidemiology and prevalence of pelvic organ prolapse. Curr Opin Urol. 2013;23(4):293–8.
2. Fornell EU, Wingren G, Kjølhede P. Factors associated with pelvic floor dysfunction with emphasis on urinary and fecal incontinence and genital prolapse: an epidemiological study. Acta Obstet Gynecol Scand. 2004;83(4):383–9.
3. Altman D, Forsman M, Falconer C, Lichtenstein P. Genetic influence on stress urinary incontinence and pelvic organ prolapse. Eur Urol. 2008;54(4):918–23.
4. Buchsbaum GM, Duecy EE, Kerr LA, Huang LS, Perevich M, Guzick DS. Pelvic organ prolapse in nulliparous women and their parous sisters. Obstet Gynecol. 2006;108(6):1388–93.
5. Bump RC, Norton PA. Epidemiology and natural history of pelvic floor dysfunction. Obstet Gynecol Clin North Am. 1998;25(4):723–46.
6. Bortolini MAT, Rizk DEE. Genetics of pelvic organ prolapse: crossing the bridge between bench and bedside in urogynecologic research. Int Urogynecol J. 2011;22(10):1211.
7. Jack GS, Nikolova G, Vilain E, Raz S, Rodríguez LV. Familial transmission of genitovaginal prolapse. Int Urogynecol J Pelvic Floor Dysfunct. 2005;17(5):498–501.
8. Nikolova G, Lee H, Berkovitz S, Nelson S, Sinsheimer J, Vilain E, et al. Sequence variant in the laminin gamma1 (LAMC1) gene associated with familial pelvic organ prolapse. Hum Genet. 2006;120(6):847–56.
9. Twiss C, Triaca V, Rodríguez LV. Familial transmission of urogenital prolapse and incontinence. Curr Opin Obstet Gynecol. 2007;19(5):464–8.
10. Dietz HP. Do Asian women have less pelvic organ mobility than Caucasians? Int Urogynecol J. 2003;14(4):250–3.
11. Mallo M, Wellik DM, Deschamps J. Hox genes and regional patterning of the vertebrate body plan. Dev Biol. 2010;344(1):7–15.
12. Du H, Taylor HS. The role of Hox genes in female reproductive tract development, adult function and fertility. Cold Spring Harb Perspect Med. 2016;6(1):a023002.
13. Taylor H. The role of HOX genes in the development and function of the female reproductive tract. Semin Reprod Med. 2000;18(01):08190.
14. Ma Y, Guess M, Datar A, Hennessey A, Cardenas I, Johnson J, et al. Knockdown of Hoxa11 in vivo in the uterosacral ligament and uterus of mice results in altered collagen and matrix metalloproteinase activity. Biol Reprod. 2012;86(4):100.
15. Connell KA, Guess MK, Chen H, Andikyan V, Bercik R, Taylor HS. HOXA11 is critical for development and maintenance of uterosacral ligaments and deficient in pelvic prolapse. J Clin Invest. 2008;118(3):1050–5.
16. Scott V, Morgan EA, Stadler HS. Genitourinary functions of Hoxa13 and Hoxd13. J Biochem. 2005;137(6):671–6.
17. Connell KA, Guess MK, Tate A, Andikyan V, Bercik R, Taylor HS. Diminished vaginal HOXA13 expression in women with pelvic organ prolapse. Menopause. 2009;16(3):529–33.
18. Yılmaz N, Ozaksit G, Terzi YK, Yılmaz S, Budak B, Aksakal O, et al. HOXA11 and MMP2 gene expression in uterosacral ligaments of women with pelvic organ prolapse. J Turk Ger Gynecol Assoc. 2014;15(2):104–8.
19. Gong R, Xia Z. Collagen changes in pelvic support tissues in women with pelvic organ prolapse. Eur J Obstet Gynecol Reprod Biol. 2019;234:185–9.
20. Ward RM, Edwards DRV, Edwards T, Giri A, Jerome RN, Wu JM. Genetic epidemiology of pelvic organ prolapse: a systematic review. Am J Obstet Gynecol. 2014;211(4):326–35.
21. Cartwright R, Kirby AC, Tikkinen KAO, Mangera A, Thiagamoorthy G, Rajan P, et al. Systematic review and metaanalysis of genetic association studies of urinary symptoms and prolapse in women. Am J Obstet Gynecol. 2015;212(2):199.e1–24.
22. Batista NC, Bortolini MAT, Silva RSP, Teixeira JB, Melo NC, Santos RGM, et al. Collagen I and Collagen III polymorphisms in women with pelvic organ prolapse. Neurourol Urodyn. 2020;39(7):1977–84.
23. Abulaizi A, Abula A, Ababaikeli G, Wan X, Du R, Zhakeer A. Identification of pelvic organ prolapse risk

susceptibility gene SNP locus in Xinjiang women. Int Urogynecol J. 2020;31(1):123–30.
24. dos Santos RGM, Pepicelli RGM, Batista NC, de Carvalho CV, Bortolini MAT, Castro RA. Collagen XVIII and LOXL 4 polymorphisms in women with and without advanced pelvic organ prolapse. Int Urogynecol J. 2018;29(6):893–8.
25. Ghersel F, Souto R, Gonzales E, Paulo D, Fernandes C, Oliveira E. Assessment of metalloproteinase matrix 9 (MMP9) gene polymorphisms risk factors for pelvic organ prolapse in the Brazilian population. Rev Bras Ginecol Obstet. 2019;41(03):164–9.
26. Li L, Sun Z, Chen J, Zhang Y, Shi H, Zhu L. Genetic polymorphisms in collagen related genes are associated with pelvic organ prolapse. Menopause. 2020;27(2):223–9.
27. Maeda PM, Bicudo APSL, Watanabe RTM, Fonseca TSM, do Souto RP, Fernandes CE, et al. Study of the polymorphism rs3025058 of the MMP 3 gene and risk of pelvic organ prolapse in Brazilian women. Eur J Obstet Gynecol Reprod Biol X. 2019;3:100031.
28. Dökmeci F, Tekşen F, Çetinkaya SE, Özkan T, Kaplan F, Köse K. Expressions of homeobox, collagen and estrogen genes in women with uterine prolapse. Eur J Obstet Gynecol Reprod Biol. 2018;233:26–9.
29. Chiaffarino F, Chatenoud L, Dindelli M, Meschia M, Buonaguidi A, Amicarelli F, et al. Reproductive factors, family history, occupation and risk of urogenital prolapse. Eur J Obstet Gynecol Reprod Biol. 1999;82(1):63–7.
30. Lince SL, van Kempen LC, Vierhout ME, Kluivers KB. A systematic review of clinical studies on hereditary factors in pelvic organ prolapse. Int Urogynecol J. 2012;23(10):1327–36.
31. Alcalay M, Stav K, Eisenberg VH. Family history associated with pelvic organ prolapse in young women. Int Urogynecol J. 2015;26(12):1773–6.
32. Norton PA, Allen Brady K, Cannon Albright LA. The familiality of pelvic organ prolapse in the Utah Population Database. Int Urogynecol J. 2013;24(3):413–8.
33. Allen Brady K, Norton PA, Hill AJ, Rowe K, Cannon Albright LA. Risk of pelvic organ prolapse treatment based on extended family history. Am J Obstet Gynecol. 2020;223(1):105.e1–8.
34. Miedel A, Tegerstedt G, Mæhle Schmidt M, Nyrén O, Hammarström M. Nonobstetric risk factors for symptomatic pelvic organ prolapse. Obstet Gynecol. 2009;113(5):1089–97.
35. McLennan MT, Harris JK, Kariuki B, Meyer S. Family history as a risk factor for pelvic organ prolapse. Int Urogynecol J. 2008;19(8):1063–9.
36. Segev Y, Auslender R, Feiner B, Lissak A, Lavie O, Abramov Y. Are women with pelvic organ prolapse at a higher risk of developing hernias? Int Urogynecol J. 2009;20(12):1451–3.
37. McNanley AR, Johnson AM, Flynn MK, Wood RW, Kennedy SD, Reeder JE. Inherited pelvic organ prolapse in the mouse: preliminary evaluation of a new murine model. Int Urogynecol J. 2009;20(1):19–25.
38. Allen Brady K, Norton PA, Farnham JM, Teerlink C, Cannon Albright LA. Significant linkage evidence for a predisposition gene for pelvic floor disorders on chromosome 9q21. Am J Hum Genet. 2009;84(5):678–82.
39. Tam V, Patel N, Turcotte M, Bossé Y, Paré G, Meyre D. Benefits and limitations of genome wide association studies. Nat Rev Genet. 2019;20(8):467–84.

Screening for Ehlers-Danlos Syndrome in the Pelvic Organ Prolapse Patient

12

Sherrie Palm

12.1 Introduction

Pelvic organ prolapse (POP) and Ehlers-Danlos syndrome (EDS) are diverse comorbid conditions with insufficient exploration or analysis of probability related to essential vaginal and pelvic health in women. POP evades female wellness focus. Women are seldom familiar with POP prior to diagnosis despite research estimating up to 50% prevalence and considerable physical, emotional, social, sexual, fitness, and employment quality of life (QOL) impacts [1]. EDS, a condition recognized as joint hypermobility, is one of the most frustrating co-existing intersects women with POP experience and more significantly exhibits as exceptionally stretchy or fragile skin that bruises and tears easily externally and provides little structural integrity internally.

EDS is under-recognized and is commonly undiagnosed or misdiagnosed during POP evaluation. Women experiencing the POP/EDS overlap may have difficulty capturing short-term surgical success or long-term surgical efficacy and potentially have a higher risk of surgical complications.

Ineffective EDS awareness and clinician curriculum are barriers to POP wellness. There is a considerable need to broaden understanding of the mechanism in which EDS accelerates POP manifestation and development. The focus of this investigation was to explore screening for EDS hypermobility and tissue integrity to improve treatment outcomes within the POP/EDS sector.

S. Palm (✉)
Association for Pelvic Organ Prolapse Support, Mukwonago, WI, USA

12.2 Case Study: POP/EDS (Ehlers-Danlos Syndrome) Comorbidity—Screening to Improve Treatment Outcome

A 48-h quick poll survey shared on January 2019 in a closed Facebook-based POP patient support forum captured input from members experiencing the POP/EDS comorbidity. An image provided in the survey clarified connective tissue disorder characteristics. A ten-question survey captured patient input.

Fifty-five women responded to an online survey. Mean age: under 20 (2%), 21–30 (2%), 31–40 (27%), 41–50 (22%), 51–60 (18%), 61+ (29%). EDS status indicated: dx by physician 45%, suspect EDS, not clinically validated 55%. Utilization of nonsurgical POP treatments prior to surgical intervention: utilized, did not help symptoms 48%, reduced symptoms 19%, did not use nonsurgical treatments 17%, preferred immediate surgery 9%, n/a 7%. Surgeon provided EDS screening prior to surgery: no 35%, patient mentioned to surgeon, surgeon not concerned 30%, patient mentioned to

F. Dökmeci, D. E. E. Rizk (eds.), *Insights Into Incontinence and the Pelvic Floor*,
https://doi.org/10.1007/978-3-030-94174-1_12

surgeon, surgeon concerned and discussed 15%, discovered EDS issues post-surgery 11%, n/a 9%. Polypropylene mesh surgery post-surgical status: holding off on surgery 36%, no complications post polypropylene mesh surgery 22%, despite use of poly mesh, POP returned 16%, mesh erosion post mesh surgery, trimming resolved issue 11%, pain with intimacy 5%, severe bleeding 5%, perineal tearing 3%, UTI 2%.

12.3 Discussion

People diagnosed with EDS frequently identify themselves as zebras related to the uniqueness of zebra stripes. Despite noteworthy occurrence, the intersect of EDS and POP is rarely recognized during routine women's wellness exams. Within the POP/EDS commonality, the EDS symptoms and manifestations can be distinct among patients, making diagnosis ambiguous. These intertwined conditions disrupt QOL in the female community from mid-teen through end of life and increase potential of surgical or nonsurgical treatment failure. Due to noteworthy occurrence of POP within the EDS population and insufficient patient and clinician awareness of EDS, there is considerable need to enhance screening and detection of EDS symptoms within patients who may or may not have been diagnosed with EDS but indicate unconventional symptoms during POP consultations.

While accurate incidence data is currently unattainable for EDS or POP, research estimates EDS occurs in 1 in 5000 people with 70% prevalence in females [2] and POP incidence at 1 in 2 women [1]. POP co-occurrence is a characteristic included within various EDS classifications, most notably but not exclusively hypermobility EDS (hEDS).

12.4 POP

POP has been medically documented for nearly 4000 years dating back to the Kahun Gynaecological Papyrus circa 1835 B.C.E. The pubococcygeus muscles (PC) are a trampoline-like set of muscles that sit at the base of the abdominal cavity supporting organs and structural tissues above them. POP manifests as PC muscles weaken or become damaged related to a variety of causal factors, allowing organs above to drop from a normal position, herniating into the vaginal canal. Pelvic organs may protrude outside of the vagina in higher grades of POP severity. POP types are bladder (cystocele), rectum (rectocele), intestines (enterocele), uterus (uterine), and vaginal apex (vaginal vault). Women may experience multiple types of POP simultaneously.

Accurate statistical evidence of POP pervasiveness is difficult to assess or validate. Anatomical changes do not always correlate with symptom severity. Currently standardized POP screening occurring during routine pelvic exams is insufficient. Barber et al. indicated that symptomatic POP was present in 3–6% of the female population, but when based on vaginal examination, it was present in up to 50% of women [1]. Wu et al. suggest genetic tendency toward prolapse is becoming more apparent [3]. The most prevalent indicators of POP are tissues bulging from the vagina, urinary incontinence, urine retention, chronic constipation, vaginal or rectal pressure, or inability to keep a tampon in. Additionally, women may experience fecal incontinence, pain with intercourse, lack of sexual sensation, and/or rectal/vaginal, back, or pelvic pain. The stigma of tissue bulge and incontinence may prevent women from disclosing embarrassing POP symptoms to clinicians unless specifically asked during routine pelvic examinations, distorting symptomatic data. Whether symptomatic or recognized via vaginal examination, POP statistics are not likely to become consistent until standardized POP screening occurs during routine pelvic examinations.

Beyond the established POP risk factors such as pregnancy, childbirth, age, estrogen depletion, and increased intra-abdominal pressure via chronic constipation, chronic coughing, obesity, or heavy lifting fitness activities, the concept of a genetic tendency toward prolapse needs to become more readily recognized. Women with a positive family history of POP are more likely to develop prolapse compared to women with no family history. Twin studies identify that genetic factors increase the risk of POP by 43% [3, 4].

12.5 EDS

EDS is a group of multi-systemic disorders that affect connective tissue throughout the body in diverse ways. There are 13 subtypes of EDS that include a variety of symptoms and severity. Most of the EDS categories are rare. Considered the most common systemic inheritable disorders of connective tissue, hypermobile EDS (hEDS) and the related hypermobility spectrum disorders (HSD) are estimated to embody 80–90% of EDS cases [5]. The EDS subtype hEDS is the most typical POP/EDS comorbid. The focus of this exploration is hEDS rather than the rarer subtypes of EDS.

EDS has a relatively new classification system. Estimates on the high side under the previous classification system indicated up to 2 million people in the UK have EDS, 10 million in the USA, 17 million in Europe, with estimated hEDS global figures at 255 million [2]. The new classification of hEDS is more selective; figures are lower than those previously stated [2]. Actual occurrences may be higher or lower due to the lack of EDS awareness in both the medical and lay communities.

POP and stress urinary incontinence (SUI) are common in women and may occur as young as teen years in the hEDS sector prior to pregnancy. Connective tissue manifestation within the hEDS community additionally may include joint hypermobility, skin hyperextensibility, tissue fragility, ligament laxity, hemorrhoids, hernias, digestive issues such as IBS, heartburn, constipation, varicose veins, pain, soft velvety skin, diastasis rectus abdominis (DRA), intussusception, slow wound healing, neuromuscular pain, and neuropathic pain [6]. Additional indicators of hEDS may including loose, unstable joints that dislocate easily, joint pain, clicking joints, extreme fatigue, skin that bruises easily, as well as dizziness and increased heart rate upon standing (Fig. 12.1).

The stretchy tissue of hEDS increases the risk of pelvic organ prolapse incidence and decreases nonsurgical treatment success. Women who have POP surgery may experience a heightened risk of surgical failure, particularly with native tissue repair. Uterine prolapse incidence is estimated to occur in 40% of cases [7, 8]. Recurrent hernia is

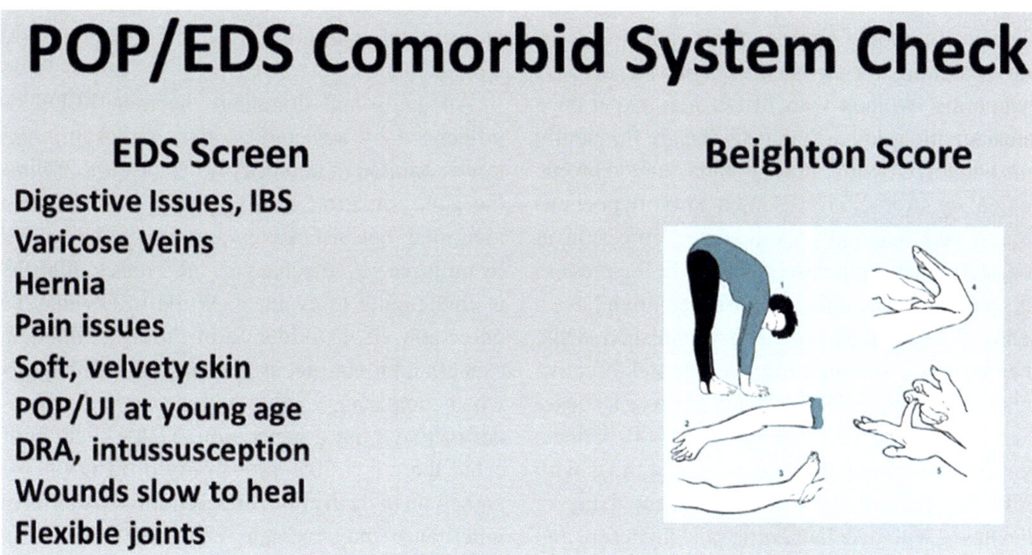

Fig. 12.1 POP/EDS comorbid system check. Courtesy of Association for Pelvic Organ Prolapse Support

an hEDS screening marker [7]. The rate of dyspareunia in EDS patients may be greater than in the general population, estimated to range between 30 and 61%, believed to be the impact of small tears in the vaginal wall and lack of appropriate vaginal secretions [5, 9–11]. Stress urinary incontinence was found in 40–70% of women with hEDS, including frequent occurrence early in life associated with bladder prolapse [8, 12]. Women with hEDS may experience painful intercourse [6]. Fecal incontinence is estimated to be 15% of hEDS patients, and rectal prolapse is more prevalent than in the general populace [8, 13]. Women with hEDS have a higher incidence of postpartum hemorrhage (19% versus 7%) and complicated perineal wounds (8% versus 0%) [8, 14]. Some of the surgical issues that may occur with POP treatment in the hEDS sector are higher rates of surgical failure in native tissue repair, mesh erosion, poor surgical wound healing, nerve entrapment, wound re-opening, greater risk of birth trauma, and extra stitches or use of steri-strip reinforcement, plus additional time needed to heal before stitch removal [7]. Substantial pain is a common occurrence with hEDS. Joint and long-term widespread pain (≥3 months) are specifically considered a part of the criteria for diagnosis of hEDS.

Indicators of hEDS occur in multiple body systems and equally confuse practitioner and patient. Women commonly go through an extensive journey searching for an accurate analysis of their symptoms. Women with hEDS may experience considerable delay in diagnosis and are frequently misdiagnosed with fibromyalgia and chronic fatigue syndrome, are assumed to be hypochondriacs, and frequently experience depression at long-term lack of precise analysis. In the process of seeing multiple clinicians, women often have a sense of being demeaned and diminished while they continue to search for answers and effective treatment. Inappropriate treatment can be a consequence. Two surveys involving 10,000 patients with 16 uncommon diseases indicated those with EDS experienced the most significant delay in diagnosis, with over half being misdiagnosed, and 70% receiving improper treatment as a result [11].

There is no precise treatment for hEDS; patients are typically advised to avoid specific activities completely, particularly those related to heavy lifting, hard foot strike, or aggressive contact athletic activities. Low-risk fitness activities such as swimming or speed-walking are recommended to reduce probability of POP occurrence.

EDS remains under-recognized and understudied. A considerable data gap exists regarding manifestation as well as recognition and understanding of comorbidity. With access to genetic testing and treatment, women with a predisposition to POP/EDS may be able to calculate increased risk [4]. We have not yet reached that platform in real-life application.

12.6 Genetics and Collagen

Genetic variants are implicated in prolapse; diminished vaginal wall resistance in each level may cause multiple organs to prolapse [12]. Collagen-associated disorders may arise from genetic defects, which can affect any spectrum of normal collagen production [15]. The most recognized inherited collagen-associated disorder is EDS [16]. While the various types of EDS have overlapping symptoms such as skin hyperextensibility, excessive bruising, and hypermobility, each type of EDS has unique characteristics that indicate the particular type of collagen most affected [7].

An autosomal dominant disorder, hEDS, is influenced by age and gender, with symptoms more common in females [6]. At the current time, the gene mutation causing hEDS has not been identified, but hEDS is understood to be caused by multiple genetic changes. Inheritance of hEDS is challenging to evaluate. While hEDS may be unrecognized in milder form during childhood, exacerbation can occur during early adult years when comparing to close relatives with the disorder or may miss a generation. Tinkle et al. indicated there is a 50% probability of hEDS being passed on to each child, but additional patterns of inheritance may indicate why hEDS occurs in particular families [6].

Collagen is a fibrous protein and is the primary element of connective tissue; it is considered one of the main determinants of biomechanical strength. Approximately 28 types of collagen have been found in the human body. Collagen produces tensile strength in skin, structural support tendons, and bone [6]. The first evidence of collagen molecules was recognized in 1930. Types I, III, and V are the primary components providing strength to soft tissue. Collagen type I is non-elastic, facilitating resistance to tensile influences. Collagen type III has an elastic quality, prevalent in more flexible tissues. Types I and III are noted in granulation tissue related to wound repair. Collagen type V is a discernible minor collagen, widely circulated in a variety of tissues [4]. An increase in collagen types III and V correlates with a decrease in mechanical strength of connective tissue due to decreased fiber size. It is generally accepted that a higher I to III ratio in tissues is indicative of greater strength, whereas a lower ratio may result in tissue laxity [7].

Numerous genetic mutations have been shown to correlate with increased prolapse predisposition. These mutations can result in disordered collagen permeation, which weakens fascial support within pelvic organ support structures [4]. Deviations in collagen metabolism may deplete fascial strength, critical support of pelvic viscera [17]. Cardinal ligament analysis indicates a 70–80% collagen composition [13]. Knuuti et al. indicated that women with joint hypermobility and recurrence of POP have significantly higher concentrations of type III collagen [17].

12.7 POP/EDS

The analysis of prolapse is multifactorial with many contributing mechanisms. Analysis predictions indicate POP will likely become more widespread and acknowledged associated with the aging population. New and refreshed evidence regarding the etiology of POP/EDS is pertinent and pivotal to women's wellness protocol and policy.

While each organ and organ system has a precise purpose, the function of the systems to address reproductive, urogenital, and defecatory function becomes less efficient when organs shift out of proper position within the pelvic cavity as POP progresses. The misalignment of organs, structural tissues, and nerves compound symptom gravity. Lack of structural tissue integrity can exacerbate symptoms, complicate care, and reduce potential for successful treatment if not recognized and analyzed appropriately before surgical treatment. Women with hEDS often experience pain more severely, both a marker prior to and concern post-surgery.

Women experiencing collagen-associated disorders such as hEDS have an increased probability of prolapse severity, more acute POP symptoms, and a predisposition to polypropylene mesh erosion. Women experiencing the POP/EDS connection have the greatest difficulty capturing surgical success of all the diverse issues women with POP navigate. They often experience a delay in diagnosis as POP progresses, are frequently misdiagnosed, and commonly receive improper treatment.

There remains a shortfall in POP/EDS exploration, with a lack of case reports and observational studies limiting insight. There is a substantial need to explore the current gap in treatment analysis and surgical complications. Identifying at-risk patients to provide improved care within the POP/EDS community is imperative. Greater understanding of POP/EDS within healthcare will provide earlier more efficient recognition of and evolution in treatment for women experiencing this life-altering combination of conditions.

12.8 QOL

Symptoms of POP/EDS can be vague or obvious, are often multi-systemic, and are equally perplexing to patient and healthcare provider. Women with hEDS typically experience a long-term diagnostic journey, visiting multiple types of clinicians in different fields of practice looking for answers to diverse symptoms. Prior to receiving a correct diagnosis of EDS, women may experience frustration, dismissal, and belittlement and are often advised to seek psychiatric counseling for physical symptoms that are very real. The chase for EDS diagnosis may go on for years before the POP/EDS connection is recognized. Frequently EDS remains undiagnosed until surgical failure occurs multiple times.

Lifestyle and behavioral activities can compound the probability or degree of POP severity. What is rarely recognized is the additional potential to impact post-surgical healing in the POP/EDS patient. Women are typically advised to return to normal activities 6 weeks post-surgery, after they have been cleared by examination. Women frequently do not feel healed at the 6-week point post-POP surgery; at 8 weeks healing is further optimized. With complex or advanced POP surgeries, 12 weeks of healing may be necessary before returning to normal activities. The POP/EDS patient requires additional time to assure weak tissue has suitably healed before resuming normal activities.

Comorbid conditions complicate care, whether or not mesh is utilized for surgical POP repair. Coexisting conditions that POP may cause or complicate such as overactive bladder, underactive bladder, dyspareunia, stress urinary incontinence, urge urinary incontinence, coital incontinence, or urinary tract infections do not always magically vanish post-POP surgery in the POP/EDS patient. Conditions that may cause or exacerbate POP such as EDS could benefit from deeper analysis.

Patient voice nearly always clarifies health and healthcare treatment reality. The following are the voices of women who have experienced POP/EDS navigation (Fig. 12.2).

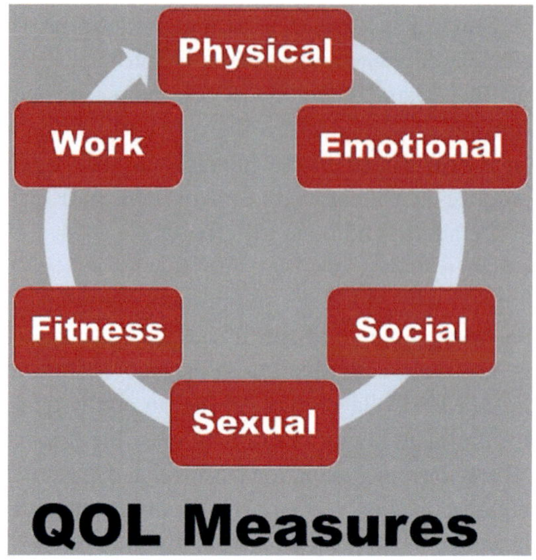

Fig. 12.2 POP/EDS quality of life measures. Courtesy of Association for Pelvic Organ Prolapse Support

> I was diagnosed EDS because of chronic pelvic pain. They discovered I had stretch marks, keloids, paper-thin scars related to EDS. The urethral prolapse and patulous urinary meatus were probably related but my doctor was unsure. It impacts my ability to sit longer than a minute, do any sort of exercise as my SI joints are constantly inflamed. I'm still very toned, just quite weak in my lower half of the body. Employment was extremely difficult related to fatigue. Also standing for hours on end nursing caused a nasty flare in vaginismus and pelvic floor pain. I can do fitness programs as long as there isn't too much stretching or working up a sweat. The 'worst' for me is honestly the pain.
> *Age 43*

> "It isn't just ONE QOL impact that is 'the worst.'" The key is for doctors to really understand how devastating this is because it severely affects *all* areas of our lives. I had light stress urine leakage my whole life and could never wear tampons, and my periods were agonizingly painful. I noticed the actual organs falling down was when I was 34 or 35. Full on rapid prolapse at 35. The unrelenting pain which impacts emotional wellbeing, sexual interactions, the inability to maintain physical fitness, also made it impossible for me to continue working. Having a BM is now a constant source of distress…painful, embarrassing, constantly worrying about fecal incontinence so I basically stay home all the time and of course worrying about leaking stool during sex is a total intimacy destroyer. The depression over the loss of myself, over the frequent doctor appointments and failed surgeries, the anger at my spouse for not making any effort to understand…all destroyed my life and my husband of 23 years left me. Can't say I blame him…I'd leave myself behind too if I could. I could write an entire chapter on how POP literally invaded every single aspect of my life. EDS was diagnosed based on the failures of my POP repairs, some minor issues I had throughput childhood, and my family history. It never caused me serious issues until the POP. And none of that was the worst…the worst is NOW at 47…dealing with horrific problems for over 10 years now with absolutely no hope for improvement in sight and I have had severe emotional and physical trauma from my experiences with the medical "professionals" that have messed many things up. The 'trigger stack-

ing' with POP/EDS is enormous, the cumulative effect of how it impacts every aspect of our lives is overwhelming.
Age 47
I have struggled with the effects of EDS all my life but did not know that the early joint problems, incredible limberness, early stretch marks meant something specific. Looking back, I suspect that POP changes started years ago but ObGyns didn't notice or didn't see the changes as harbingers of what was to come so they didn't say anything. It is hard to say what has been worse for me in terms of POP. The rectocele worsening very rapidly was frightening and the impact on daily life from the sensation of it protruding and the dragging feeling was hard to deal with. Going through the surgery (Dec 2018) with the knowledge that it will likely fail pretty quickly was hard. The prolapse has already returned to a small degree. It's psychologically challenging to live with the anticipation that whatever discomforts I have today will most likely be worse in the future. On the bright side, even at almost 65, sex remains very good. My husband and I have found ways to accommodate changes and continue to enjoy sex.
Age 64

12.9 Screening Shortfall

While the physical struggles of women navigating POP/EDS are considerable, the frustrations they experience related to clinician dismissal are often more pronounced and are usually intensified by experiencing it repetitively as they move from physician to physician. The following are the voices of women experiencing EDS within a global online FB-based POP support forum.

I've had eight POP-related surgeries since I gave birth to my daughter thirty years ago, but no one ever mentioned EDS to me.
Age 56
There was no doubt to me that I had the hypermobile type EDS (I also have the velvet skin and other characteristics), and I asked my doctor to get a referral to the proper specialists. He laughed at me.
Age 45
Could I have EDS? If yes, further surgery might be in vain. In fact, it might worsen things. Those were my thoughts based on the information from the internet. 'I guess you could have EDS,' my urogyn advised, 'but what do you want the diagnosis for? It doesn't make any difference.'
Age 34
Didn't get diagnosed with EDS until I was 38 years old. So much misinformation.
Age 44
10 years ago, at 35 I had my first symptoms, and my doctor knew I have hEDS, and brushed me off each time I mentioned my prolapse concerns and rectocele. She didn't offer any help or refer me to a urogynecologist until my uterus became a stage 3.
Age 45
I was told I couldn't have POP before they even looked because I don't have kids. Then told I should just have kids because EDS will make my prolapse severe no matter what I do.
Age 27
Diagnosed with EDS at 41 when I developed bladder, rectal, and uterine prolapse without ever having been pregnant. Went to "the best of the best" cash pay surgeons because I was desperate for a good outcome. All of them said they had operated on many EDS patients. When I asked if they did anything differently during surgery because of EDS, like suture a distinct way, they said no and acted like I was stupid for worrying. Well, I've had ruptured internal sutures twice. After one of my operations, I told every doctor I saw for a year that all the symptoms I was dealing with came on in one day, exactly two months after said surgery. I expressed concern about my history with ruptured sutures. Every single time I was dismissed until I could actually see something protruding from my vagina again. Had another operation and low and behold, the sutures from my previous surgery had ruptured. In two words I would describe my last 3 years (4 operations) for prolapse as humiliation and dismissal!!
Age 44
Check patients for possible EDS through simple clinical questions prior to operating. I was told that it is not possible to know you have a connective tissue disorder unless prolapse repairs fail. Mine failed 6 months after. Took me a year to recover from the operation. Took 6 months to recover from the second. Asking about autoimmune issues and the Brighton Scale should give the surgeon a VERY good idea of what he/she is dealing with! I was 43 at the time of surgery.
Age 50
I've had rectal prolapse since I was 19 or 20 and have never had kids. My first POP surgery was unsuccessful, and I had to have a second one a year ago with mesh (I am 26 now). So far it has been successful. No one mentioned EDS to me, my first surgeon said during surgery my collagen appeared 'stretchy.' I have some symptoms of connective tissue disorder but have never been diagnosed. Other than connective tissue and constipation/disordered eating, I have no other explanation for the prolapse issues I will be struggling with for the rest of my life.
Age 26

12.10 Conclusion

POP is a compelling and quickly evolving area of women's health in need of research expansion to address unmet needs. EDS is a significant group of tissue integrity conditions that may reduce the effectiveness of nonsurgical treatments and increase the risk of surgical complications in women experiencing POP. The diverse nature of the POP/EDS intersect often results in medical personnel failing to recognize the issues, resulting in patients experiencing surgical treatment complications, negatively impacting clinician/patient relationships, and generating resentment and distrust in healthcare.

While studies express concerns regarding the anticipated significant growth pattern of POP in the aging population, there currently exists a tsunami of young women experiencing health consequences with inadequate screening for POP due to less than adequate curriculum provided to diagnostic clinicians. The same lack of curriculum related to EDS at the subspecialist level creates a similar practice gap of the POP/EDS comorbidity. This shortfall of awareness and conception of the POP/EDS model impedes treatment in women with these overlapping conditions.

It is imperative EDS screening become consistent in patients who indicate atypical system, lifestyle, or behavioral abnormalities, to reduce surgical complication risk. Clinicians unfamiliar with EDS may assume pain is imagined when in fact hEDS can cause significant pain. The invalidation of patient pain may have a deeply negative impact on the relationship between clinician and patient as well as the quality of life of the patient.

Every woman's individual POP/EDS experience is unique and may not necessarily mirror another woman's experience given the zebra-like nature of EDS. Developing and optimizing care strategies must be based on individual needs. As awareness and de-stigmatization of POP increases in the coming decade, a wealth of vision will usher in fresh treatment protocol and evolved surgical procedures. Ideally POP/EDS protocol will advance as well.

It takes a specializing surgeon to repair POP within the complex female pelvic cavity, a diverse mass of multiple organ systems, soft tissue, muscle, tendons, ligaments, boney structures, and nerves interwoven tightly within a very compact compartment. To complicate the complexity of prolapse surgery, women with POP typically have more than one type of POP in need of simultaneous repair, and women with EDS often lack the tissue integrity to assure repair will have long-term efficacy. POP procedures truly should be left to the experts, even more so POP/EDS.

Patients and their families indicate that when surgeries go wrong, they are routinely met with a wall of silence, hostility, or denial. Under these circumstances, patients will quickly lose confidence and trust in their surgeons. In addition to physical impact, patients suffer emotionally knowing that they have been harmed.

Every surgical procedure comes with risk, thus the significance of appropriate surgical training, selective patient screening, and evaluation of the most suitable treatment to optimize patient satisfaction and results. Surgical complications are far from patients' thoughts when they consult with physicians. Patients hope and expect their clinicians to provide safe and appropriate care. Increased awareness is crucial within both patient and practitioner sectors to enable evolution of POP/EDS screening and best practice. Women with POP/EDS simply want their clinicians to listen to them, to believe them, and to treat them with the same respect given to healthcare providers—even if what is they are sharing flies in the face of what their medical education has taught them.

Acknowledgment This research has no financial disclosures or conflicts of interest.

References

1. Barber MD, Maher C. Epidemiology and outcome assessment of pelvic organ prolapse. Int Urogynecol J. 2013;24(11):1783–90.
2. Demmler JC, Atkinson MD, Reinhold EJ, Choy E, Lyons RA, Brophy ST. Diagnosed prevalence of Ehlers-Danlos syndrome and hypermobility spectrum disorder in Wales, UK: a national electronic cohort

study and case–control comparison. BMJ Open. 2019;9(11):e031365.
3. Lim VF, Khoo JK, Wong V, Moore KH. Recent studies of genetic dysfunction in pelvic organ prolapse: the role of collagen defects. Aust N Z J Obstet Gynaecol. 2014;54(3):198–205.
4. Segev Y, Auslender R, Feiner B, Lissak A, Lavie O, Abramov Y. Are women with pelvic organ prolapse at a higher risk of developing hernias? Int Urogynecol J Pelvic Floor Dysfunct. 2009;20(12):1451–3.
5. Pezaro DS, Pearce DG, Reinhold DE. Understanding hypermobile Ehlers-Danlos syndrome and Hypermobility Spectrum Disorders in the context of childbearing: an international qualitative study. Midwifery. 2020;88:102749.
6. Hein LC, DeGregory CB, Umari F. Ehlers-danlos syndrome: it's not your normal hoofbeats. J Nurse Pract. 2019;15(4):277–81.
7. Kökçü A, Yanik F, Cetinkaya M, Alper T, Kandemir B, Malatyalioglu E. Histopathological evaluation of the connective tissue of the vaginal fascia and the uterine ligaments in women with and without pelvic relaxation. Arch Gynecol Obstet. 2002;266(2):75–8.
8. Castori M, Camerota F, Celletti C, Grammatico P, Padua L. Quality of life in the classic and hypermobility types of Ehlers-Danlos syndrome [corrected]. Ann Neurol. 2010;67(1):145–6; author reply 146–7.
9. Kerkhof MH, Hendriks L, Brölmann HAM. Changes in connective tissue in patients with pelvic organ prolapse—a review of the current literature. Int Urogynecol J Pelvic Floor Dysfunct. 2009;20(4):461–74.
10. Gilliam E, Hoffman JD, Yeh G. Urogenital and pelvic complications in the Ehlers-Danlos syndromes and associated hypermobility spectrum disorders: a scoping review. Clin Genet. 2020;97(1):168–78.
11. Castori M, Morlino S, Dordoni C, Celletti C, Camerota F, Ritelli M, et al. Gynecologic and obstetric implications of the joint hypermobility syndrome (a.k.a. Ehlers-Danlos syndrome hypermobility type) in 82 Italian patients. Am J Med Genet A. 2012;158A(9):2176–82.
12. Tinkle BT. A guide for the issues & management of Ehlers-Danlos syndrome hypermobility type and the hypermobility syndrome. Niles: Left Paw Press, LLC; 2010. Joint Hypermobility Handbook.
13. Arunkalaivanan AS, Morrison A, Jha S, Blann A. Prevalence of urinary and faecal incontinence among female members of the Hypermobility Syndrome Association (HMSA). J Obstet Gynaecol. 2009;29(2):126–8.
14. Lind J, Wallenburg HCS. Pregnancy and the Ehlers-Danlos syndrome: a retrospective study in a Dutch population: Ehlers-Danlos syndrome and pregnancy. Acta Obstet Gynecol Scand. 2002;81(4):293–300.
15. Lammers K, Lince SL, Spath MA, Kempen LC, Hendriks JC, et al. Pelvic organ prolapse and collagen-associated disorders. Int Urogynecol J. 2012;23(3):313–9. https://doi.org/10.1007/s00192-011-1532-y.
16. Knuuti E, Kauppila S, Kotila V, Risteli J, Nissi R. Genitourinary prolapse and joint hypermobility are associated with altered type I and III collagen metabolism. Arch Gynecol Obstet. 2011;283(5):1081–5.
17. Wu M-P. Regulation of extracellular matrix remodeling associated with pelvic organ prolapse. J Exp Clin Med. 2010;2(1):11–6.

13 Obstructive Defecatory Symptoms with Pelvic Organ Prolapse

Şerife Esra Çetinkaya, Mehmet Murat Seval, Elif Nazlı Çetindağ, and Fulya Dökmeci

13.1 Introduction

Pelvic organ prolapse is a well-known condition defined as "the descent of one or more of the anterior vaginal wall, posterior vaginal wall, the uterus (cervix), or the apex of the vagina (vaginal vault or cuff scar after hysterectomy)" [1]. Pelvic organ prolapse may lead to a variety of clinical presentations, such as protrusion, bulge, lower urinary tract symptoms, sexual symptoms, and defecatory symptoms according to its severity [2]. Nearly every urogynecology society recommends the POPQ system as the only validated method for the objective assessment of prolapse in all three (anterior, apical, and posterior) compartments of the vagina [3, 4]. Nevertheless, prolapse has been considered symptomatic when the leading edge is beyond the hymen, with increased urinary tract, sexual, defecatory, and prolapse symptoms [5, 6].

Ş. E. Çetinkaya · F. Dökmeci
Department of Obstetrics and Gynecology, Ankara University School of Medicine, Ankara, Turkey

M. M. Seval (✉)
Department of Obstetrics and Gynecology, Ankara University School of Medicine, Cebeci Hospital, Ankara, Turkey
e-mail: seval@ankara.edu.tr

E. N. Çetindağ
Department of Obstetrics and Gynecology, Lösante Children's and Adult Hospital, Ankara, Turkey

Defecatory dysfunction is a heterogeneous condition that includes any difficulty with defecation and constitutes one of the two main components of anorectal dysfunction, together with anal incontinence [7]. Obstructed defecation is a subtype of defecatory dysfunction presenting with symptoms of straining to defecate, feeling of incomplete bowel evacuation, splinting, and manual evacuation/digitation. Obstructed defecation can be caused by anatomical defects such as rectal or pelvic organ support defects, or functional conditions such as defecatory dyssynergia. Posterior compartment prolapse and perineal descent are the leading pelvic organ support defects in women presenting with obstructive defecatory symptoms.

The terminology and classification of female anorectal dysfunction symptoms were updated in the 2017 joint report of the International Urogynecological Association (IUGA)/International Continence Society (ICS). In this report, defecatory and post-defecatory symptoms were classified with the inclusion of the new symptoms of splinting, digitation, and sensation of blockage, in addition to straining to defecate, feeling incomplete bowel evacuation, and constipation. Moreover, the definition of constipation was updated and classified as slow transit and obstructive defecation [8]. As constipation is a commonly used definition for women with obstructive defecatory symptoms by both patients and healthcare providers, it is noteworthy to

F. Dökmeci, D. E. E. Rizk (eds.), *Insights Into Incontinence and the Pelvic Floor*,
https://doi.org/10.1007/978-3-030-94174-1_13

emphasize that it should be questioned in detail whether constipation would be due to infrequent bowel motions and delays in transit of bowel contents to reach the rectum or difficulty in evacuation.

Population-based studies reported that the prevalence of constipation varies from 2 to 27% due to different diagnostic criteria of the defecatory dysfunctions considered in different studies [9]. However, obstructive defecatory symptoms can be more common in women with pelvic organ prolapse.

The prevalence of pelvic organ prolapse (for any compartment) was reported to be 41.1% for women with a uterus and 38% for hysterectomized women in a large-scale cross-sectional analysis in the Women's Health Initiative Hormone Replacement Therapy Clinical Trial. The prevalence of posterior compartment prolapse was also reported to be approximately 18% of all women included in this study with approximately one in five participants having prolapse at ≥2 sites [10]. It was demonstrated that 73% of women had complaints of at least one obstructive defecatory symptom of any degree of bother and 36% with at least one bothersome defecatory symptom (responding moderately or quite a bit) in a nationwide longitudinal cohort study with women undergoing pelvic organ prolapse surgery. More than 50% of these women had reported splinting, straining, or incomplete evacuation prior to prolapse surgery in this study (53%, 52%, and 59%, respectively) [11].

13.2 Literature Review

There are many studies investigating the relationship between posterior vaginal compartment prolapse and obstructive defecatory symptoms in the literature. However, almost all of these studies have presented conflicting findings regarding this relationship, probably due to differences in patient populations, various assessment methods of pelvic organ prolapse, and the use of different standardized symptom scales.

In a very recent longitudinal cohort study examining the pre- and postoperative defecatory symptoms in 3515 women undergoing pelvic organ prolapse surgery, it has been demonstrated that posterior prolapse is a contributing factor for obstructed defecation in women. They also found a linear correlation between obstructive symptoms such as splinting, straining, and incomplete evacuation with increasing stages of posterior vaginal wall prolapse, from Stage 0 to Stage 2. However, there was an inconsistency between the obstructive symptoms and posterior prolapse in women with advanced stages (Stages 3–4). Nevertheless, an improvement in obstructive symptoms has also been observed after posterior vaginal wall prolapse surgery [11].

In another study, 265 women were divided according to the presence of posterior vaginal wall prolapse using POPQ stages (POPQ Stage ≥2 vs. <2). Although posterior vaginal prolapse was found to be significantly related to age, body mass index, number of pregnancies, and number of births, no clear association was demonstrated between posterior prolapse and defecatory dysfunction [12].

Saks et al. performed a cross-sectional study to determine whether the presence of obstructive defecatory symptoms is associated with the site and severity of pelvic organ prolapse in 260 women with grade ≥2 prolapse according to the Baden-Walker halfway system. They concluded that obstructive bowel symptoms were significantly associated with posterior vaginal prolapse, without any association with the severity [13]. Digesu et al. assessed the relationship of vaginal prolapse severity to symptoms and quality of life in a prospective observational study including 355 women and found a strong relationship between posterior prolapse and bowel symptoms [14].

Erekson et al. conducted a cross-sectional study to estimate the association between posterior vaginal prolapse and obstructive bowel symptoms, such as splinting, straining, or incomplete bowel emptying, in 721 women. Although the authors found no association between posterior vaginal prolapse and bothersome straining or incomplete evacuation, they were only able to demonstrate an association with Stage II or greater posterior vaginal prolapse and bothersome symptoms of splinting alone [15]. In another study including 237 women with symptomatic pelvic organ prolapse, symptoms of incomplete evacuation and digital manipulation of the Pelvic Floor Distress Inventory-20 (PFDI-20) (items 8 and 4, respectively) were found to be weakly correlated with advanced posterior vaginal wall prolapse [16].

Collins et al. evaluated defecatory symptoms similarly using items 4 (splinting) and 8 (incomplete evacuation) of the PFDI-20, specifically with pb and Bp POP-Q points in a database including 1663 women. A significant relationship was found only with the Bp point measurement [17]. Neto et al. evaluated only constipation as the obstructive defecatory symptom, using the Cleveland Clinic Constipation Score (CCCS) with POPQ measurement points of Bp, Pb, and Gh in 613 women with pelvic floor disorders. They accepted constipation as positive in women with a score ≥7 and found no association between constipation and the presence of posterior prolapse and GH measurement. However, they found a positive correlation with constipation and the POPQ measurement of Pb [18].

Understanding the relationship between prolapse and pelvic floor symptoms is crucial in the management of patients, as reviewed in the literature above. Somehow, there appears to be a relationship between obstructive defecatory symptoms and posterior vaginal support in women. Herein, a study will be presented investigating both the comparison and the correlation of obstructed defecation (splinting, straining, and incomplete evacuation) with the presence and staging of posterior vaginal prolapse.

13.3 Case Study: The Relation of Posterior Vaginal POP-Q Points with Obstructive Defecatory Dysfunction Symptoms

(a) **Aim and Scope**

In this study, the impact of posterior vaginal prolapse on obstructed defecation was examined in women with pelvic floor disorders.

(b) **Study Design and Material Methods**

The data of women presenting with pelvic floor disorders (n = 363) was reviewed. As prolapse is clinically more symptomatic when the leading edge approaches the hymen [19], patients were grouped using Bp point of Pelvic Organ Prolapse Quantification (POPQ) system (Group 1, Bp above −1 cm, n = 117; Group 2, Bp below −1 cm, n = 246). Obstructive defecatory symptoms, including splinting, straining, and the sensation of incomplete evacuation, were assessed using answers to subgroups of the Pelvic Floor Distress Inventory-20 (PFDI-20). Patients who splint or manually assist in the evacuation of stool from the rectum were identified with question number 4 of the PFDI-20, which is "Do you ever have to push on the vagina or around the rectum to have or complete a bowel movement?" The intensive need to strain was assessed with question number 7 of the PFDI-20, which is "Do you feel you need to strain too hard to have a bowel movement?" The sensation of incomplete evacuation was identified with question number 8 of the PFDI-20, which is "Do you feel you have not completely emptied your bowels at the end of a bowel movement?" A comparison was made according to the presence of posterior vaginal wall prolapse, with respect to the clinical characteristics and the aforementioned items of PFDI-20 evaluating obstructed defecation. Additionally, each point in the posterior vaginal wall according to the POPQ system (points Ap, Bp, D, and perineal body (pb)) was also assessed for correlation with obstructive defecatory symptoms, using these items in all women.

(c) **Results of the Study**

Of the 363 women with pelvic floor disorders, the Bp point was below −1 cm in 246 women (67.7%, stage ≥2 posterior vaginal wall prolapse) and above −1 cm in 117 women (32.3%, stage <2 posterior vaginal wall prolapse). As shown in Table 13.1, the women with stage ≥2 posterior prolapse had a significantly higher body mass index (p = 0.011). No significant differences were

Table 13.1 Baseline characteristics, presence of obstructive defecatory dysfunction symptoms, and scores for related questions of the PFDI-20

	Posterior POP-Q Bp above −1 cm (stage < 2) *n* = 117	Posterior POP-Q Bp below −1 cm (stage ≥ 2) *n* = 246	*P*
Baseline characteristics			
Age (years), mean ± SD	56 ± 12	54 ± 12	0.282
Post-menopausal status, *n* (%)	84 (71)	152 (61)	0.061
Parity, mean ± SD	2.8 ± 1.7	3.1 ± 1.8	0.092
Body-mass index (kg/m^2), mean ± SD	28 ± 5	30 ± 6	**0.011**[a]
Tobacco use	17 (14)	33 (13)	0.773
Comorbidities			
Diabetes, *n* (%)	23 (19)	63 (25)	0.212
Hypertension, *n* (%)	54 (46)	107 (43)	0.633
Coronary artery disease, *n* (%)	17 (14)	43 (17)	0.479
Obstructive airway disease, *n* (%)	19 (16)	36 (14)	0.690
Vaginal delivery, *n* (%)	110 (94)	236 (95)	0.418
Vaginal delivery of macrosomic baby, *n* (%)	29 (88)	53 (21)	0.490
Pelvic surgery, *n* (%)	9 (7)	23 (9)	0.602
Symptoms			
Women with at least one obstructed defecatory symptom, *n* (%)	91 (77)	196 (79)	0.678
PFDI-20 Q4, median (IQR)	0 (0–2)	1 (0–3)	**0.001**[b]
PFDI-20 Q7, median (IQR)	1 (0–2)	2 (0–3)	**0.012**[b]
PFDI-20 Q8, median (IQR)	1 (0–2)	1 (0–3)	0.451

Student-t test, Mann-Whitney U test, and Chi-square tests were used as appropriate. *P* values <0.05 were considered significant

[a] Student-t test

[b] Mann-Whitney U test. PFDI-20 Q4: "Do you ever have to push on the vagina or around the rectum to have or complete a bowel movement?"; PFDI-20 Q7: "Do you feel you need to strain too hard to have a bowel movement?"; PFDI-20 Q8: "Do you feel you have not completely emptied your bowels at the end of a bowel movement?"

observed between the groups regarding age, parity, comorbidities, number of vaginal deliveries, vaginal deliveries of macrosomic babies, or histories of pelvic surgery. Straining and splinting were more common in women with stage ≥2 posterior prolapse. Table 13.2 shows the correlation of symptom bother with prolapse severity. There was a significant but weak correlation between splinting and points Ap and Bp (rho 0.186 and 0.189, respectively, $p < 0.001$). Straining was weakly correlated with Pb measurement and Bp point (rho 0.133 and 0.103, respectively, $p < 0.011$). Incomplete bowel evacuation was not correlated with any of the posterior vaginal POPQ points, and point D was not correlated with any of the obstructive defecatory symptoms.

In this case study, straining and splinting were found to be more common in women with posterior prolapse than women without posterior prolapse, and a statistically significant but weak correlation was found between posterior vaginal descent and these obstructive defecatory symptoms. More specifically, both straining and splinting increased with the descent of the Bp point. In addition, splinting was also correlated with the Ap point, and Pb measurement was correlated only with straining. However, the "feeling of incomplete bowel evacuation" did not demonstrate any correlation with any of the pos-

Table 13.2 Correlation of posterior wall POP-Q points with items of the PFDI-20

Scores		Ap	pb	Bp	D
Splinting PFDI-20 Q4	rho	0.186**	−0.004	0.189**	0.019
	p	< 0.001	0.933	< 0.001	0.723
Straining PFDI-20 Q7	rho	0.064	0.133*	0.104*	0.074
	p	0.223	0.011	0.049	0.158
Incomplete PFDI-20 Q8	rho	0.012	0.050	0.009	−0.049
	p	0.827	0.346	0.861	0.348

PFDI-20: Pelvic Floor Distress Inventory-20. Spearman's correlation analyses were used to evaluate the correlation. * *P* values <0.05 were considered significant, ** *P* values <0.001 were considered highly significant
PFDI-20 Q4: "Do you ever have to push on the vagina or around the rectum to have or complete a bowel movement?"; PFDI-20 Q7: "Do you feel you need to strain too hard to have a bowel movement?"; PFDI-20 Q8: "Do you feel you have not completely emptied your bowels at the end of a bowel movement?"

terior POPQ measurements, and point D showed no association with any of the obstructive defecatory symptoms.

13.4 Discussion

As stated previously, the discrepancies in the methodology of the studies examining the association of posterior vaginal prolapse with obstructed defecation performed so far lead to heterogeneous and conflicting results in the literature. In the present case study, all three questions regarding obstructed defecation of the PFDI-20 (items 4, 7, and 8) have been evaluated with all posterior vaginal wall POPQ points. The most consistent finding in the literature together with this case study is the association of point Bp with splinting. Similarly, straining seems to be associated with the Pb measurement. Thus, restoration of a rectocele and perineal body may improve symptoms in patients with symptoms of splinting and straining, as shown in the study of Karjalainen, P.K. et al. On the other hand, to the best of our knowledge, obstructed defecation and points Ap and D have not been evaluated before, and in this study, they seem to have no relationship [11]. The feeling of incomplete bowel emptying also seems to be associated with posterior prolapse in the literature. However, this could not be demonstrated in this study.

The routinely used assessment methods of the posterior vaginal wall, such as the POPQ Bp point and Pb measurement, may be insufficient to demonstrate the anatomical defect. Moreover, this insufficiency might probably be one of the reasons for the discrepancies and weak correlations. Thus, the evaluation of the posterior wall support using imaging methods, such as ultrasound or magnetic resonance imaging, and functional examinations, might provide a promising holistic approach for the comprehension of anorectal dysfunction.

13.5 Conclusion

Although it is well accepted that anatomical problems, such as posterior vaginal wall prolapse, lead to obstructed defecation, the probable underlying functional causes in women are still poorly understood. The impact of contributing factors such as aging, hormonal status, and vaginal delivery on anatomical defects and dysfunctional problems add to the complexity of the relationship between defecatory and post-defecatory symptoms with posterior prolapse. In this context, future studies are needed.

References

1. Haylen BT, de Ridder D, Freeman RM, Swift SE, Berghmans B, Lee J, et al. An International Urogynecological Association (IUGA)/International Continence Society (ICS) joint report on the terminology for female pelvic floor dysfunction. Int Urogynecol J. 2010;21(1):5–26.
2. Grimes CL, Lukacz ES. Posterior vaginal compartment prolapse and defecatory dysfunction: are they related? Int Urogynecol J. 2012;23(5):537–51.
3. Practice Bulletin No. 176: pelvic organ prolapse. Obstet Gynecol. 2017;129(4):e56–72.
4. Pham T, Burgart A, Kenton K, Mueller ER, Brubaker L. Current use of pelvic organ prolapse quantification by AUGS and ICS members. Female Pelvic Med Reconstr Surg. 2011;17(2):67–9.
5. Swift SE, Tate SB, Nicholas J. Correlation of symptoms with degree of pelvic organ support in a general population of women: what is pelvic organ prolapse? Am J Obstet Gynecol. 2003;189(2):372–7.
6. Gutman RE, Ford DE, Quiroz LH, Shippey SH, Handa VL. Is there a pelvic organ prolapse threshold that predicts pelvic floor symptoms? Am J Obstet Gynecol. 2008;199(6):683.e1–7.
7. Brown H, Grimes C. Current trends in management of defecatory dysfunction, posterior compartment prolapse, and fecal incontinence. Curr Obstet Gynecol Rep. 2016;5(2):165–71.
8. Sultan AH, Monga A, Lee J, Emmanuel A, Norton C, Santoro G, et al. An International Urogynecological Association (IUGA)/International Continence Society (ICS) joint report on the terminology for female anorectal dysfunction. Int Urogynecol J. 2017;28(1):5–31.
9. American College of Gastroenterology Chronic Constipation Task Force. An evidence-based approach to the management of chronic constipation in North America. Am J Gastroenterol. 2005;100:S1–4.
10. Hendrix SL, Clark A, Nygaard I, Aragaki A, Barnabei V, McTiernan A. Pelvic organ prolapse in the women's health initiative: gravity and gravidity. Am J Obstet Gynecol. 2002;186(6):1160–6.
11. Karjalainen PK, Mattsson NK, Nieminen K, Tolppanen A-M, Jalkanen JT. The relationship of defecation symptoms and posterior vaginal wall prolapse in women undergoing pelvic organ prolapse surgery. Am J Obstet Gynecol. 2019;221(5):480.e1–480.e10.
12. Augusto KL, Bezerra LRPS, Murad-Regadas SM, Neto JAV, Vasconcelos CTM, Karbage SAL, et al. Defecatory dysfunction and fecal incontinence in women with or without posterior vaginal wall prolapse as measured by pelvic organ prolapse quantification (POP-Q). Eur J Obstet Gynecol Reprod Biol. 2017;214:50–5.
13. Saks EK, Harvie HS, Asfaw TS, Arya LA. Clinical significance of obstructive defecatory symptoms in women with pelvic organ prolapse. Int J Gynecol Obstet. 2010;111(3):237–40.
14. Digesu GA, Chaliha C, Salvatore S, Hutchings A, Khullar V. The relationship of vaginal prolapse severity to symptoms and quality of life. BJOG. 2005;112(7):971–6.
15. Erekson EA, Kassis NC, Washington BB, Myers DL. The association between stage II or greater posterior prolapse and bothersome obstructive bowel symptoms. Female Pelvic Med Reconstr Surg. 2010;16(1):59–64.
16. Ellerkmann RM, Cundiff GW, Melick CF, Nihira MA, Leffler K, Bent AE. Correlation of symptoms with location and severity of pelvic organ prolapse. Am J Obstet Gynecol. 2001;185(6):1332–8.
17. Collins SA, O'Sullivan DM, Lasala CA. Correlation of POP-Q posterior compartment measures with defecatory dysfunction. Int Urogynecol J. 2012;23(6):743–7.
18. Neto JAV, Vasconcelos CTM, Regadas SMM, Bezerra LRPS, Lustosa KA, Karbage SAL. Clinical impact of bowel symptoms in women with pelvic floor disorders. Int Urogynecol J. 2017;28(9):1415–20.
19. Kahn MA, Breitkopf CR, Valley MT, Woodman PJ, O'Boyle AL, Bland DI, et al. Pelvic Organ Support Study (POSST) and bowel symptoms: straining at stool is associated with perineal and anterior vaginal descent in a general gynecologic population. Am J Obstet Gynecol. 2005;192(5):1516–22.

Surgical Treatment of Posterior Compartment Defects

14

Traian Enache, Andreea Enache, Marcel Moisa, and Mihai Ionica

Transvaginal meshes have been in use for the last 20 years, so during this period of time all techniques evolved and changed. Like any other new method, many adjustments have been needed, and yet almost nothing is final. In the first years, the surgeons tried to find the most suitable way to insert meshes, and also that time we had a great number of complications [1]. A few practitioners and companies persisted in vaginal mesh surgery in spite of FDA warning and legal and media risks. Correcting the errors of the past and since 2011, we have a substantial number of publications that have begun to demonstrate scientifically the efficacy and low morbidity of these techniques [2, 3]. There are also prospective and retrospective studies with significant follow-up that confirm the good results of transvaginal meshes [4, 5].

In surgical cure of posterior compartment defects, one of the major steps is apical repair [6]. There are many techniques that restore the apical suspension, but there is no consensus on the most efficient one. We are proposing a new approach using a small patch of polypropylene mesh.

Based on the analysis of the posterior transvaginal mesh, which offers a good support has more complications and has a quite bad reputation, we tried to develop a much safer way to insert the mesh. We found that the part of the mesh located caudally from the plane of levator ani muscles is functionally inert, its presence at the level of ischioanal fossa being only the consequence of the insertion technique. Also, most associated complications are due to the mesh passage through the anatomical space mentioned above. Thus, we propose a new technique through which only the fragment of mesh between the two sacrospinous anchors is kept and the distal fragments of the mesh are abandoned. In addition, a polypropylene "patch" is inserted at the level of the transverse vaginal incision and the two sacrospinous wires are passing through the lateral sides of it [7].

This polypropylene "patch" is made intraoperatively from a larger piece of mesh. Most often it has a rectangular shape with dimensions of 4 × 2 cm. Depending on the particularities of each case, its shape may undergo minor changes.

In cases of vaginal vault prolapse, we left some extensions in the cranial parts, bilateral, where we anchored the sacrospinous wires to compensate for the lack of substance due to the absence of the cervix. In patients who also associated rectocele and where it required its cure with posterior "bridge," we created a lower triangular or semicircular extension with a maximum size of 1.5 cm from the lower edge of the "patch" (Fig. 14.1). Physiologically, the uterosacral ligaments provide the posterior vector compo-

T. Enache (✉) · A. Enache · M. Moisa
Clinical Hospital of Obstetrics and Gynecology "Prof. Dr. Panait Sarbu", Bucharest, Romania

M. Ionica
Clinical Emergency Hospital "Floreasca", Bucharest, Romania

F. Dökmeci, D. E. E. Rizk (eds.), *Insights Into Incontinence and the Pelvic Floor*, https://doi.org/10.1007/978-3-030-94174-1_14

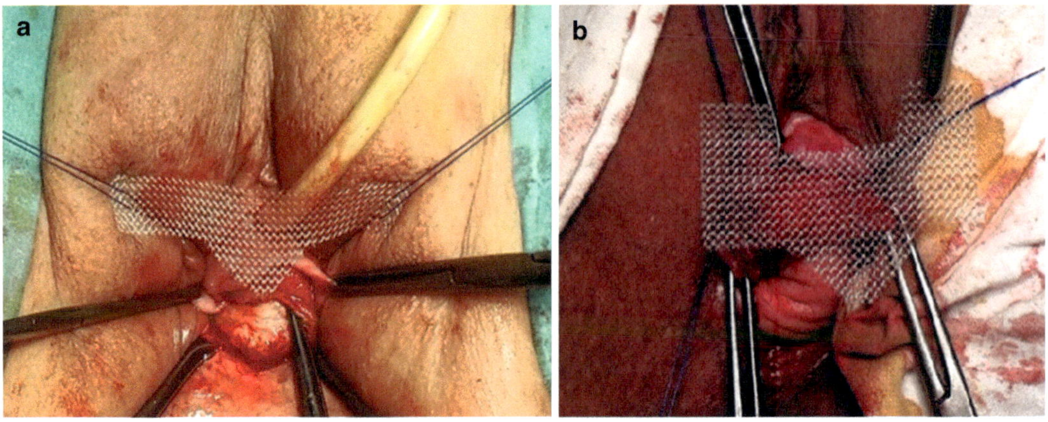

Fig. 14.1 (**a**) Posterior "*patch*" with sacrospinous fixation in a patient in whom a posterior "bridge" is associated (from the archive of Enache T.). (**b**) Posterior "patch" with sacrospinous fixation in a patient with vaginal vault prolapse and rectocoele

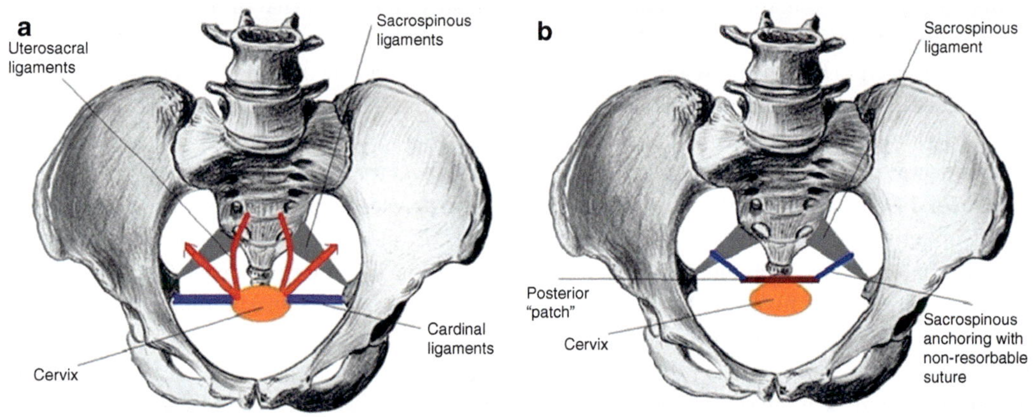

Fig. 14.2 Disposition of cardinal and uterosacral ligaments. (**a**) Vector analysis. The arrow is the vector result of the "tension in the wire" in the cardinal and uterosacral ligaments. (**b**) Postoperative position of the posterior "patch" with sacrospinous fixation

nent of the cervix, and the cardinal ligaments provide the lateral component. Transposed in biomechanical language, we are talking about a "tension in the wire" that is opposed to the displacement of the cervix, one oriented posteriorly and the other one laterally.

The result of these forces is a vector with posterolateral orientation (Fig. 14.2a).

In the case of the posterior "patch," the sacrospinous anchoring wires also have a posterolateral direction, similar to that of the two ligament components (Fig. 14.2b).

Thus, from a biophysical point of view, the posterior "patch" fixed sacrospinously has the prospect of a pathogenic correction of the defective anchoring of the cervix and the elitrocele. In the case of uterine prolapse, we preferred an additional technique depending on the possible pelvic floor disorders associated. For the cases in which an anterior vaginal prolapse coexisted, we preferred the four-arm surgical cure, two passed transobturator, and two laterocervical, subsequently fixed to the sacrospinous wires, thus also realizing the anchoring of the cervix. To the extent that there is no cystocele associated and there is only an apical defect, damage to uterosacral and cardinal ligaments, we practiced a pericervical cerclage with the anchoring of the edges of the mesh to the two sacrospinous wires. Vaginal vault prolapse benefits from the same surgical technique, the etiopathogeny being identical to that of uterine prolapse.

Surgical Steps

1. A transverse incision is made at the level of posterior vaginal mucosa, at 2 cm below its insertion on the cervix.
2. Digital dissection is performed with the index finger of the same hand posterolateral to the ischial spine and bilaterally.
3. The marking of sacrospinous ligaments with the index finger, bilateral, medial, and in contact with the ischial spine.
4. Passing a 2/0 non-resorbable monofilament wire through each sacrospinous ligament using a special anchoring device approximately halfway to the sacrospinous ligament, somehow more lateral than in the case of posterior mesh anchoring and marking the ends of the wires with an autostatic spreading forceps. The maneuver is performed by positioning the instrument's handle in the hand opposite to the side of the patient operated on. Holding takes place so that the thumb is in contact with the plunger of the sliding needle of the instrument.

   The instrument is inserted with the same hand corresponding to the side of the patient operated on, the index finger being in contact with the sacrospinous ligament at about 2 cm lateral to the ischial spine. The tip of the instrument is positioned so that the concavity is oriented inferiorly towards the sacrospinous liagament. The tip of the instrument will be pressed on the ligament with the index finger. At this point, with the thumb of the contralateral hand, the plunger is activated to the tip, so that the sliding needle will pierce the ligament and will meet the wire that is passed over the end of the instrument.

   The retraction of the plunger follows, also meaning the retraction of the needle that has the wire, thus realizing the anchoring of the wire to the sacrospinous ligaments. By retracting the instrument, both ends of the wire are at the level of the vaginal incision.
5. The insertion of the polypropylene "patch," passing the ends of the wires anchored sacrospinously through the loops of the mesh, in the lateral sides, bilaterally.
6. Fixing the "patch" to the insertion on the cervix of sacrospinous ligaments, the wires will be located medial to the sacrospinous ones. In the case of patients with a history of total hysterectomy, the fixation of the "patch" is done at the posterior vaginal mucosa, 1 cm below the postoperative scar.
7. Tying the ends of the wires anchored sacrospinous with one another, with consequent reduction of uterine prolapse and elitrocele. The sutures should not be strained excessively, thus avoiding overcorrection. A part of the wire will remain suspended, as mentioned above.
8. Suture of the vaginal cut. If there are additional steps, these will be made separately.

   The technique described above has two advantages: it avoids most of the complications and it is simpler. The "in vivo" provision of the "patch" with sacrospinous fixation represents a technical solution that respects the vector distribution, thus providing the premises for the restoration of pelvic organ physiology. The patient is mesh-covered for 24 h postoperatively, the discharge being made at 48 h at the latest if no complications occur.

The results at 3 years are favorable, with a relapse rate of less than 1% in a group of 150 patients, but a statistical confirmation at 5 years is required. However, prospects are encouraging. The method was registered at the State Office for Inventions and Trademarks (OSIM) in Romania with the title "Surgical kit and method for elitrocele correction vaginally" and the Patent No. 130607/29.11.2016 was obtained [8].

In the following, we will offer examples of the application of the method in some cases that associated the apical defect and its correction by the abovementioned method.

14.1 Case Study: Pelvic Floor Disorders: A New Perspective (A New Surgical Technique with a Polypropylene Patch for Posterior Compartment Defect)

Case 1: A 57-year-old patient presented with posterior vaginal fornix symptomatology, nocturia, urge incontinence, dyspareunia, and medium pelvic pains. The clinical examination revealed a posterior compartment defect at all three levels: elitrocele with minimal uterine prolapse, rectocele, and perineal body defect. The surgical correction was performed with a "patch" posteriorly fixed to the sacrospinous ligaments and, additionally, the cure of rectocele with posterior "bridge" (Fig. 14.3).

At 6 months, the patient returned with a satisfactory anatomical result and a significant clinical improvement; however, nocturia was still persistent, but with a lower frequency from six to three episodes per night. Moreover, a significant reduction of hemorrhoidal disease was observed, which the patient also noticed.

Case 2: A 54-year-old patient presented for a formation that came out from the vaginal introitus, nocturia, and urge incontinence, which she declared was however variable. The objective examination revealed a second-degree uterine prolapse, elitrocele, and third-degree rectocele (Fig. 14.4).

Surprisingly, the anterior wall did not present any pelvic floor disorder. Surgical treatment consisted in mounting a posterior "patch" with sacrospinous fixation, which reconstructed the cardinal and uterosacral ligaments vectorally. A more difficult moment was the dissection of the hernial sac and the reduction of enterocoele (Fig. 14.4b). In this case, a patch with a particular shape was made (Fig. 14.4c) with two extensions anteriorly and laterally, and through their loops, the sacrospinous wires were passed, and, with an inferior and median extension, the posterior "bridge" was attached for the correction of rectocele (Fig. 14.4d). Postoperative progression was favorable at 6 months, with the disappearance of symptoms and the restoration of the anatomy.

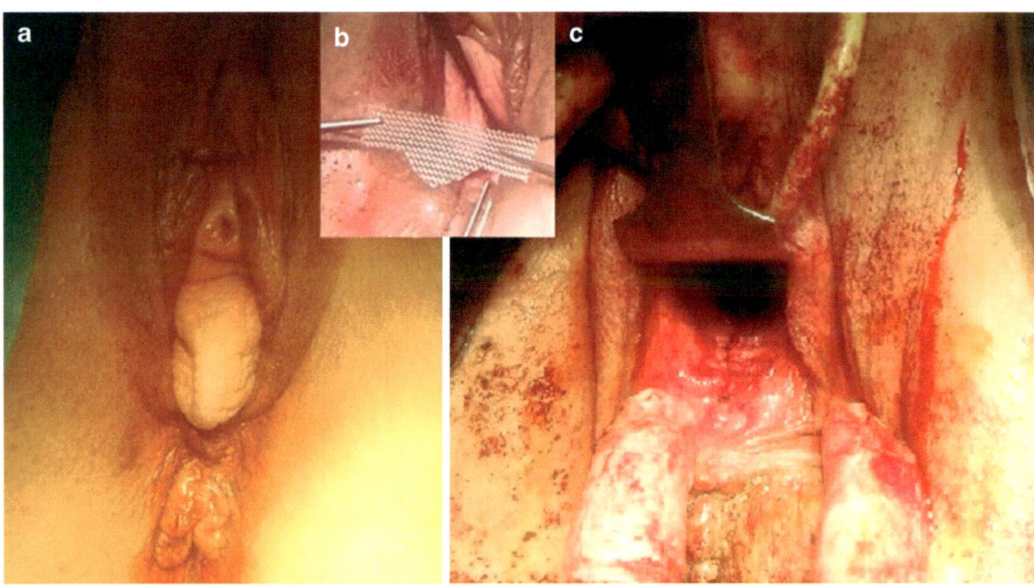

Fig. 14.3 Posterior vaginal prolapse—rectocele and elitrocele. (**a**) Preoperative aspect, (**b**) intraoperative aspect, (**c**) postoperative aspect (from the archive of **Enache T.**)

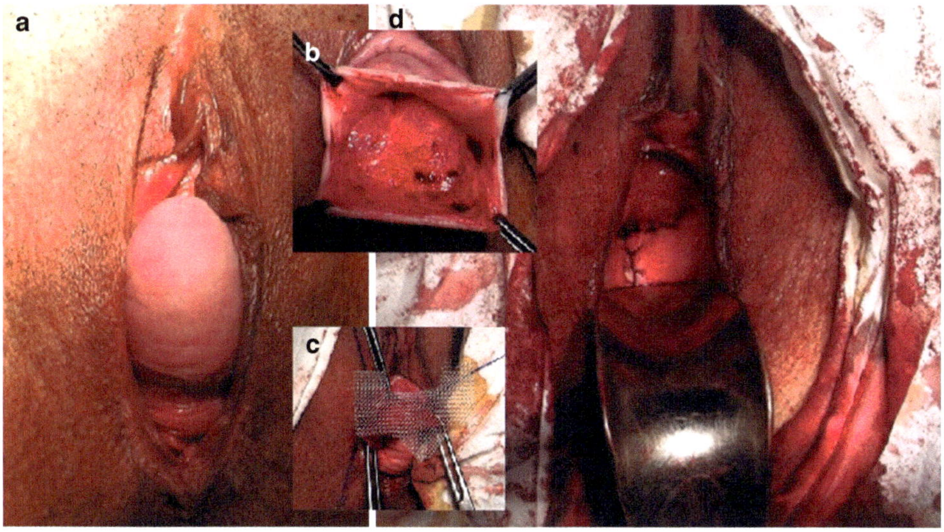

Fig. 14.4 Posterior uterine and vaginal prolapse. (**a**) Preoperative aspect, (**b**, **c**) intraoperative aspect, (**d**) postoperative aspect (from the archive of **Enache T**.)

In order to verify statistically the new method, we performed a prospective study that took place in the Clinical Hospital of Obstetrics and Gynaecology "Prof. Dr. Panait Sîrbu" in Bucharest, between 2012 and 2016 involving 95 patients with pelvic floor dysfunction consisting in pelvic floor disorders with posterior defects among others. We have divided all patients in two subgroups: in the first one, with 37 patients, we used surgical methods with native tissue repair. We used the perineal and vaginal approach, with posterior colpoperineorrhaphy, McCall suture when enterocoele coexisted, or even Amreich-Richter technique in two cases of vaginal vault prolapse.

The second subgroup consisted 58 patients where we used posterior patch with sacrospinous fixation technique to cure posterior compartment defects, associating different other methods like posterior bridge for treatment of rectocoele.

We analyzed both subgroups before and 6 months after surgery. All patients completed a pre- and postoperative questionnaire, beneficiated of clinical examination, preoperative urodynamics, and pre- and postoperative echography.

All patients presented symptoms like frequency, urgency and nocturia, pelvic pains, or hemorrhoids. We studied the preoperative and postoperative dynamics of these variables within each group. We quantified frequency and nocturia with number of episodes per day and urgency, hemorrhoids, and pelvic pains on a scale ranging from 0 to 3 in intensity as perceived by the patient (Table 14.1).

After statistical analysis, we found a postoperative improvement in some symptoms, in both groups. Analyzing the uterine artery velocimetry, we found a significant lowering of resistivity index in the second subgroup. A primary conclusion might be that this procedure significantly increases pericervical blood circulation.

Comparing the surgical outcome in these patients, we discovered a significant improvement of nocturia, frequency, and hemorrhoids in the second subgroup, with $p < 0.01$. All the other parameters taken into the discussion did not differ significantly.

The anatomical results were satisfactory in both groups immediately postoperative and 6 months after. There were no serious complications either.

Table 14.1 Statistical analysis of patients' variables. *M* mean value, *SD* standard deviation, *MSD* mean standard deviation, *p* probability

Variable	Probabilistic invariants	First subgroup		Second subgroup	
		Pre	Post	Pre	Post
Frequency	M	8.12	6.06	9.57	6.79
	SD	3.84	1.85	5.09	1.99
	MSD	0.66	0.32	0.96	0.38
	p	4.18E		0.000554	
Nocturia	M	2.03	1.24	3.0	1.32
	SD	1.59	0.87	3.37	0.94
	MSD	0.28	0.15	0.64	0.18
	p	1.2		0.00783	
Urgency	M	1.67	0.58	1.82	0.89
	SD	1.19	0.61	1.12	0.8
	MSD	0.21	0.1	0.21	0.15
	p	6.15E − 07		8.5E − 05	
Hemorrhoids	M	0.91	0.42	0.57	0.18
	SD	0.88	0.61	0.63	0.39
	MSD	0.15	0.1	0.12	0.07
	p	0.000214		0.00529	
Pelvic pains	M	1.03	0.17	0.82	0.25
	SD	0.73	0.27	0.55	0.52
	MSD	0.127	0.52	0.10	0.1
	p	4.84E − 08		5.68E − 05	
Right uterine artery RI	M	0.84	0.83	0.88	0.83
	SD	0.1	0.08	0.06	0.05
	MSD	0.02	0.02	0.01	0.01
	p	0.465224		0.000134	
Left uterine artery RI	M	0.84	0.83	0.88	0.84
	SD	0.08	0.08	0.07	0.05
	MSD	0.01	0.02	0.02	0.01
	p	0.325242		0.00924	

14.2 Conclusion

There are some symptoms related to the posterior compartment defect that significantly improve after vaginal surgery. Apparently, correcting anatomy we may achieve restoration of function. We may conclude that when these symptoms associate with pelvic floor disorders, they are surgically curable. Posterior patch with sacrospinous fixation proved to be an easy way of correcting level I defect, with minimum complications. It also provides a satisfactory anatomical result.

Posterior patch with sacrospinous fixation might have a better result in pelvic and pericervical blood circulation. The better cure of hemorrhoids and the improvement of uterine velocimetry plead for that idea.

References

1. Delorme E. What transvaginal meshes surgery tells us about conflict of interests. J Gynecol Obstet Hum Reprod. 2020;49(1):101636. https://doi.org/10.1016/j.jogoh.2019.101636. Epub 2019 Sep 11.
2. Stanford EJ, Moore RD, Roovers JP, Courtieu C, Lukban JC, Bataller E, Liedl B, Sutherland SE. Elevate anterior/apical: 12-month data showing safety and efficacy in surgical treatment of pelvic organ prolapse. Female Pelvic Med Reconstr Surg. 2013;19(2):79–83.
3. Rivaux G, Fatton B, Letouzey V, Cayrac M, Boileau L, de Tayrac R. Utero-vaginal suspension using a bilateral vaginal anterior sacrospinous fixation with mesh. Preliminary results. Prog Urol. 2012;22(17):1077–83.
4. Chang CP, Hsu FK, Lai MJ, Chang WH, Lee NR, Lee HL, Horng HC, Wang PH. Uterine-preserving pelvic organ prolapse surgery using the UPHOLD LITE vaginal support system: the outcomes of 291 patients.

Medicine (Baltimore). 2019;98(14):e15086. https://doi.org/10.1097/MD.0000000000015086.
5. Duport C, Duperron C, Delorme E. Anterior and middle pelvic organ prolapse repair using a six tension-free strap low weight transvaginal mesh: long-term retrospective monocentric study of 311 patients. J Gynecol Obstet Hum Reprod. 2019;48(3):143–9. https://doi.org/10.1016/j.jogoh.2018.11.008. Epub 2018 Nov 30.
6. Weintraub AY, Friedman T, Baumfeld Y, Neymeyer J, Neuman M, Krissi H. Long term functional outcomes following mesh-augmented posterior vaginal prolapse repair. Int J Gynaecol Obstet. 2016;135(1):107–11. https://doi.org/10.1016/j.ijgo.2016.04.005. Epub 2016 Jun 16.
7. Enache T, Enache A, Moisa M, Ionica M. Surgical management of posterior compartment defect in patients with pelvic floor dysfunction. Pelviperineology. 2016;35(2):37–9.
8. Enache T, Mueller-Funogea I-A, Enache A, Moisa M. Enache T Sr. "Surgical kit and method for elitrocele correction vaginally" and the Patent No. 130607/29.11.2016. State Office for Inventions and Trademarks (OSIM).

15 Sacropexy of the Vagina and Rectum with a Single Mesh

Kristina Drusany Starič, Urška Eržen Rupnik, Adolf Lukanović, and Gregor Norčič

15.1 Pelvic Organ Prolapse

Pelvic organ prolapse (POP) is a condition that drastically alters a patient's quality of life [1] and can negatively affect her social life due to urinary, anorectal, and sexual dysfunctions [2]. The goal of POP surgical therapy is to restore normal anatomy of the vagina and prolapsed organs, to reduce or eliminate prolapse-related symptoms, and to restore physiological functions [3].

Vaginal vault prolapse and apical uterine prolapse are defined as the descent of the vaginal cuff, cervix, or uterus below a point which is 2 cm less than the total vaginal length above the plane of the hymen [4]. Seventy-two percent of pelvic organ prolapses are associated with other pelvic floor defects: cystocele, rectocele, or enterocele [5]. The incidence of pelvic floor prolapse is 30% in women between the ages 20 and 59 and over 50% in women over 50. The likelihood of surgery for POP is 19% and 30% for reoperation. This makes POP not only a significant healthcare problem but also a non-negligible expense for the healthcare system [6].

The most common risk factors for POP are parity and mode of delivery, child birthweight, age, menopausal status (estrogen deficiency), congenital collagen disorders (type IV Ehlers-Danlos syndrome, Marfan syndrome), race, previous surgeries to correct pelvic organ prolapse (colposuspension, sacrospinous fixation, hysterectomy), and chronic conditions that increase intra-abdominal pressure (chronic constipation, pulmonary disease, obesity, prolonged heavy lifting). The role and mechanism of some factors are not yet well elucidated [6–9].

The symptoms of POP can be divided into five major groups:

1. Vaginal symptoms such as the sensation of vaginal bulging, a visible or palpable bulge, feeling of pressure in the vagina, and bloody or purulent discharge.
2. Urinary symptoms manifested by incontinence, frequency, urgency, weak or prolonged urinary stream, feeling of incomplete bladder emptying, the need for manual reduction of prolapse to ensure complete voiding, and the need for a change of position to ensure complete voiding or start voiding.
3. Bowel symptoms which include incontinence, flatulence, liquid or solid stool, urgency, feel-

K. D. Starič (✉) · A. Lukanović
Division of Gynecology and Obstertrics, Department of Gynecology, Medical Faculty, University Medical Centre Ljubljana, University of Ljubljana, Ljubljana, Slovenia
e-mail: kristina.drusany@kclj.si; adolf.lukanovic@guest.arnes.si

U. E. Rupnik
Community Health Centre Idrija, Idrija, Slovenia

G. Norčič
Division of Surgery, Department of University of Ljubljana, University Medical Centre Ljubljana, Ljubljana, Slovenia
e-mail: gregor.norcic@kclj.si

F. Dökmeci, D. E. E. Rizk (eds.), *Insights Into Incontinence and the Pelvic Floor*,
https://doi.org/10.1007/978-3-030-94174-1_15

ing of incomplete emptying and splinting (pushing on or around the vagina or perineum), and need to start or complete defecation ("digitation").
4. Sexual symptoms which include dyspareunia, decreased sensitivity, and incontinence during intercourse.
5. Other symptoms which include low back pain (reduced or resolved in the supine position) and abdominal pain or feeling of pressure [8, 9].

The diagnosis of POP involves taking patient's medical history and clinical examination where the POP-Q system (Pelvic Organ Prolapse Quantification System) is most commonly used to objectify prolapse [9]. Depending on the symptoms, diagnostics may include imaging and urodynamic diagnostic examinations [10].

The management for POP is indicated in symptomatic patients. Conservative treatment is the first choice in women with POP and involves pelvic floor muscle training and the use of pessaries [11]. There are no data supporting the use of local estrogen as primary therapy for POP [12]. Surgical treatment is suitable for patients where conservative treatment has been unsuccessful or rejected. Various surgical approaches are in use—abdominal or transvaginal. Patient's own tissues or artificial materials are used for prolapse correction. The uterus can be spared in POP repair, or concomitant hysterectomy can be performed. Meta-analyses have shown that surgical treatment of pelvic organ prolapse improves the patients' quality of life [13]. Today we can compare success rates of surgical procedures and risk factors, thanks to numerous studies of POP; however, we are still unable to prevent frequent POP recurrences or onset of new symptoms using current surgical techniques [14].

15.2 Rectoanal Intussusception

Rectoanal intussusception (RI) (also called internal rectal prolapse) is an invagination of the rectum into itself during defecation. RI was found in 12–31% of patients with defecation disorders by some authors [15, 16] and as high as 50% even in asymptomatic patients by others [17]. The exact ethology of RI is unknown. Structural abnormalities of the pelvic floor, rectal wall connective tissue dysfunction, and functional causes leading to increased intra-abdominal pressure have all been associated with RI. The course of RI is also not clear since the progression to external prolapse is variable or slow [18]. The cardinal symptom in patients with symptomatic RI is a feeling of incomplete fecal evacuation/tenesmus, in some patients also constipation and a burning sensation toward the sacrum, which is exacerbated when straining; fecal incontinence is also a common symptom [19].

The gold standard for RI diagnostics is defecography, the results of which must be interpreted critically in relation to the clinical picture [20]. Dynamic magnetic resonance imaging (DPMRI) is an alternative to defecography and has the advantage of absence of ionizing radiation as well as better spatial resolution of the structure. The disadvantages of the method are mainly its poorer specificity and high costs [18]. Dynamic transperineal ultrasound (DTP-US) is a means of diagnosis that allows us to evaluate all compartments within the pelvis in real time and their relationship at rest and during straining and defecation [21]. Clinical examination correlates well with the diagnosis of intussusception when the segment is longer than 3 cm and is less reliable for shorter segments [22].

Initial therapy of symptomatic RI is always conservative with dietary measures, laxatives, suppositories, enemas, and biofeedback therapy [23]. Conservative biofeedback therapy is a form of anal EMG (electromyography) that uses probe connected to a computer. It is successful in 37–100% in obstructive defecation and 50–90% in fecal incontinence [24]. Surgical treatments most used for RI include various methods of abdominal rectopexy, a stapled trans-anal rectal resection (STARR) procedure for trans-anal anteroposterior rectotomy, and the Delorme procedure [18, 22]. There is no data yet that clearly show the advantage of one surgical technique over another based on randomized trials [18].

15.3 Case Study: Feasibility of Correcting Vaginal Vault Prolapse and Intussusception with One Y Mesh (First Results)

Urška Eržen Rupnik, Kristina Drusany Starič, Gregor Norčič and Adolf Lukanović

Department of Gynecology, University Medical Centre Ljubljana, Ljubljana, Slovenia
Department of Abdominal Surgery, University Medical Centre Ljubljana, Ljubljana, Slovenia

The study deals with pelvic organ prolapse, rectoanal intussusception, and apical uterine prolapse in nine patients. For the first time, using a single Y mesh a total of nine procedures were performed for the repair of pelvic organ prolapse and rectoanal intussusception between January 2016 and September 2018 at the University Medical Centre Ljubljana. Preoperatively, the diagnosis of POP and RI was confirmed by clinical examination, perineal ultrasound, and defecography (Fig. 15.1).

The surgery itself was performed interdisciplinary, as collaboration between a gynecologist and an abdominal surgeon. After establishing pneumoperitoneum, the preparation of the vaginal vault (or cervix), rectum, and sacrum followed. The distal end of the posterior arm of the Y mesh was sutured to the rectum at the level of the puborectalis muscle. Anterior wall of the extraperitoneal rectum was attached to the mesh using single resorbable sutures. The mesh itself was fixated to the sacrum using an endo-tracker. Additionally, the posterior arm of the Y mesh was also sutured to the posterior wall of the vaginal vault, and the anterior arm of the Y mesh was sutured to the anterior wall of the vaginal vault. The mesh was then completely covered with peritoneum. A modified form of the procedure—hystero-recto-sacropexy—was performed in two uterus-preserved patients. Establishing pneumoperitoneum and the standard placement of an optic trocar through the navel and three working trocars (one on each side in the lower quadrant of the abdomen and one suprapubically) was followed by the preparation of the anterior longitudinal ligament, later followed by the opening of the peritoneum toward the rectum and dissection of the peritoneum between the bladder and the uterus. An opening was made into the left and right round ligaments (Lat. Lig. Rotundum) through which a halved anterior arm of the polypropylene mesh was later inserted. The posterior arm of the Y mesh was attached at the level of the puborectalis muscle to the rectum with absorbable sutures and to the sacrum with titanium tacks using an endo-tracker. Both halves of the anterior arm of the mesh, which were inserted through the openings through the round ligaments, were sutured to the anterior portion of the cervix. The mesh was completely covered with peritoneum. A schematic representation of the steps of both procedures is summarized in Fig. 15.2. A video was also taken showing key steps in the procedure (Fig. 15.3). The surgery took on average 2 h and 15 min. Patients were discharged to home care on the third postoperative day. During hospitalization none of the patients reported postoperative complications.

15.4 Discussion

POP and RI are often presented concurrently to different extents in the same patient. This fact has been recognized and respected with the introduction of laparoscopic surgical techniques that address both issues simultaneously. Already in the first description of the laparoscopic ventral mesh rectopexy by D'Hoore et al., the fixation of the vagina to the mesh has also been performed [25]. Similar procedure with laparoscopic mesh rectopexy and concomitant sacrocolpopexy has been described by Slawik et al. [26]. Even in open surgery, the combined procedure has been advocated at the time by Lim et al. [27]. The unresolved issues to date remain, however, whether the concomitant procedure as such is associated with more complications as each of them alone, regarding the technical details of each procedure and the clinical importance of RI as opposed to overt rectal prolapse.

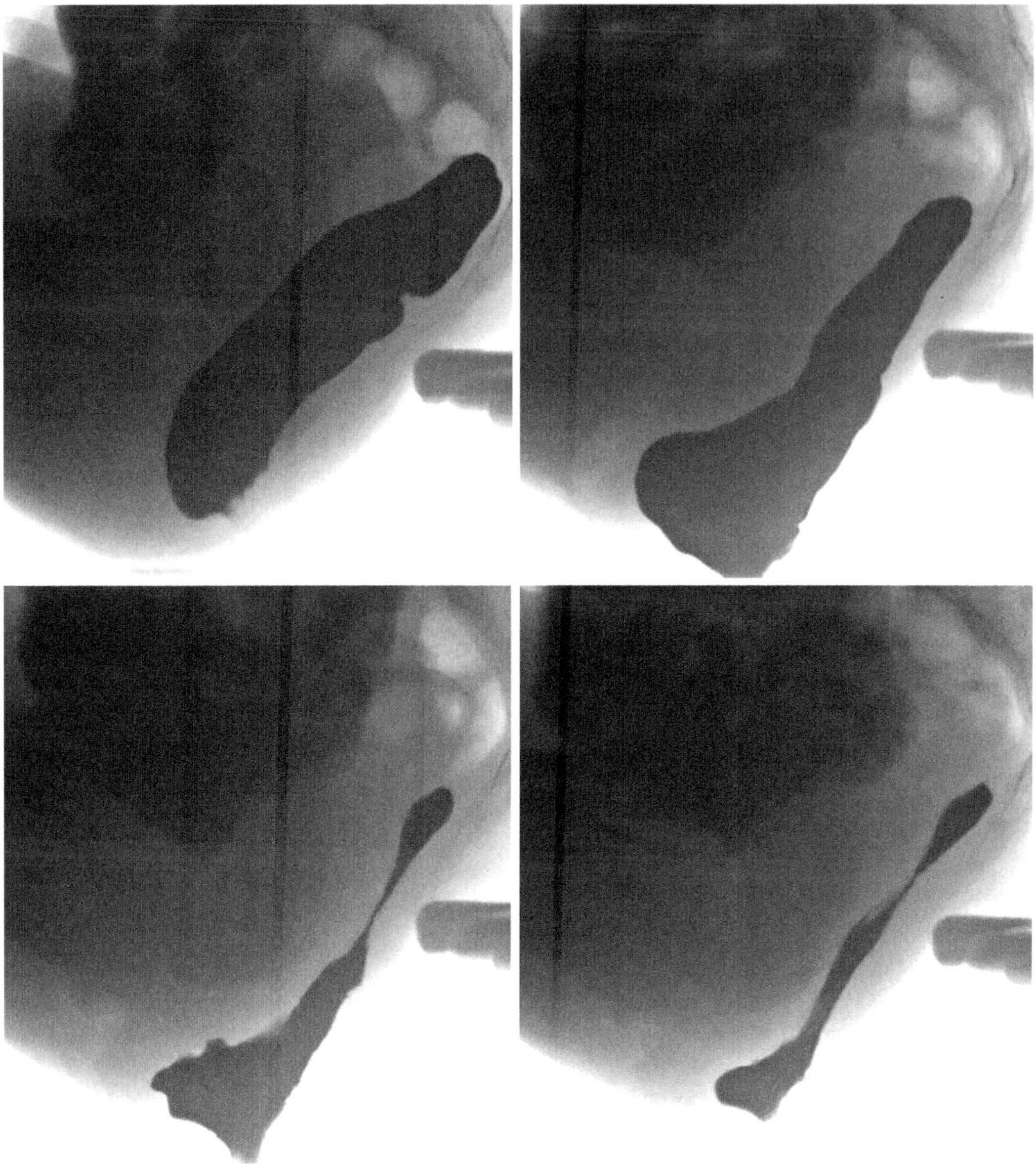

Fig. 15.1 Anterior rectocele, intra-anal intussusception, and rectal prolapse diagnosed using defecography (accurate assessment of the rate of prolapse is not possible using this test)

One of the rare publications that report increased incidence of postoperative complications with addition of rectopexy to sacrocolpopexy is the retrospective study of Unger et al. [28]. In their comparison of robotic and laparoscopic sacrocolpopexy in 406 patients between 2006 and 2012, they have found higher risk of blood transfusions, abscess formation, and osteomyelitis in 36 patients with concomitant rectopexy. On the other hand, a much larger clinical database analysis of laparoscopic sacrocolpopexies, laparoscopic rectopexies, and combined procedures (7232, 1560, and 123 patients, respectively) performed between 2013 and 2016 has found no difference in major complications between these groups of patients [29]. The authors concluded that the combined procedure might be appropriate in selective patients.

Fig. 15.2 Steps in laparoscopic colpo-recto-sacropexy (left) and hystero-recto-sacropexy (right)

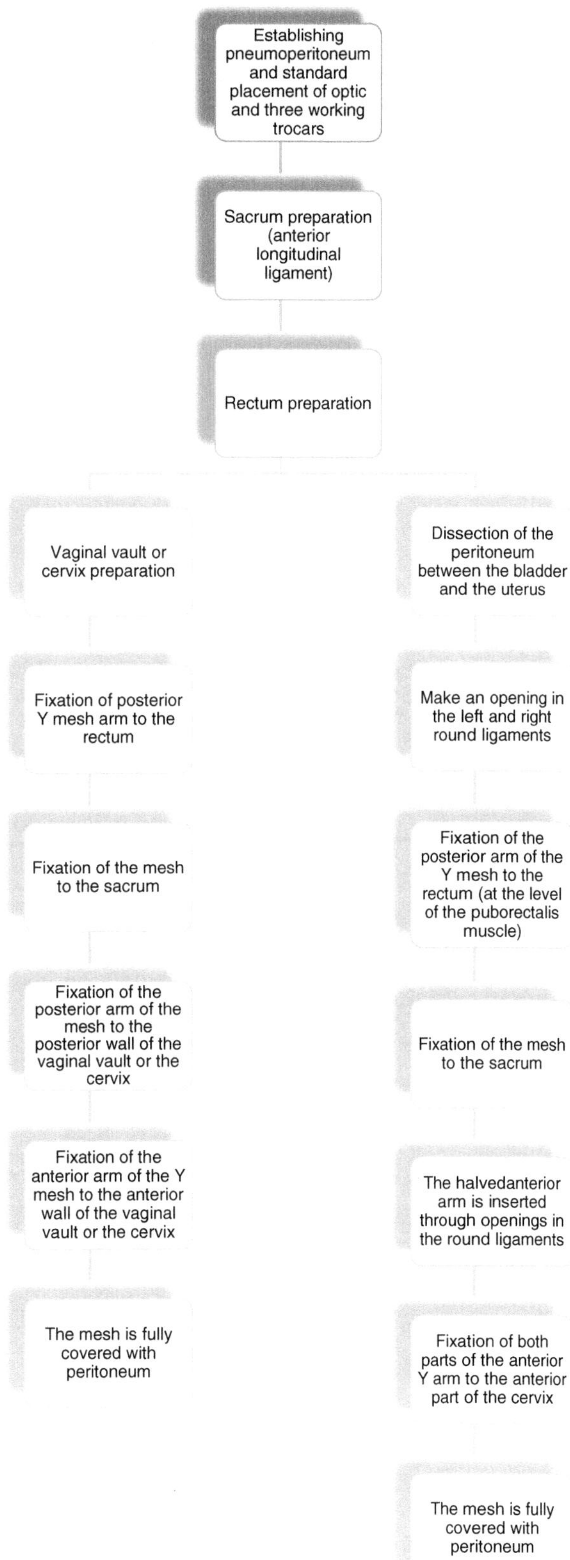

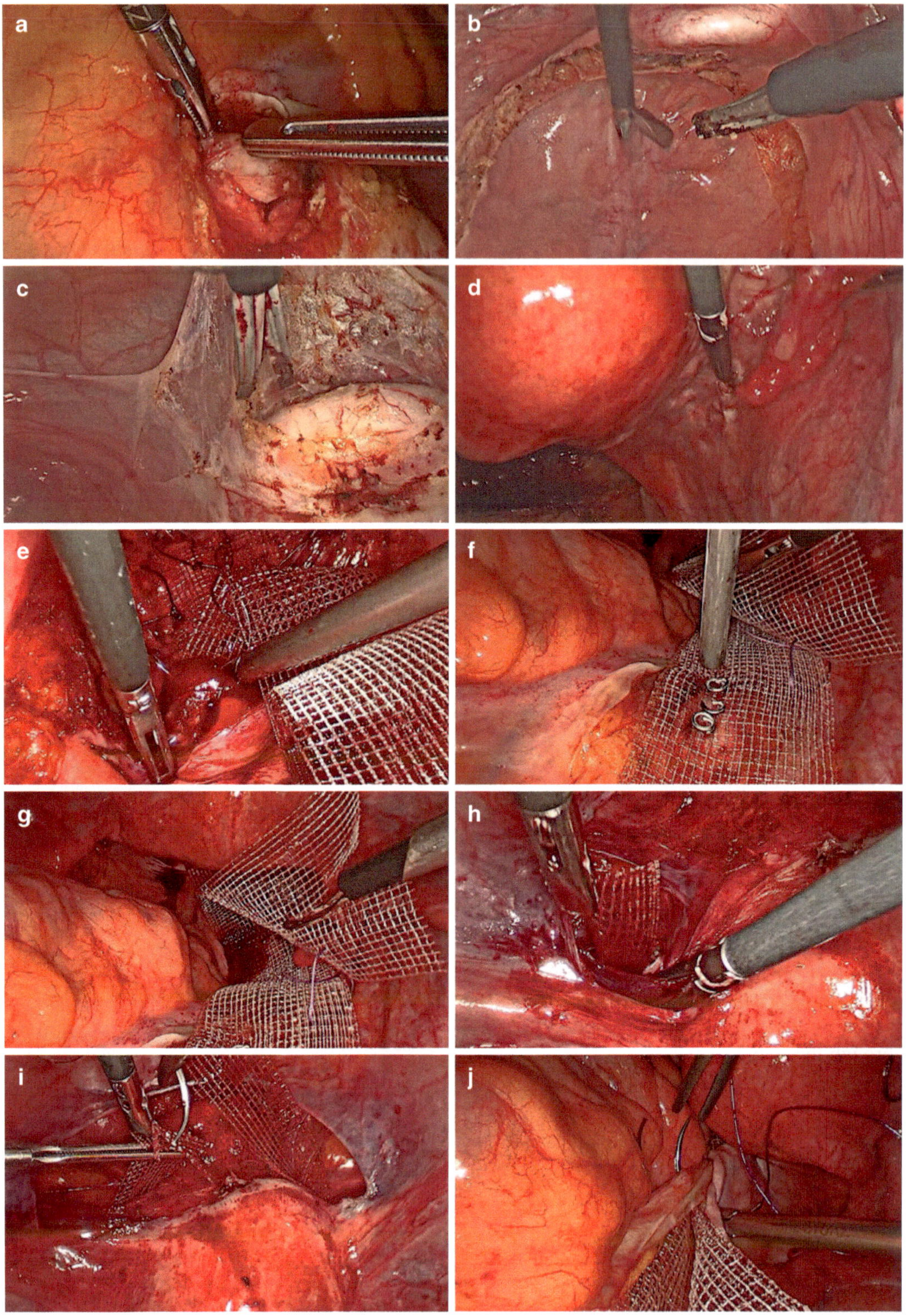

Fig. 15.3 Laparoscopic and hystero-recto-sacropexy. (**a**) Sacrum preparation, (**b**) rectum preparation, (**c**) dissection of the peritoneum between the bladder and the uterus, (**d**) opening in the round ligaments, (**e**) fixation of the posterior Y mesh arm to the rectum, (**f**) fixation of the mesh to the sacrum, (**g**) halved anterior arm of the mesh, (**h**) both parts of the anterior arm inserted through each openings in the left and right round ligaments, (**i**) fixation of both parts of the anterior Y arm to the anterior part of the cervix, (**j**) mesh fully covered with peritoneum

Another analysis of 3394 rectopexies and 206 combined procedures has also found no difference in operative morbidity by adding sacrocolpopexy to rectopexy [30]. These results are in concordance with our findings that show very low morbidity in our nevertheless small group of patients.

The biggest problem of literature analysis on rectopexy and/or laparoscopic POP surgery lies in the fact that technical details of performed procedures differ substantially between various authors. Some authors use only one mesh that is fixated to the rectum as well as to the fornix of the vagina on one side and to the sacral promontory on the other side [25, 26]. Others use two meshes that are fixated separately on both organs and to the sacral promontory [31]. Variability within the group of patients that underwent rectopexies derived from databases is therefore quite substantial since many different surgical techniques are performed (posterior and/or anterior rectal mobilization, suture rectopexies with or without associated sigmoid resection or mesh rectopexies alone) [29, 32]. Even greater is the variation of the material of the meshes used, the number and/or the material of the sutures used to fixate the mesh to the target organ, and regarding the fixation of the mesh to the sacral promontory (i.e., using tackers or sutures). In our study, we have used the standard laparoscopic rectopexy technique as described by D'Hoore et al. The uniqueness of our technique lies in the sacrocolpopexy part of procedure in those subgroups of patients that still had their uterus preserved. In these cases, we have split the second arm of the single mesh in half and inserted both parts through the round ligaments in order to fixate it on anterior upper part of the previously dissected vesiculo-vaginal septum, thus reinforcing the middle compartment reliably with minimal amount of additional mesh material.

The reports on concurrent procedure due to POP and RI exclusively are rare. Some authors only report on concurrent procedure for POP and overt (or complete) rectal prolapse [32]. The majority of the reports are however on the not further specified or mixed group of patients regarding their colorectal pathology, combined of patients with overt rectal prolapse as well as some cases of RI (internal rectal prolapse) [33–35]. In the latter group, authors mainly report of functional complaints in the form of obstructive defecation syndrome or fecal incontinence. In the majority of publications on concurrent procedure, the surgery resulted in significant improvement of the reported constipation and/or fecal incontinence [25, 26, 31–35]. These results are in concordance with our findings, where only one patient reported of persistence of constipation.

In the article a novel technique is described. Short-term results of laparoscopic correction of apical prolapse and rectoanal intussusception with a single Y mesh are particularly good; however, the limitation of the study is small number of patients, which is due to the very rare indications for this procedure.

The outcomes of the surgery were monitored with follow-up visit at 6–12 weeks after the patient was discharged from the hospital. All patients had improved anatomy of the pelvic organs, the obstruction was resolved in eight cases and in one case the obstruction remained, and further diagnostics was initiated. Cecum-level obstruction, which could be the result of the procedure, was confirmed; nevertheless, further tests will be needed to confirm the causal relationship. All patients were subjectively satisfied with the procedure and have reported an improved quality of life. The results are consistent with a study done at UMC Ljubljana in 2016 [14] that monitored complications after laparoscopic sacropexy with a polypropylene mesh between 2013 and 2015 in 38 patients. One of the patients experienced pain in the coccyx area after the procedure, which eventually resolved on its own, while another patient experienced problem with defecation; there were no other postoperative complications. Also, patient satisfaction with the intervention was high. The duration of the procedure was 90–180 min, which means that the fixation of the rectum did not significantly prolong the average duration of laparoscopic colpo-recto-sacropexy or hystero-recto-sacropexy—135 min—compared to only sacropexy.

Moreover, we have particularly good first long-term results of patients treated in the first half of 2016, where there are no mesh-related complications or recurrence of genital prolapse/problems with defecation.

15.5 Conclusion

In this chapter we described the advantage of a new technique: laparoscopic correction of POP and rectal intussusception using a single Y mesh with very favorable results. The new procedure firstly uses less foreign material in the body and thus has lower likelihood of associated complications. The interdisciplinary approach enables the merging of two otherwise separate surgeries into one, with its consequently reduced risk of complications due to surgery and anesthesia itself. We present a step by step approach of sacropexy of the vagina and rectum using a single Y mesh.

In conclusion, we believe that based on our own experience and on the results of the published literature, the concomitant laparoscopic procedure of POP and RI using one mesh is feasible with low postoperative morbidity and good functional outcome.

References

1. Dowell CJ, Bryant CM, Moore KH, Simons AM. Calculating the direct cost of urinary incontinence: a new test instrument. BJU Int. 1999;83(6):596–606.
2. Hendrix SL, Clark A, Nygaard I, Aragaki A, Barnabei V, McTiernan A. Pelvic organ prolapse in the Women's Health Initiative: gravity and gravidity. Am J Obstet Gynecol. 2002;186(6):1160–6.
3. Bojahr B, Tchartchian G, Waldschmidt M, Schollmeyer T, De Wilde RL. Laparoscopic sacropexy: a retrospective analysis of perioperative complications and anatomical outcomes. JSLS. 2012;16(3):428–36.
4. Abrams P, Cardozo L, Fall M, et al. The standardisation of terminology of lower urinary tract function: report from the standardisation sub-committee of the international continence society. Neurourol Urodyn. 2002;21(2):167–78.
5. Sederl J. Zur operation des prolapses der blind endigenden sheiden. Geburtshilfe Frauenheilkd. 1958;18:824–8.
6. Aytan H, Ertunç D, Tok EC, Yaşa O, Nazik H. Prevalence of pelvic organ prolapse and related factors in a general female population. Turk J Obstet Gynecol. 2014;11(3):176–80.
7. Uzoma A, Farag KA. Vaginal vault prolapse. Obstet Gynecol Int. 2009;2009:275621.
8. Doshani A, Teo RE, Mayne CJ, Tincello DG. Uterine prolapse. BMJ. 2007;335(7624):819–23.
9. Persu C, Chapple CR, Cauni V, Gutue S, Geavlete P. Pelvic Organ Prolapse Quantification System (POP-Q)—a new era in pelvic prolapse staging. J Med Life. 2011;4(1):75–81.
10. Thakar R, Stanton S. Management of genital prolapse. BMJ. 2002;324(7348):1258–62.
11. Giarenis I, Robinson D. Prevention and management of pelvic organ prolapse. F1000Prime Rep. 2014;6:77. Published 2014 Sep 4.
12. Rahn DD, Good MM, Roshanravan SM, et al. Effects of preoperative local estrogen in postmenopausal women with prolapse: a randomized trial. J Clin Endocrinol Metab. 2014;99:3728.
13. Doaee M, Moradi-Lakeh M, Nourmohammadi A, Razavi-Ratki SK, Nojomi M. Management of pelvic organ prolapse and quality of life: a systematic review and meta-analysis. Int Urogynecol J. 2014;25:153–63.
14. Drusany Starič K, et al. Outcome of laparoscopic sacropexy with polypropylene mesh. Eur J Obstet Gynecol Reprod Biol. 2011;206:253–4.
15. Agachan F, Pfeifer J, Wexner SD. Defecography and proctography. Results of 744 patients. Dis Colon Rectum. 1996;39(8):899–905.
16. Mellgren A, Bremmer S, Johansson C, et al. Defecography. Results of investigations in 2,816 patients. Dis Colon Rectum. 1994;37(11):1133–41.
17. Shorvon PJ, McHugh S, Diamant NE, Somers S, Stevenson GW. Defecography in normal volunteers: results and implications. Gut. 1989;30(12):1737–49.
18. Blaker K, Anandam JL. Functional disorders: rectoanal intussusception. Clin Colon Rectal Surg. 2017;30(1):5–11.
19. Christiansen J, Zhu BW, Rasmussen OO, Sorensen M. Internal rectal intussusception: results of surgical repair. Dis Colon Rectum. 1992;35:1026–9.
20. Jorge JMN, Habr-Gama A, Wexner SD. Clinical applications and techniques of cinedefecography. Am J Surg. 2001;182:93–101.
21. Weiss EG, McLemore EC. Functional disorders: rectoanal intussusception. Clin Colon Rectal Surg. 2008;21(2):122–8.
22. Karlbom U, Graf W, Nilsson S, Pahlman L. The accuracy of clinical examination in the diagnosis of rectal intussusception. Dis Colon Rectum. 2004;47(9):1533–8.
23. Cariou de Vergie L, Venara A, Duchalais E, Frampas E, Lehur PA. Internal rectal prolapse: definition, assessment and management in 2016. J Visc Surg. 2017;154(1):21–8.
24. Hwang YH, Person B, Choi JS, et al. Biofeedback therapy for rectal intussusception. Tech Coloproctol. 2006;10:11–6.
25. D'Hoore A, Penninckx F. Laparoscopic ventral recto(colpo)pexy for rectal prolapse: surgical tech-

nique and outcome for 109 patients. Surg Endosc. 2006;20(12):1919–23.
26. Slawik S, Soulsby R, Carter H, Payne H, Dixon AR. Laparoscopic ventral rectopexy, posterior colporrhaphy and vaginal sacrocolpopexy for the treatment of recto-genital prolapse and mechanical outlet obstruction. Color Dis. 2008;10(2):138–43.
27. Lim M, Sagar PM, Gonsalves S, Thekkinkattil D, Landon C. Surgical management of pelvic organ prolapse in females: functional outcome of mesh sacrocolpopexy and rectopexy as a combined procedure. Dis Colon Rectum. 2007;50(9):1412–21.
28. Unger CA, Paraiso MF, Jelovsek JE, Barber MD, Ridgeway B. Perioperative adverse events after minimally invasive abdominal sacrocolpopexy. Am J Obstet Gynecol. 2014;211(5):547.e1–8.
29. Weinberg D, Qeadan F, McKee R, Rogers RG, Komesu YM. Safety of laparoscopic sacrocolpopexy with concurrent rectopexy: peri-operative morbidity in a nationwide cohort. Int Urogynecol J. 2019;30(3):385–92.
30. Geltzeiler CB, Birnbaum EH, Silviera ML, Mutch MG, Vetter J, Wise PE, Hunt SR, Glasgow SC. Combined rectopexy and sacrocolpopexy is safe for correction of pelvic organ prolapse. Int J Color Dis. 2018;33(10):1453–9.
31. Campagna G, Panico G, Caramazza D, Anchora LP, Parello A, Gallucci V, Vacca L, Scambia G, Ercoli A, Ratto C. Laparoscopic sacrocolpopexy plus ventral rectopexy as combined treatment for multicompartment pelvic organ prolapse. Tech Coloproctol. 2020;24(6):573–84.
32. Yang SJ, Yoon SG, Lim KY, Lee JK. Laparoscopic vaginal suspension and rectopexy for rectal prolapse. Ann Coloproctol. 2017;33(2):64–9.
33. Martín Del Olmo JC, Toledano M, Martín Esteban ML, Montenegro MA, Gómez JR, Concejo P, Rodríguez de Castro M, Del Rio F. Outcomes of laparoscopic management of multicompartmental pelvic organ prolapse. Surg Endosc. 2019;33(4):1075–9.
34. Lauretta A, Bellomo RE, Galanti F, Tonizzo CA, Infantino A. Laparoscopic low ventral rectocolpopexy (LLVR) for rectal and rectogenital prolapse: surgical technique and functional results. Tech Coloproctol. 2012;16(6):477–83.
35. Watadani Y, Vogler SA, Warshaw JS, Sueda T, Lowry AC, Madoff RD, Mellgren A. Sacrocolpopexy with rectopexy for pelvic floor prolapse improves bowel function and quality of life. Dis Colon Rectum. 2013;56(12):1415–22.

Repair of Pelvic Organ Prolapse with Mesh Surgery

16

Cristina Margarita Fernández-Ávila, Rodrigo García-Baquero, Blanca Madurga-Patuel, and José Luis Álvarez-Ossorio

16.1 Introduction

The human being is the only mammal capable of walking and simultaneously maintaining an upright position. This fact, greatly affected by the law of gravity, implies somewhat unfavorable repercussions for the pelvic region that must support the weight of the abdominal organs. Therefore, throughout evolution, fundamental modifications have emerged in the pelvic skeleton, and in the surrounding muscles and ligaments, to offset the negative effect of the law of gravity. A prime example of the aforementioned adverse effects of the standing position are pelvic organ prolapses (POP).

The prevalence of this pathology is clearly on the rise: it is estimated that the number of women with pelvic organ prolapse will rise from 3.3 million women in 2010 to 4.9 million in 2050. Pelvic floor dysfunction is considered to be underdiagnosed, affecting 50% of women, although only 10–20% will seek assistance [1]. More than 60% of the patients affected by this condition present more than one pathology as the pelvic floor organs constitute a functional and organic unit [2]. It is estimated that a woman's risk of undergoing surgery related with POP during her life varies from 6.3 to 19%, with 30% requiring one or more surgical interventions due to recurrence [3]. Some authors have reported re-intervention rates for recurrence after primary reconstructive surgery of between 43 and 58% [4].

The anatomical support of the pelvic viscera is provided mainly by the levator ani and the connective tissue junctions of the pelvic organs: vaginal support arises from the connective tissue junctions between the vagina and the pelvic lateral wall, the vaginal wall and levator ani muscles [5].

In 1994, Delancey had already introduced the concept of the division of the support of the pelvic connective tissue in three levels (I–III) that represent apical, mid-vaginal, and distal support, respectively. The upper portion of the paracolpium (Level I) consists of a lamina from which the vagina is suspended attaching it to the pelvic wall and is responsible for suspending the apex of the vagina after hysterectomy. In the middle third of the vagina, the paracolpium joins the vagina laterally to the tendinous arch and the fascia of the elevator ani muscles (Level II). This stretches the vagina transversally between the bladder and the rectum. The structural layer that supports the bladder (pubocervical fascia) is made up of the anterior vaginal region and its attachment through the endopelvic fascia to the pelvic wall. Similarly, the posterior vaginal wall and endopelvic fascia (rectovaginal fascia) form the containing layer that prevents protrusion of the rectum toward its anterior surface. The lower third of the vagina (Level III) fuses with the peri-

C. M. Fernández-Ávila (✉) · R. García-Baquero
B. Madurga-Patuel · J. L. Álvarez-Ossorio
Hospital Universitario Puerta Del Mar, Urology, Cádiz, Spain

F. Dökmeci, D. E. E. Rizk (eds.), *Insights Into Incontinence and the Pelvic Floor*, https://doi.org/10.1007/978-3-030-94174-1_16

neal membrane, levator ani muscle, and the perineal body. Defects in the mid-level vaginal base (pubocervical and rectovaginal fascia) result in cystocele and rectocele, while the loss of upper suspensory fibers of the paracolpium and parametrium is responsible for the development of vaginal and uterine prolapse and these defects of combined form [6].

During examination, the prolapse of the anterior compartment is the most frequently reported site of prolapse, and it is diagnosed twice as frequent as the defects of the posterior compartment and three times more common than apical prolapse [7]. After hysterectomy, 6–12% of women will develop a prolapse of the vaginal vault [8], and in two thirds, multicompartmental prolapse will be present.

The etiology of POP is believed to be multifactorial with contributions from both environmental and genetic risk factors. The environmental factors that contribute to POP include vaginal delivery and newborn weight, chronic increases in intra-abdominal pressure, obesity, advanced age, and estrogen deficiency [9].

Not all prolapses are clinically symptomatic, and finding mild asymptomatic prolapses during pelvic floor examination is common. If symptoms are present, the most frequent complaints include a sensation of pressure, a lump or protrusion, and with evidence upon physical examination of a second degree or greater anterior and/or posterior and/or central vaginal wall prolapse. Ellkermann et al. found that in 237 women evaluated for POP, 73% reported urinary incontinence, 86% urinary urgency and/or frequency, 34–62% voiding dysfunction, and 31% fecal incontinence [10]. Evaluation of a patient with vaginal prolapse requires a comprehensive review of the full spectrum of pelvic floor symptoms and an assessment of how these symptoms affect her quality of life.

16.2 Literature Review

POP surgery is an increasingly important therapeutic aspect in clinical practice due to the aging of our population and is increasingly prevalent as a therapeutic option, despite surgical and hospitalization times that are three times longer compared to other surgeries related to the pelvic floor such as continence surgery. Given the increasing time and resources that will be required for POP surgery in the future, it is paramount that we perform effective, long-lasting, and cost-effective interventions with minimal morbidity.

Historically, most studies evaluating the treatment of POP have focused exclusively on anatomic success without considering other important aspects such as symptoms, vaginal accommodation, and quality of life. In fact, for a patient, individually, the most important result of a surgical procedure is the relief of their symptoms and improvement of their quality of life [11]. However, until recently these areas have been ignored. The objectives of pelvic floor reconstruction are to relieve symptoms, restore anatomy, improve or preserve function, prevent actions that alter other compartments, and improve quality of life [12].

Anterior colporrhaphy was the standard procedure in the management of the prolapsed anterior compartment. That said, in the early 2000s, there was a movement toward the use of prosthetics to increase the efficacy of native tissue repair in reconstructive gynecology. This was due to the articles published by Olsen et al. [13] where they reported a reoperation rate of 29% after prolapse or continence surgery and Weber et al. [14] who reported a 70% failure rate of native tissue anterior compartment repair. Recent reassessment of the same demographic 10 years later revealed a significantly lower reoperation rate of 17% [15]. More importantly, Weber et al. [14] and Sand et al. [16] reported in randomized controlled clinical trials that anterior colporrhaphy was successful in managing cystocele in only 30%. A recent re-analysis of the latter data, using the hymen as the threshold for objective success, reported considerably better results, with only 10% anatomic recurrence beyond the hymen, 5% symptomatic recurrence, and a lower reoperation rate of 1% at 23 months of follow-up [17]. During the decade between these initial and later publications, surgeons introduced a large number of biologic and mesh grafts to improve the outcomes of prolapse surgery. In later studies such as that of Julian et al. [18], it was shown that patients with several vaginal repairs had better results with a new repair with prosthetic material, in this case a Marlex® mesh (Bard, Covington, GA), compared to previous colporrhaphy, although follow-up reported an erosion rate of up to 25%.

The 2016 Cochrane Review also reported on 16 trials that evaluated nearly 2000 women with the aim of comparing anterior colporrhaphy versus permanent polypropylene mesh POP repair. The meta-analysis showed that recurrence of anterior wall prolapse (RR 0.34, 95% CI 0.25–0.46) and reoperation for prolapse (RR 0.44, 95% CI 0.24–0.46) was significantly less common after mesh repair compared to colporrhaphy. There were no differences between the groups in terms of quality of life outcomes or dyspareunia rates. However, the transvaginal polypropylene mesh group had higher rates of reoperation due to mesh exposure, stress urinary incontinence or prolapse (RR 1.62, 95% CI 1.15–2.28), and prolapse in the apical or posterior compartment (RR 1.85, 95% CI 1.01–3.37) compared to anterior colporrhaphy. Surgical time (MD 17.9 min, 95% CI 10.0–25.8), transfusion rate (RR 2.37, 95% CI 1.32–4.24), cystotomy (RR 4.65, 95% CI 1.22–17.77), and de novo stress urinary incontinence (RR 1.55, 95% CI 1.02–2.35) were higher after use of transvaginal polypropylene mesh compared to colporrhaphy. The mesh erosion rate was 11.5%, and 7% underwent surgical correction for repair [19].

One fact that we must take into account is that recently, most of the products made with polypropylene meshes evaluated in this meta-analysis have been withdrawn by the manufacturers due to the ongoing litigation regarding the use of this type of material vaginally. Because of this, new transvaginal polypropylene prosthetic products have emerged that have been introduced to decrease the rate of complications, specifically mesh erosion. Altman et al. [20] based on a multicenter prospective case series, which evaluated 207 women with apical prolapse undergoing the Uphold® pelvic floor system (Boston Scientific, USA), reported a subjective success rate of 90% per year and a reoperation rate for mesh exposure of 1.3%. Similarly, De Tayrac et al. found at 3 years, in 79 women with grade 3–4 cystocele, an anatomical success rate of 95%, a satisfaction rate of 98%, and a mesh exposure rate of 1.3% using a mesh of lightweight (28 g/m^2) polypropylene (Surgimesh® Prolapse Xlight, Aspide Medical, France) [21].

Studies where the device used was Restorelle® (Coloplast, Minneapolis, USA) report rates of absence of postoperative complications of 98.2%. The most frequent complications included urinary retention (8.7%), urinary tract infections (5.5%), and hematoma (2.7%). Other complications related to neighboring organs (bladder, rectum, and ureters) were very rare (<1%). A total of 2.8% of the patients had grade III complications according to the Clavien-Dindo classification (mesh extrusion). 80.3% did not present complications during the 3 months of study follow-up. Despite these promising data, the follow-up time of this study is short to ensure the absence of complications within a longer follow-up period [22]. Despite the current negative sentiment around transvaginal mesh, these new lightweight mesh products require further reassessment.

In the 2016 Cochrane meta-analysis of grafts vs native tissue repairs for vaginal prolapse, only one case of reoperation for dyspareunia or pain was reported in the nearly 1000 cases of transvaginal mesh evaluated [19]. However, pain and dyspareunia were the main causes of adverse events that triggered the 2011 FDA (Food and Drug Administration) warnings on the safety of transvaginal mesh [23]. These findings raise the possibility that pain and dyspareunia after transvaginal mesh surgery may be underreported and possibly only identified in trials with longer-term evaluation.

Alternatively, autologous material was considered as a possible option to synthetic prosthetic grafts with a lower risk of host rejection or infection. Gandhi et al. reported preliminary results of a randomized control trial comparing anterior colporrhaphy alone vs fascia lata graft for cystoceles [24]. In 1 year they could not demonstrate that the addition of the fascia lata graft improved the success rate compared to anterior colporrhaphy alone, being 71% compared to 82% (p 0.07); however, the rate of recurrent anterior prolapse in examination was lower after biological graft repair compared to anterior colporrhaphy (RR 0.74, 95% CI 0.55–0.99 $n = 646$, $I^2 = 29\%$, low-quality evidence), being the operative time for colporrhaphy shorter than the biological graft procedure (MD −10.35, 95% CI −14.45 to −6.24).

Reoperation after POP surgery for recurrence is an important measure of the effectiveness of the procedure. It is important to note that reoperation rates represent the "tip of the iceberg" in terms of surgical failures, as there are women with recurrent symptomatic prolapse who do not wish to undergo another operation. However, repeat surgery for recurrent POP is always an undesirable result that should, in most cases, be considered as a failed surgical procedure. Reoperation rates after POP surgery vary widely in the literature, largely due to different definitions and timelines. In a meta-analysis of 258 studies evaluating the reoperation rate after apical prolapse repairs, Diwadkar et al. reported a reoperation rate of 3.9% (95% CI: 3.5–4.4%) for traditional vaginal vault suspensions (sacrospinal ligament suspension and uterosacral vault suspensions) after a mean of 32 months, 2.3% (95% CI 1.9–2.7%) for sacrocolpopexy with follow-up mean 26 months and 1.3% (95% CI 1.0–1.7%) after transvaginal mesh procedures with a mean follow-up of 17 months. In particular, the total reoperation rate, including reoperations for recurrent POP and complications, was higher in the transvaginal mesh group (8.5%) [25].

The reoperation rate after POP surgery was defined in the joint report by the ICS (International Continence Society) and the IUGA (International Urogynecological Association), making a clear distinction between additional surgeries after primary surgical correction of POP, as the character of these can be very heterogeneous. The classification of these surgeries was established as follows:

- Primary prolapse/different compartment surgery—prolapse in a new compartment after previous surgery in a different compartment.
- Repeat surgery—a repeat operation for prolapse that arises from the compartment that was previously operated on.
- Surgery for complications (e.g., exposure or extrusion of the mesh, pain, or hemodynamic compromise of the patient, hemorrhage).
- Surgery for conditions not related to prolapse (e.g., subsequent surgery for stress urinary incontinence or fecal incontinence).

Recently, Ow et al. retrospectively compared 237 women who underwent 185 native tissue repairs and 161 transvaginal mesh repairs for recurrent prolapse. The transvaginal mesh group had significantly lower follow-up rates of symptomatic prolapse, prolapse upon examination, and reoperation for prolapse than the native tissue repairs group. However, the mesh exposure rate (anterior 15%, posterior mesh 21%) and associated reoperation (anterior 9%, posterior 15%) were significantly higher [26]. Trials such as this one show that in women with recurrent prolapse, transvaginal mesh has significant advantages and disadvantages compared to native tissue repairs and this profile is similar to that described for primary repairs, except that the exposure rates of the mesh appear to be higher in recurrent POP surgery.

Another surgical alternative on the rise in the last decade is laparoscopic or robotic sacrocolpopexy. This was born with the purpose of maintaining the existing good results of abdominal sacrocolpopexy but with the advantages of minimally invasive surgery. The case series demonstrate adequate acceptance in the short and medium term, with success rates of 91% (range: 60–100%), subjective success rates of 79–98% [27, 28], and a mean reoperation rate of 5.6%. In a meta-analysis, it was concluded that, in general, a large group of vaginal surgery with and without mesh is associated with a higher risk of prolapse recurrence upon examination (RR 1.9 95% CI 1.3–2.7), reoperation for prolapse recurrence (RR 2.3 95% CI 1.2–4.3), postoperative stress urinary incontinence (RR 1.9 95% CI 1.2–2.9), and dyspareunia (RR 2.5 95% 1.2–5.5) compared with sacrocolpopexy [29]. However, sacrocolpopexy was associated with a higher rate of paralytic ileus or small bowel obstruction (2.7% vs 0.2%, $p < 0.01$), complications related to intraperitoneal mesh or suture (4.2% vs 0.4%,

$p < 0.01$), and thromboembolic disease (0.6% vs 0.1%, $p = 0.03$) [30].

The robotic sacrocolpopexy is currently the latest version of this technique. The robotic approach is associated with objective cure rates of 84–100%, subjective cure rates of 92–95%, and a mesh erosion rate of 2% (range: 0–8%). In general, we can find postoperative complications in this meta-analysis in up to 11% (range: 0–43%), with serious complications in 2% and with a conversion rate of <1% to open surgery (range: 0–5%) [31].

Traditionally, researchers have defined surgical success using anatomical results (POP-Q stages 0–1, Table 16.1) and defined surgical failure as POPQ stage 2 or greater. More recently it is suggested that these anatomical definitions are too strict as more than 75% of women presenting for annual gynecological exams with no symptoms of pelvic organ prolapse would not be found in the definition of "optimal anatomical result" and almost 40% would not meet the definition of "satisfactory anatomical result" [32]. The absence of symptoms of vaginal protrusion postoperatively has a significant relationship with the patient's evaluation of general improvement and improvement in quality of life after surgery, while anatomical success alone does not, and thus vaginal protrusion symptoms are of great importance when evaluating the surgical outcome of POP [11]. Another possible factor to take into account in the different studies is the concept of success used together with the POP classification used. Some authors have used the Baden-Walker prolapse classification system instead of the POP-Q; other studies have used a combination of anatomical criteria and the presence or absence of symptoms to define the success of the treatment. Such variability makes it difficult to compare the results between the different studies.

Table 16.1 POP-Q staging criteria

Pelvic organ prolapse quantification system (POP-Q)	
Stage	Description
0	No prolapse, anterior and posterior points are all −3 cm, and C or D is between -TVL and -(TVL-2) cm
1	The criteria for stage 0 are not met, and the most distal prolapse is more than 1 cm above the level of the hymen (less than −1 cm)
2	The most distal prolapse if between 1 cm above and 1 cm below the hymen (at least one point is −1, 0, or +1)
3	The most distal prolapse is more than 1 cm below the hymen but no further than 2 cm less than TVL
4	Represents complete procidentia or vault eversion; the most distal prolapse protrudes to at least (TVL-2) cm

16.3 Case Study: Use of Unique Incision Mesh for Pelvic Organ Prolapse Repair (Real-World Experience)

(a) **Aim and Scope**

In this study we will show the results obtained at our center with one of the most recent devices for the transvaginal correction of female POP, the Restorelle® single-incision mesh (Coloplast, USA). This product was later withdrawn from the market along with other transvaginal prosthetic devices for the correction of POP (April 2019), following its ban by the FDA.

Restorelle® Direct Fix Mesh products incorporate SmartMesh® technology (physiologically compatible ultralight mesh). It provides long-term strength while maintaining the vaginal elasticity of natural tissue. Its placement allows for an anterior sacrospinous ligament approach, using a disposable device (Digitex®) designed to place sutures without direct visualization. The proximal arms of the mesh are sutured to the anterior sacrospinous ligament, and the distal arms of the mesh are sutured to the arch of the pelvic tendinous fascia.

(b) **Study Design, Material, and Methods**

In a retrospective study of patients who underwent surgical correction of POP in the same center between January 2016 and December 2017 with the Restorelle® device, we analyzed demographic variables, prolapse characteristics, associated symptoms, gynecological history, recurrence, and degree of satisfaction taken from the existing medical history. The degree of POP was evaluated according to the Baden-Walker classification. The surgical indication was symptomatic patients with grade ≥2 POP (primary or recurrent). All interventions were performed by a single surgeon after an antibiotic prophylaxis protocol.

(c) **Results of the Study**

We retrospectively analyzed 78 patients operated on at our center with a mean age of 64.2 years (48–78). The comorbidities evaluated were diabetes mellitus (DM), arterial hypertension, and body mass index (BMI), being 21%, 48%, and 27.5 kg/m^2, respectively, and a mean parity of 2.2 births (1–5). Thirty-six percent of our patients had a history of gynecological surgical, the most prevalent being hysterectomy in up to 50% of the operated patients. The most frequently treated prolapse was anterior (72%), followed by posterior (12%), and mixed anterior-posterior (12%), with only one case of apical and posterior prolapse. Of these, four were recurrent prolapses. The most common grade of prolapse was III and IV with a frequency of 54% and 42%, respectively (Table 16.2).

Regarding the functional and clinical results, 50% of the sexually active patients had preoperative dyspareunia, which persisted after the intervention in two patients. Preoperative UI (urinary incontinence) was present in 48%, with urgency, stress UI, and mixed UI in 37%, 31%, and 19%, respectively. Eighteen percent of these patients resolved their UI and 12% had postoperative UI (Table 16.3). We obtained a success rate of 92%, understood as absence of extrusion (6%), pain (3%), or functional recurrence (3%) 6 months after surgery. The anatomic recurrence rate was 9%. The total Clavien-Dindo IIIa complication rate was the most prevalent with 6.4% (extrusion), followed by grade II (3.8%). There were none in group IV or V. Cases of extrusion were resolved on an outpatient basis with local anesthesia. The mean follow-up time was 13.5 months. In general, the patients were satisfied (57.7%) or very satisfied (36%), and only 6.4% of the patients were dissatisfied and none were very dissatisfied.

Table 16.2 Demographic variables and clinical characteristics before surgery

Demographics	Variable value (n = 78)
Age (years)	64.2 (48–78)
BMI (kg/m^2)	27.5 (21.9–33.3)
<25	13 (16.7%)
25–29.9	46 (59%)
>30 27	19 (24.4%)
DM	17 (21.8%)
Arterial hypertension	38 (48.7%)
Clinical history	
Parity	2.2 (1–5)
Previous gynecological operation	28 (36%)
Previous hysterectomy	14 (18%)
Previous POP surgery	4 (5.1%)
Pelvic organ prolapse	
Cystocele	57 (73.1%)
Rectocele	9 (11.5%)
Apex	1 (1.3%)
Mixed	11 (14.1%)
Grade	
Stage 2	2 (2.6%)
Stage 3	43 (55.1%)
Stage 4	33 (42.3%)

Values are presented as median [range] or number (%); *BMI* body mass index, *POP* pelvic organ prolapse

Table 16.3 Results and complications during follow-up

Results	Preoperative	Postoperative
Dyspareunia	21 (26.9%)	2 (2.6%)
Urinary incontinence:	38 (48%)	24 (30.7%)
Urgency	29 (37.2%)	27 (34.6%)
Stress	24 (30.8%)	12 (15.4%)
Mixed	15 (19.2%)	8 (10.3%)
Unmasked UI		9 (11.5%)
Complications		
Extrusion	5 (6.4%)	
Pain	3 (3.8%)	
Functional recurrence	3 (3.8%)	
Anatomical recurrence	7 (9%)	

16.4 Discussion

Surgical techniques can be performed using an abdominal or vaginal approach, depending on the medical history, physical examination, and experience of the surgeon. Laparoscopic sacrocolpopexy is an adequate therapeutic option with a high success rate in 80–100% of cases [33, 34]. However, this technique is not always appropriate, especially for patients who are at high risk for anesthesia, have a multi-operated abdomen, or are in recurrent prolapse. In these cases, a vaginal approach offers an interesting surgical alternative. Transvaginal mesh was developed to maintain the advantage of a vaginal procedure while reducing the risk of recurrent prolapse compared to native tissue repair.

In the short and medium term, our results are similar to the articles published in relation to the success rate of studies with the same device and implantation route (92% in our series vs 80.3%) [22] and different prosthetic devices but with the same implantation route (91.3%) [35], although its comparison is difficult due to the existence of different follow-up times. In our series, the minimum follow-up time was 6 months, while in studies such as the one published by Ferry et al., they only had 3 months of follow-up. We could say that our success rate is slightly higher, despite a longer follow-up. Our good results may be due to the fact that all surgeries were performed by a single surgeon with extensive experience in vaginal POP correction surgery with mesh interposition. If we compare other techniques with a recent boom, such as laparoscopic or robotic sacrocolpopexy [27, 28], there are also no great differences with respect to the success rate, 92% in our series versus 80–100% in those mentioned.

Our anatomical correction rate at 6 months of follow-up was 91%, similar to that found in other studies with this same device, 87.9% [22], or other lightweight devices with the same implantation route, which oscillates between 79 and 96.5% [35–37], although their comparison is equally difficult due to different follow-up times. This same mesh surgery with the same anatomical correction rate criterion was 98.7% at 36 months for De Tayrac et al. [21] and 93.7% for Denancé et al. [38]. Most of the published studies are retrospective [39], and those that are prospective have a follow-up period that is too short. If we compare other techniques such as robotic sacrocolpopexy [27], we find similar rates of absence of anatomic recurrence (95%).

Regarding the complications observed, the mesh extrusion rate in our series was 6.4% compared to 1.3–11.5% published in other studies with lightweight vaginal mesh (28 g/m^2) [19, 21]. In a study published with the Restorelle® device, an extrusion rate of 2.8% was observed, lower than that obtained at our center. Again, this difference can be justified because the postsurgical follow-up at our center was more than double that of the referenced study [22]. Furthermore, in general, we can affirm that it is difficult to compare our data with the literature, as there is great diversity of previously available prosthetic products.

The functional results obtained are similar to those published to date. We can find postoperative dyspareunia in 1.76% of patients in some existing studies after the use of transvaginal mesh [36, 40], a rate very similar to that of our study with only two existing cases. In the case of laparoscopic sacrocolpopexy, there seems to be a lower risk of dyspareunia compared to the transvaginal implantation device (RR 0.39, 95% CI 0.18) [41, 42]. Incontinence rates were lower after correction of the prolapse, mainly stress urinary incontinence improved [40, 43], and 12% of new cases appeared. On the other hand, the appearance of de novo stress urinary incontinence is common in the treatment of prolapse with the use of prosthetic material (RR 1.55, 95% CI 1.02–2.35—anterior colporrhaphy versus use of transvaginal mesh), a fact that patients undergoing this surgery should always be advised of. However, our rate of de novo urinary incontinence with the use of transvaginal mesh is similar to that published with the laparoscopic colposacropexy technique (12%) [41].

Our study presents several limitations. The first of these is the retrospective and nonrandomized nature of our study. Furthermore, all the interventions were carried out by the same surgeon with great experience, which makes it difficult to reproduce these results in other centers and makes it difficult to compare them with other studies. On the other hand, the results of the treatments of non-oncological pathologies usually respond to very high expectations on behalf of the patients, so we can consider a limitation of our study the absence of quality of life questionnaires that assess the impact of success obtained after surgery and possible complications during follow-up.

16.5 Conclusion

In our experience, the Restorelle® device and its transvaginal placement is a safe procedure, with low morbidity and a high satisfaction rate in properly selected patients and in the hands of expert surgeons. Complications are rare and can be resolved by outpatient surgery.

Considering long-term complications is essential to properly weigh the risk-benefit ratio of each procedure, which is why more studies with a longer follow-up period than those currently available in the literature are necessary to judge this type of device with more evidence.

Acknowledgments We have no conflicts of interest.

In this chapter I want to thank the doctors Ph. García-Baquero, Ph. Madurga Patuel, and Ph. Álvarez-Ossorio for their participation as well as the doctors Ph. Ojeda Claro, Ph. Flor Peña, Ph. Agüera Bitaubé, Ph. Ruiz Guerrero, Ph. Rosety Rodríguez, Ph. León Delgado, Ph. Soto Delgado, and Ph. Ledo Cepero for their participation in the related case presented.

References

1. Phillips CH, Anthony F, Benyon C, Monga AK. Collagen metabolism in the uterosacral ligaments and vaginal skin in women with uterine prolapse. BJOG. 2006;113:39–46.
2. Hodgkinson CP. Metallic bead-chain urethrocystography in preoperative and postoperative evaluation of gynecologic urologic problems. Clin Obstet Gynecol. 1978;21:725–30.
3. Barski D, Otto T, Gerullis H. Systematic review and classification of complications after anterior, posterior, apical, and total vaginal mesh implantation for prolapse repair. Surg Technol Int. 2014;24:217.
4. European Commission, Directorate General for Health & Consumers. Opinion on the safety of surgical meshes used in urogynecological surgery. [Internet]. Luxembourg: European Commission; 2015 [citado 12 de octubre de 2019]. Disponible en: http://bookshop.europa.eu/uri?target=EUB:NOTICE:NDAS14005:EN:HTML.
5. Norton PA. Pelvic floor disorders: the role of fascia and ligaments. Clin Obstet Gynecol. 1993;36(4):926–38.
6. DeLancey JO. The anatomy of the pelvic floor. Curr Opin Obstet Gynecol. 1994;6(4):313–6.
7. Handa VLGE, Hendrix S, et al. Progression and remission of pelvic organ prolapse: a longitudinal study of menopausal women. Am J Obstet Gynecol. 2004;190(1):27–32.
8. Aigmueller T, Dungl A, Hinterholzer S, Geiss I, Riss P. An estimation of the frequency of surgery for posthysterectomy vault prolapsed. Int Urogynecol J. 2010;21:299–302.
9. Brown JS, et al. Pelvic organ prolapse surgery in the United States, 1997. Am J Obstet Gynecol. 2002;186(4):712–6.
10. Ellerkmann RM, Cundiff GW, Melick CF, Nihira MA, Leffler K, Bent AE. Correlation of symptoms with location and severity of pelvic organ prolapse. Am J Obstet Gynecol. 2001;185(6):1332–7; discussion 7–8.
11. Barber MD, Brubaker L, Nygaard I, Wheeler TL 2nd, Schaffer J, Chen Z, et al. Defining success after surgery for pelvic organ prolapse. Obstet Gynecol. 2009;114(3):600–9.
12. Madurga Patuel M, et al. Documento de consenso de la asociación española de urología sobre la utilización de mallas en la cirugía del prolapso de órganos pélvicos [Internet]. Spain: Asociación Española de Urología; 2019 [Citado Octubre 2019]. https://www.aeu.es/UserFiles/files/DocuAeuMallasCxPOP2019.pdf.
13. Olsen AL, Smith VJ, Bergstrom JO, Colling JC, Clark AL. Epidemiology of surgically managed pelvic organ prolapse and urinary incontinence. Obstet Gynecol. 1997;89(4):501–6.
14. Weber AM, Walters MD, Piedmonte MR, Ballard LA. Anterior colporrhaphy: a randomized trial of three surgical techniques. Am J Obstet Gynecol. 2001;185(6):1299–304.
15. Denman MGW, Boyles S, Smith V, Edwards R, Clark A. Reoperation rate 10 years after surgically managed pelvic organ prolapse and urinary incontinence. Am J Obstet Gynecol. 2008;198:555.
16. Sand PK, Koduri S, Lobel RW, Winkler HA, Tomezsko J, Culligan PJ, et al. Prospective randomized trial of polyglactin 910 mesh to prevent recurrence of cystoceles and rectoceles. Am J Obstet Gynecol. 2001;184(7):1357–62.
17. Chmielewski L, Walters MD, Weber AM, Barber MD. Reanalysis of a randomized trial of 3 techniques of anterior colporrhaphy using clinically rel-

evant definitions of success. Am J Obstet Gynecol. 2011;205(1):69.e1–8.
18. Julian TM. The efficacy of Marlex mesh in the repair of severe, recurrent vaginal prolapse of the anterior midvaginal wall. Am J Obstet Gynecol. 1996;175(6):1472–5.
19. Maher C, Feiner B, Baessler K, Christmann-Schmid C, Haya N, Marjoribanks J. Transvaginal mesh or grafts compared with native tissue repair for vaginal prolapse. Cochrane Database Syst Rev. 2016;2:CD012079.
20. Altman D, Mikkola TS, Bek KM, Rahkola-Soisalo P, Gunnarsson J, Engh ME, et al. Pelvic organ prolapse repair using the Uphold Vaginal Support System: a 1-year multicenter study. Int Urogynecol J. 2016;27(9):1337–45.
21. De Tayrac R, Brouziyne M, Priou G, Devoldere G, Marie G, Renaudie J. Transvaginal repair of stage III-IV cystocele using a lightweight mesh: safety and 36-month outcome. Int Urogynecol J. 2015;26(8):1147–54.
22. Ferry P, Bertherat P, Gauthier A, Villet R, Del Piano F, Hamid D, Fernandez H, Broux PL, Salet-Lizée D, Vincens E, Ntshaykolo P, Debodinance P, Pocholle P, Thirouard Y, de Tayrac R. Transvaginal treatment of anterior and apical genital prolapses using an Ultra lightweight mesh: Restorelle® Direct Fix™. A retrospective study on feasibility and morbidity. J Gynecol Obstet Hum Reprod. 2018;47(9):443–9.
23. FDA. Urogynecologic surgical mesh: update on the safety and effectiveness of transvaginal placement for pelvic organ prolapse 2011 15/10/2013; (13 July 2011). p. 1–15. http://www.fda.gov/downloads/MedicalDevices/Safety/AlertsandNotices/UCM262760.pdf.
24. Gandhi S, Goldberg RP, Kwon C, Koduri S, Beaumont JL, Abramov Y, et al. A prospective randomized trial using solvent dehydrated fascia lata for the prevention of recurrent anterior vaginal wall prolapse. Am J Obstet Gynecol. 2005;192(5):1649–54.
25. Diwadkar GB, Barber MD, Feiner B, Maher C, Jelovsek JE. Complication and reoperation rates after apical vaginal prolapse surgical repair: a systematic review. Obstet Gynecol. 2009;113(2 Pt 1):367–73.
26. Ow LL, Lim YN, Dwyer PL, Karmakar D, Murray C, Thomas E, et al. Native tissue repair or transvaginal mesh for recurrent vaginal prolapse: what are the long-term outcomes? Int Urogynecol J. 2016;27(9):1313–20.
27. Higgs PJ, Chua HL, Smith AR, editors. Long term review of laparoscopic sacrocolpopexy. England; 2005.
28. Rivoire C, Botchorishvili R, Canis M, Jardon K, Rabischong B, Wattiez A, et al., editors. Complete laparoscopic treatment of genital prolapse with meshes including vaginal promontofixation and anterior repair: a series of 138 patients. United States; 2007.
29. Maher C, Feiner B, Baessler K, Christmann-Schmid C, Haya N, Brown J. Surgery for women with apical vaginal prolapse. Cochrane Database Syst Rev. 2016;10(10):CD012376.
30. Siddiqui NY, Grimes CL, Casiano ER, Abed HT, Jeppson PC, Olivera CK, et al. Mesh sacrocolpopexy compared with native tissue vaginal repair: a systematic review and meta-analysis. Obstet Gynecol. 2015;125(1):44–55.
31. Serati M, Bogani G, Sorice P, Braga A, Torella M, Salvatore S, et al. Robot-assisted sacrocolpopexy for pelvic organ prolapse: a systematic review and meta-analysis of comparative studies. Eur Urol. 2014;66(2):303–18.
32. Swift S, Woodman P, O'Boyle A, Kahn M, Valley M, Bland D, et al. Pelvic Organ Support Study (POSST): the distribution, clinical definition, and epidemiologic condition of pelvic organ support defects. Am J Obstet Gynecol. 2005;192(3):795–806.
33. Lucot J-P, Fritel X, Debodinance P, Bader G, Cosson M, Giraudet G, et al. Étude randomisée comparant la promontofixation coelioscopique à la chirurgie prothé tique par voie vaginale pour le traitement des cystocé les: PROSPERE (PROSthetic PElvic organ prolapse REpair). J Gynécol Obstét Biol Reprod. 2013;42(4):334–41.
34. Park Y-H, Yang SC, Park ST, Park SH, Kim HB. Laparoscopic reconstructive surgery is superior to vaginal reconstruction in the pelvic organ prolapse. Int J Med Sci. 2014;11(11):1082–8.
35. Laso-García IM, Rodríguez-Cabello MA, Jiménez-Cidre MA, Orosa-Andrada A, Carracedo-Calvo D, López-Fando L, Burgos-Revilla FJ. Prospective long-term results, complications and risk factors in pelvic organ prolapse treatment with vaginal mesh. Eur J Obstet Gynecol Reprod Biol. 2017;211:62–7.
36. Hinoul P, Ombelet WU, Burger MP, Roovers J-P. A prospective study to evaluate the anatomic and functional outcome of a transobturator mesh kit (prolift anterior) for symptomatic cystocele repair. J Minim Invasive Gynecol. 2008;15(5):615–20.
37. Khan ZA, Thomas L, Emery SJ. Outcomes and complications of trans-vaginal mesh repair using the ProliftTM kit for pelvic organ prolapse at 4 years median follow-up in a tertiary referral centre. Arch Gynecol Obstet. 2014;290(6):1151–7.
38. Denancé M, Quiboeuf E, Hocké C. Results, safety and patient satisfaction at 6 months of vaginal anterior wall prolapse surgery by transvaginal repair with mesh use. Prog Urol. 2016;26(10):582–8.
39. Unger CA, Barber MD. Vaginal mesh in pelvic reconstructive surgery: controversies, current use, and complications. Clin Obstet Gynecol. 2015;58(4):740–53.
40. Duport C, Duperron C, Delorme E. Anterior and middle pelvic organ prolapse repair using a six tension-free strap low weight transvaginal mesh: long-term retrospective monocentric study of 311 patients. J Gynecol Obstet Hum Reprod. 2019;48(3):143–9.
41. Wei D, Wang P, Niu X, Zhao X. Comparison between laparoscopic uterus/sacrocolpopexy and total pelvic floor reconstruction with vaginal mesh for the treat-

ment of pelvic organ prolapse. J Obstet Gynaecol Res. 2019;45(4):915–22.
42. Coolen AWM, van IJsselmuiden MN, van Oudheusden AMJ, Veen J, van Eijndhoven HWF, Mol BWJ, Roovers JP, Bongers MY. Laparoscopic sacrocolpopexy versus vaginal sacrospinous fixation for vaginal vault prolapse, a randomized controlled trial: SALTO-2 trial, study protocol. BMC Womens Health. 2017;17(1):52.
43. Van Raalte HM, Lucente VR, Molden SM, Haff R, Murphy M. One-year anatomic and quality-of-life outcomes after the Prolift procedure for treatment of posthysterectomy prolapse. Am J Obstet Gynecol. 2008;199(6):694.e1–6.

17

Sacrouterine Ligament Augmentation with Vaginal Approach

Marijan Lužnik and Jan Lužnik

17.1 Introduction

The paired uterosacral ligaments (USLs; or Latin 'ligamenta sacro-uterina') are the centre of numerous pathophysiological considerations, most notably in relation to chronic pelvic pain syndrome (CPPS) and pelvic floor dysfunction (PFD) due to pelvic organ prolapse (POP) [1–4].

Classical vaginal surgical techniques with loose USLs plication have an increasing failure rate with time [5]. In a follow-up study evaluating the long-term results of several classical vaginal surgical techniques, the reported recurrence rate of POP was around 30% [6]. Moreover, the authors concluded that for CPPS, the long-term surgical outcomes were superior if the USLs were reinforced with a polypropylene tape, which was precisely inserted into the position of the USLs [7]. Based on this knowledge, we developed a vaginal surgical technique for USLs augmentation using anterior transobturator-tapes (ATOTs) (Fig. 17.1) for correction of apical and anterior vaginal prolapse (Figs. 17.2a and 17.6a). With ATOTs and uterosacral ligaments augmentation (USLA), we are able to restore the physiologic natural anatomy using a minimally invasive approach.

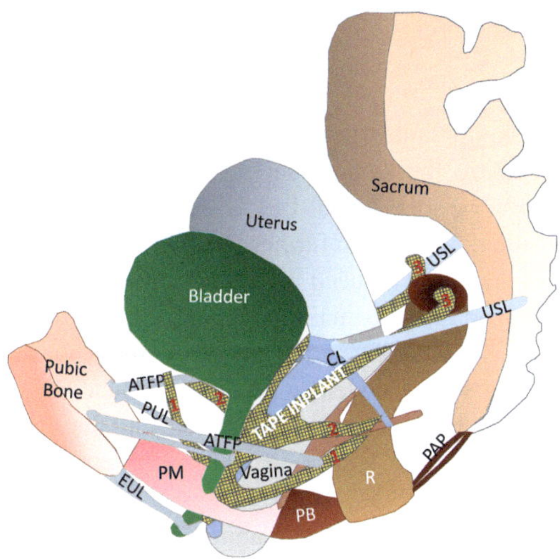

Fig. 17.1 Schematic representation showing postoperative mesh position; arcus tendineus fascia pelvis (ATFP), cardinal ligament (CL), external urethral ligament (EUL), perineal body (PB), perineal membrane (PM), postanal plate (PAP), pubourethral ligament (PUL), rectum (R), uterosacral ligament (USL)

17.2 Surgical Method Description

Rupnik, Starič, Norčič and Lukanović

Ljubljana, Slovenia

Based on our extensive surgical experience with 600 vaginal procedures using individually cut

M. Lužnik (✉)
General Hospital Slovenj Gradec, Slovenj Gradec, Slovenia
e-mail: marijan@mediarh.si

J. Lužnik
University Medical Centre, Maribor, Slovenia
e-mail: jan.luznik@ukc-mb.si

F. Dökmeci, D. E. E. Rizk (eds.), *Insights Into Incontinence and the Pelvic Floor*,
https://doi.org/10.1007/978-3-030-94174-1_17

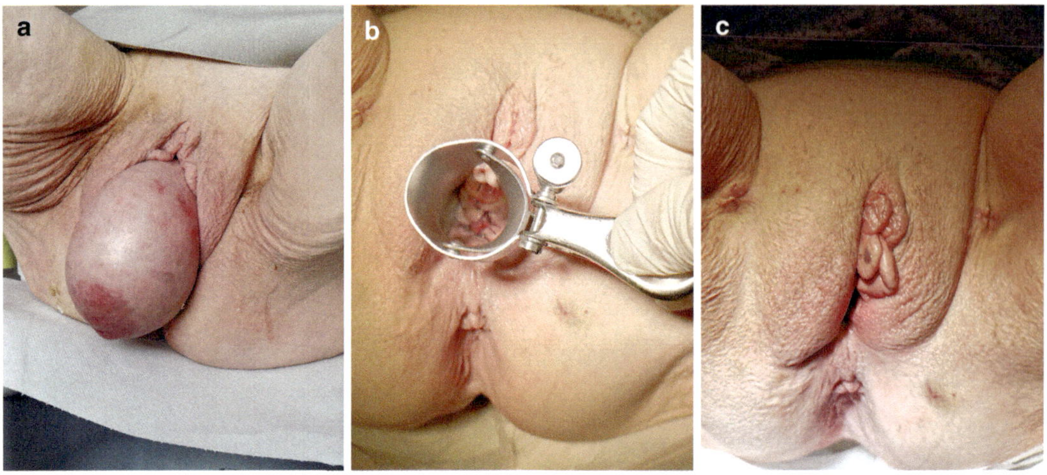

Fig. 17.2 Patient with total utero-vaginal prolapse before (**a**) and after pelvic floor reconstruction (**b**, **c**) (total vaginal hysterectomy and USLA with ATOTs)

mesh implants (performed between 2000 and 2016 by the same surgeon) for correction of POP, we developed the USLA with ATOTs method. In order to further improve our method, we gradually reduced the mesh size and in 2016 dropped the proximal (deep) pair of transobturator arms, which were then used for augmentation of USLs. The Slovenian National Medical Ethics Committee approval was obtained, and the study followed the tenets of the Declaration of Helsinki.

The correction of vaginal prolapse with ATOTs and USLA is performed with a simultaneous obliteration of cavum Douglasi (cD) and with an excision of redundant peritoneum, which is often performed after a total vaginal hysterectomy that is made in the same procedure. When ATOTs with USLA is used for correction of vaginal cuff prolapse, it is important to perform culdotomy with obliteration of cD and excision of redundant peritoneum. In cases without hysterectomy, 50% of the prolapse correction of the uterus and anterior vaginal wall was made with simultaneous excision of elongated cervix uteri and in some cases also with culdotomy and obliteration of cD with excision of redundant peritoneum. Non-absorbable polypropylenes mesh (60 g/m^2) 10 cm × 15 cm was used to create individually cut tape implants (Fig. 17.3a–c). Two pairs of tapes were inserted transobturatorly (under urethra and bladder neck) through 1 dermal incision in the femoral-genital folds on each side (Figs. 17.4 and 17.6l–n), and both pairs of transobturator tapes are completely separated by a tissue septum, until a colpotomy opening under the urethra and a colpotomy opening under the bladder neck is performed (Fig. 17.4a, b). Two apical tapes for USLA had been individually moved laterally into the vesicovaginal space before being inserted completely tension free in the direction of both uterosacral ligaments (Figs. 17.5 and 17.6o, p).

17.3 Clinical Outcomes

Between January 2017 and August 2020, 63 corrections of apical and anterior vaginal prolapse stage II–IV by ICS system (median age 61 years [36–79 years]) were performed with ATOTs and USLA by the same experienced surgeon. The preoperative vaginal status was assessed as stage II–

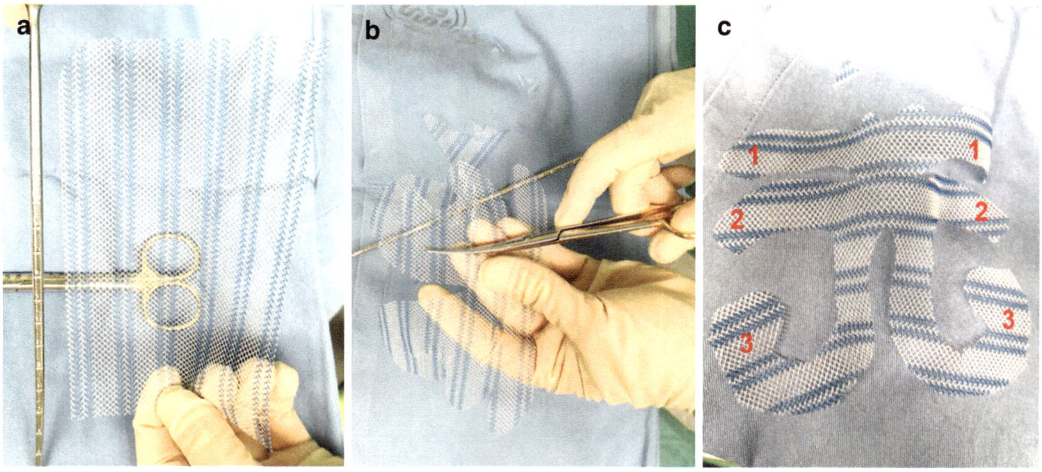

Fig. 17.3 Non-absorbable polypropylenes mesh (60 g/m^2) 10 cm × 15 cm (**a**). Cutting of tapes (**b**). Self-cut tapes (**c**)

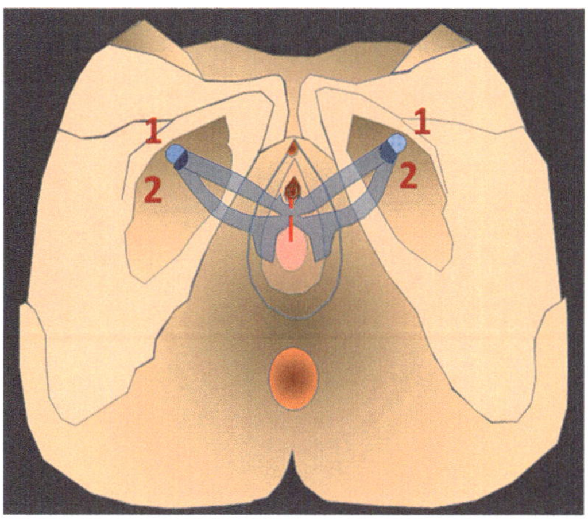

Fig. 17.4 Two pairs of tapes were inserted transobturatorly

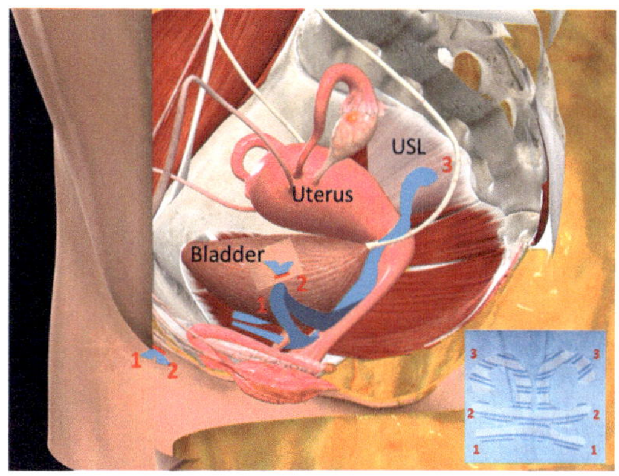

Fig. 17.5 Left apical tape (3) in lateral vesicovaginal space and inserted in the direction of left uterosacral ligament

IV by the ICS system. ATOTs with USLA were used with or without vaginal hysterectomy (49 and 8 cases, respectively). In six cases, ATOTs with USLA were used for correction of vaginal cuff prolapse (Table 17.1). The postoperative ICS stage was assessed on day 5, 3 months, and 12 months after surgery. Urine, faecal continence, and sexual function were evaluated using a questionnaire 12 months postoperatively.

All patients had an ICS stage zero (Fig. 17.2b, c) on postoperative day 5. Sixty out of 63 patients (95%) had an ICS stage zero 3 months after surgery (4 patients had not yet had a postoperative examination after 3 months). Fifty out of 63 patients (79%) have already completed 1 year follow-up and remained ICS stage zero, without any pelvic pain. During the first year of follow-up, no serious complications were observed. We did not have any intraoperative complication. Until now no recurrence of POP was observed. In three cases (5%), postoperative complications were observed (two implant material exposures and one patient developed de novo overactive bladder (OAB) symptoms with borderline urine retention (60 mL)). A small denuded tape part was excised under local anaesthesia and left open

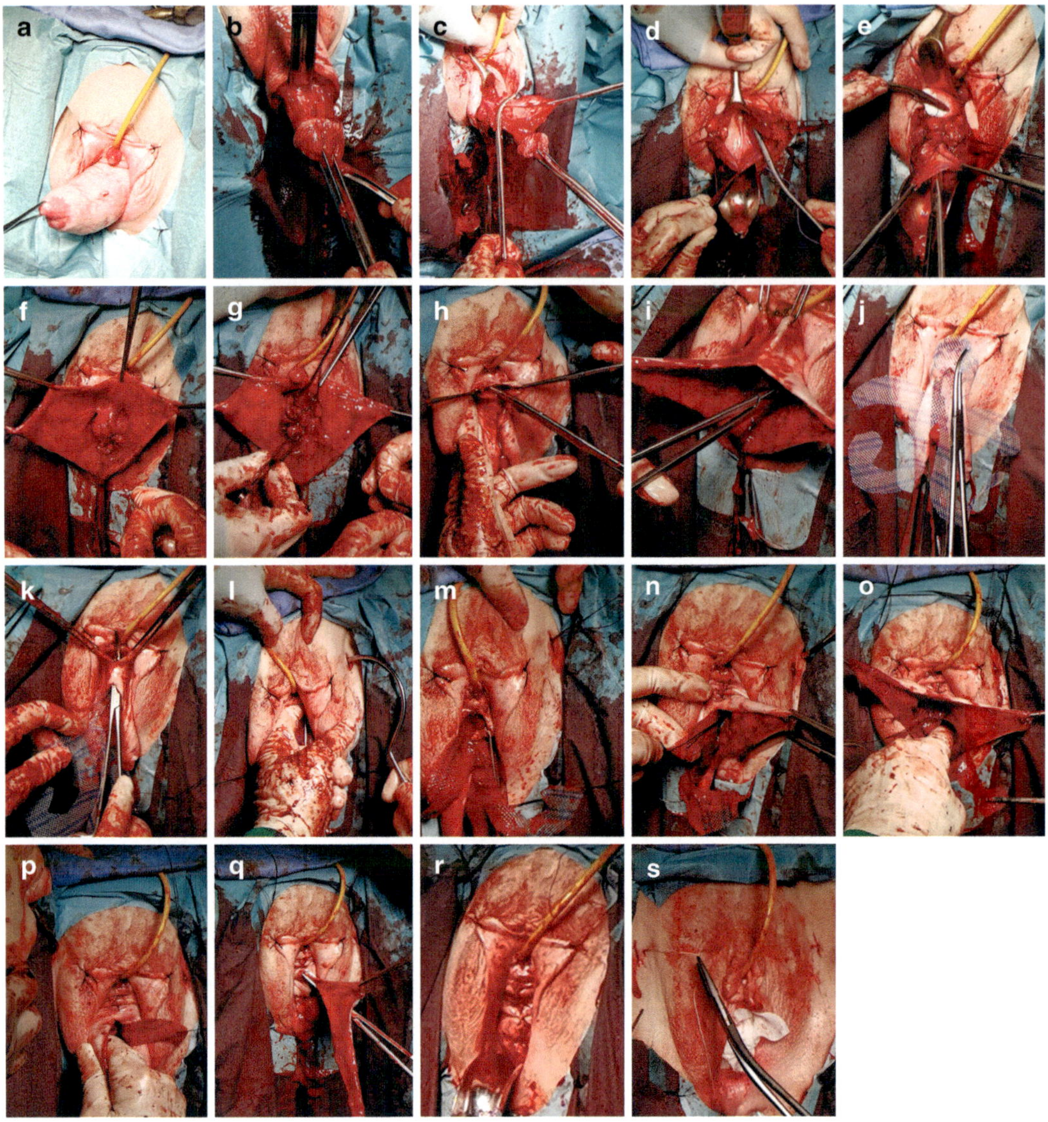

Fig. 17.6 Patient with total utero-vaginal prolapse at the beginning of the procedure (**a**); dissection of cervix uteri (**b**); hysterectomy (**c**). The first needle puncture of circular suture of peritoneum is placed cranially and away from the edge of the operative wound (**d**). Excision of redundant peritoneum of cavum Douglasi (**e**). The last layer of vesical sutures—cystorrhaphy (**f**). Sutures of endopelvic membrane of cavum Douglasi (**g**). After excision of urethral caruncle follows 10 mm long suburethral incision of vagina and the dissection of the anterior vaginal wall between urethra and the pubic ramus on the right site to create tunnel for tape 1 (**h**). The dissection of the anterior vaginal wall was continued between the bladder and the pelvic side wall in a blunt or sharp way laterally until the tendinous arch of the pelvic fascia on left site to create a tunnel for tape 2 (**i**). Self-cut tape implant before insertion (**j**). Insertion of both tapes 1 (left and right) in suburethral incision (**k**). Puncture 'outside in' with a metal-eyed needle hook transobturatorly for insertion of tape 1 on left (**l**). Left tape 1 was inserted transobturatorly (**m**). Suburethral incision is sutured after both tapes 1 are inserted. Follows puncture with a metal hook transobturatorly for tape 2 on left (**n**). Both tapes 1 and 2 are inserted. Follows blunt dissection of the left USL away from the surrounding subperitoneal tissue with index finger (**o**). Dissection of the subperitoneal tissue in direction of right USL and insertion of tapes 3 (**p**). Excision of redundant vagina wall (**q**). Incision of vagina is sutured (**r**). Suture of right cutaneous incision on the left side is already done (**s**)

Table 17.1 The number of ATOTs + USLA performed for POP correction

	Vaginal cuff prolapse	Without hysterectomy	With hysterectomy	Together
ATOTs + USLA	6	8	49	63
Median age	66	50	62	61
Range	**54–77**	**42–62**	**36–79**	**36–79**

USLA Uterosacral ligament augmentation, *ATOTs* Anterior transobturator tapes

to heal spontaneously (no vaginal sutures were used). The OAB symptoms and urine retention were successfully managed by mechanically cutting the suburethral tape. After intervention, urine incontinence symptoms did not reoccur.

17.4 Interpretation of Clinical Outcomes

In contrast to other currently used methods for the treatment of pelvic organ prolapse, where the apical tapes are attached directly, around or through the sacrospinal ligament, reconstruction of the vagina and strengthening of the uterosacral ligaments [7] with ATOTs is performed by completely tension-free insertion of two apical tapes in the direction of both uterosacral ligaments. Therefore, during sexual intercourse, tape implants remain far away from the sacrospinal ligaments (outside the penetration line during sexual intercourse), which not only successfully reduces the risk of postoperative dyspareunia but also reduces the rate of other postoperative complications (e.g. extrusion of tape material) to rate of TVT-O procedures. The aesthetic advantage of our procedure is provided by one skin incision or a stab wound hidden in the femoral-genital folds on the left and right side. Both pairs of transobturator tapes are inserted separately through the same skin incision on the right and left sides and then are completely separated by a tissue septum, until colpotomy opening under the urethra and under the bladder neck (Figs. 17.4 and 17.5). It is important that the suburethral and subvesical part of two anterior tapes remain in the medial part connected. This connection is covered by the vaginal wall, which was not interrupted at the anterior colpotomy, which is performed with two incisions. Therefore, the suburethral and subvesical portions of both anterior tapes retain flattened in the shape of the tape and cannot be twisted into a cord until they pass through the inner transobturator membrane and muscle. This provides excellent support to the urethra and eliminates the risk of postoperative stress urinary incontinence in cases of occult urethral insufficiency [8]. Transobturator tapes connect both tendon arches (arcus tendineus fascia pelvis) and serve as a good anchor for apical tapes that run individually laterally in the paravesical space before being inserted loosely upward, parallel to the USLs (Figs. 17.1 and 17.5). Vaginal reconstruction by strengthening the USLs can also be successfully used to support the pelvic organs in the case of a lateral defect to the pubocervical fascia and in the case of damage to the apical cardinal and uterosacral ligaments. Reinforcement of level 1 also with simultaneously obliteration of cavum Douglasi and excision of redundant peritoneum is a good prevention against enterocele. Reconstruction of abnormalities on level 2 and 3 with classical colpoperineoplasty and rectorrhaphy is rarely necessary to be used to restore the natural anatomy.

17.5 Conclusion

Apical and anterior vaginal prolapse repair with self-cut ATOTs with USLA is safe and offers excellent short- and long-term anatomical and functional results. Further studies are required to assess the long-term effectiveness of the approach.

Acknowledgement Both authors contributed to the chapter and to the presented case.

Conflict of Interest None.

Financial Support None.

References

1. Martius H. Lerbuch der Gynäkologye. Stuttgart: Thieme; 1946.
2. Petros PE, Ulmsten U. The posterior fornix syndrome: a multiple syndrome complex of pelvic pain and abnormal urinary symptoms deriving from laxity in the posterior fornix. Scand J Urol Nephrol. 1993;27(Suppl 153 part IV):89–93.
3. Petros PE. Severe chronic pelvic pain in women may be caused by ligamentous laxity in the posterior fornix of the vagina. Aust N Z J Obstet Gynaecol. 1996;36(3):351–4.
4. Abendstein B, Brugger BA, Furtschegger A, Rieger M, Petros PE. Role of the uterosacral ligaments in the causation of rectal intussusception, abnormal bowel emptying, and fecal incontinence—a prospective study. J Pelviperineology. 2008;27:118–21.
5. Margulies RU, Rogers MA, Morgan DM. Outcomes of transvaginal uterosacral ligament suspension: systematic review and meta-analysis. Am J Obstet Gynecol. 2010;202(2):124–34.
6. Olsen A, Smith V, Bergstrom JO, Colling JC, Clark AL. Epidemiology of surgically managed pelvic organ prolapse and urinary incontinence. Obstet Gynecol. 1997;89:501–6.
7. Goeschen K. Role of uterosacral ligaments in the causation and cure of chronic pelvic pain syndrome. Pelviperineology. 2015;34:2–17.
8. Matsuoka PK, Pacetta AM, Baracat EC, Haddad JM. Should prophylactic anti-incontinence procedures be performed at the time of prolapse repair? Systematic review. Int Urogynecol J. 2015;26(2):187–93.

The Manchester-Fothergill Operation

18

Marino Romero Ramírez, Gemma López Gómiz, Jordi Moreno Sánchez, Beatriu Roca Comella, and Albert Font Vilamitjana

Pelvic organ prolapse (POP) is a very common disfunction that affects up to 50% of the women around the world [1]. It could have a huge impact on their quality of life. Advanced age, number of deliveries, vaginal delivery mode and high body mass index are the most important risk factors for POP [2]. Different vaginal compartments can be involved in POP, being the prolapse of anterior vaginal wall (cystocele) the most common form, followed by posterior vaginal prolapse (rectocele) and apical prolapse (uterine or vaginal vault prolapse).

Manchester-Fothergill procedure is an old technique to treat the POP described for the first time at the end of XIX century by Dr. Archibald Donald. At the beginning, this procedure consisted on the amputation of the cervix associated to an extensive anterior colporrhaphy and a colpoperineorrhaphy. In 1921, Dr. W.E. Fothergill proposed a modified technique consisting on the suture of the paracolpos and cardinal ligaments in front of the cervix, leading to a better suspension of the stump of the cervix [3].

The main indications of this procedure are (1) women with cervical elongation with few or no significative uterine body prolapse and (2) premenopausal women who want to preserve their uterus or their reproductive function.

In spite of being a fast technique with no admission required, with good results and few complications, it has been abandoned in many hospitals, probably due to a generational replacement issue.

M. Romero Ramírez (✉) · G. López Gómiz
J. Moreno Sánchez · B. Roca Comella
A. Font Vilamitjana
Department of Obstetrics and Gynecology, Consorci Sanitari de Terrassa, Terrassa, Spain
e-mail: mromeror@cst.cat; glopez@cst.cat; 30761jms@comb.cat; broca@cst.cat; afont@cst.cat

18.1 Case Study: The Manchester Operation—Our Experience at Regional Hospital of Terrassa

A 3 years follow-up of the Manchester-Fothergill procedure for cervical elongation treatment.

We designed a retrospective observational study with a cohort of 45 women who underwent the Manchester-Fothergill procedure (MP) at Consorci Sanitari de Terrassa (Barcelona, Spain) from 2013 to 2016. We did a 3-year follow-up.

We included women that consulted to our pelvic floor unit because of a symptomatic POP. All of these women were evaluated by an expert clinician specialist in pelvic floor disfunctions by pelvic examination with vaginal speculum and bimanual exam. The main criteria to propose to the patient a MP was the presence of a third grade apical prolapse due to cervical elongation but with mild or inexistent uterine body prolapse in absence of uterine pathology. We also included patients who, besides MP, required an anterior

F. Dökmeci, D. E. E. Rizk (eds.), *Insights Into Incontinence and the Pelvic Floor*,
https://doi.org/10.1007/978-3-030-94174-1_18

and/or a posterior colporrhaphy and/or a tension-free vaginal tape for stress urinary incontinence. Moreover, one of the patients also underwent a laparoscopic bilateral tubal occlusion as a contraceptive method.

All the patients were operated on in our outpatient surgical unit. No admission was initially required because of the kind of surgery they underwent.

In our hospital we are performing a modified Manchester-Fothergill technique: (1) permeabilization of cervical canal with a paediatric Foley catheter; (2) pericervical incision and dissection of the vaginal mucosa from the cervix; (3) anterior colpotomy and liberation of vesicouterine ligaments; (4) clamping, section and ligature of both uterosacral and cardinal ligaments; (5) amputation of the cervix; (6) Sturmdorf suture covering the posterior lip of the amputated cervix with the vaginal flap; (7) fixation of both uterosacral ligaments with a suture to the anterior surface of the cervix; (8) Sturmdorf suture covering the anterior lip of the amputated cervix; and (9) anterior and/or posterior colpoperineorrhaphy if required.

The aim of this study is to evaluate the clinical characteristics, effectiveness and complications of the surgical treatment of cervical elongation through MP.

All data was collected in a Microsoft Access 2007® database. We used SPSS Statistics version 26 (Microsoft®) for the statistical analysis. For the descriptive analysis, we calculated percentages and absolute values for the nominal variables and average, median, standard deviation, ranks, percentiles and 95% confidence interval for ordinal variables.

We included 45 patients who underwent a MP. The demographic and characteristics of the participants is summarized in Table 18.1. Mean age was 47.9 ± 8.2 years, parity 1.9 ± 0.7 births, and average body mass index 25.8 kg/m^2 (Table 18.1).

All patients underwent ambulatory surgery, except one of them who was admitted because of an auricular fibrillation detected during the intervention, being the only intraoperative complication we had which was not related with the technique.

Table 18.1 Demographic and characteristics of the participants and the Manchester-Fothergill procedure intervention (percent or mean ± standard deviation)

Women (*n*)	45
Age (years)	47.9 ± 8.23
Body mass index (kg/m^2)	25.8 ± 6.35
Parity (births)	1.9 ± 0.72
Length of surgery (min)	49 ± 16.63
Ambulatory surgery (*n* (%))	
Yes	44 (97.8%)
No	1 (2.2%)
Kind of anaesthesia (*n* (%))	
Spinal	30 (66.7%)
General balanced with gases	11 (24.4%)
General intravenous	4 (8.9%)

The average length of the surgery was 49 min. From all surgeries, 71.1% were a MP alone, while the rest were associated with a colpoperineorrhaphy (20.0%), a tension-free vaginal tape (6.7%) and a laparoscopic tubal sterilization (2.2%).

Regarding the kind of anaesthesia, 66.7% of the women received spinal anaesthesia, 24.4% general balanced with gases and 8.9% general intravenous anaesthesia.

As shown in Fig. 18.1, 1 month after the surgery ($n = 45$), we found that 31 patients (68.8%) had no complications and 14 (31.1%) had minor postoperative complications from which 6 of them reported pain. This pain may be related with the plicature of the uterosacral ligaments. Two reported few and limited vaginal bleeding (no intervention needed to stop the bleeding) and two stress urinary incontinence (one of them was one of the suburethral tape which failed, and the other one was an anterior colporrhaphy with an occult stress incontinence). Two women presented low urinary tract infection. One of them had a mild urinary retention and another one a surgical wound infection which was solved with topical antibiotics.

At the 6-month check-up, 32 patients came to the follow-up visit. From them, 84.3% were totally asymptomatic, two of them still reported pain, two had surgical wound granuloma in the

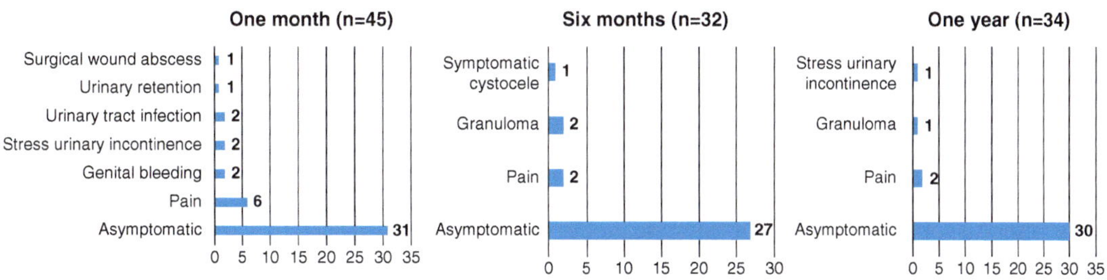

Fig. 18.1 Follow-up after procedure

stump of the cervix that was cauterized with silver nitrate, and one had a symptomatic third grade cystocele.

At the annual check-up (n = 34), 91.2% were asymptomatic, two patients reported persistence of pain (which finally was solved with pelvic floor rehabilitation in few months), one had a persistence of asymptomatic granuloma in the cervical stump, and one reported persistence of stress urinary incontinence.

At 2 years check-up (n = 17) and 3 years check-up (n = 10), all patients reported being asymptomatic and satisfied with the results of the surgery.

No case of cervical stenosis was observed.

18.2 Discussion

Manchester-Fothergill procedure was described for the first time in late nineteenth century and perfectioned in the early twentieth century [3]. This classic technique for the surgical treatment of POP has been abandoned in many hospitals because it has been considered obsolete. However, it is still included in most of the current guidelines as a successful technique to treat the middle compartment prolapse [4, 5] and is a technique that we are still using nowadays in our hospital.

A recent meta-analysis compared uterine preservation surgery versus hysterectomy in pelvic organ prolapse treatment. They concluded that MP should be chosen over vaginal hysterectomy with native tissue suspension because it resulted in a shorter surgery length and less estimated blood loss (grade of recommendation 2B) [6]. In our study, the average length of the surgery was 49 min. Other authors that compared MP with vaginal hysterectomy for the treatment of POP concluded that MP seems to be an effective procedure in terms of anatomical outcomes as compared with vaginal hysterectomy for POP caused by true cervical elongation [7]. Recognizing a true cervical elongation is a challenge, and this is the reason why it is essential to perform an accurate pelvic examination using the Pelvic Organ Prolapse Quantification (POP-Q).

Beyond the fact that MP provides adequate mid-compartment support [8], a prospective study concluded that MP has excellent subjective results without significative impact in the sexual outcomes, especially in dyspareunia de novo [9]. From this cohort, 96% reported being asymptomatic at the annual check-up. We found that only two patients reported pain at the annual check-up, probably because of the suture of uterosacral ligaments. This pain was solved by pelvic floor rehabilitation.

Regarding the risk of cervical and uterine malignancies during follow-up after MP, Engelbredt et al. found in a cohort of 299 women who underwent a MP that only 10 women (3.3%) needed hysterectomy after MP for different reasons. They all had normal histology. From the 159 women who underwent Pap smear tests after MP, only 1 of them was diagnosed of a cervical intraepithelial neoplasia 1 (CIN 1), which had turned normal after 6 months [10]. No cases of malignance histology were observed in the anatomopathological evaluation of the patients from our study.

18.3 Conclusion

Manchester-Fothergill operation is a fast and safe technique not requiring admission. The only intraoperative complication that was observed was not related with the technique. There were only minor short- and long-term complications that were completely solved in all cases within the first 2 years. No case of cervical stenosis was observed.

Manchester procedure showed good results and few and minor complications. This technique should be considered and offered for the treatment of uterine prolapse in selected patients who wish to keep their uterus.

Acknowledgements Marino Romero Ramírez, Gemma López Gómiz, Jordi Moreno Sánchez and Albert Font Vilamitjana contributed to the presented case and chapter. We acknowledge the contribution of Beatriu Roca Comella to this chapter.

Conflict of Interests The authors certify that no actual or potential conflict of interest in relation to this article exists.

References

1. Cooper J, Annappa M, Dracocardos D, Cooper W, Muller S, Mallen C. Prevalence of genital prolapse symptoms in primary care: a cross-sectional survey. Int Urogynecol J. 2015;26(4):505–10.
2. Vergeldt TFM, Weemhoff M, IntHout J, Kluivers KB. Risk factors for pelvic organ prolapse and its recurrence: a systematic review. Int Urogynecol J. 2015;26(11):1559–73.
3. Fothergill BWE, Edin MD. The end results of vaginal operations for genital prolapse. J Obs Gyn Brit Emp. 1921;28:251–5.
4. National Institute for Health and Care Excellence (NICE). Urinary incontinence and pelvic organ prolapse in women: management. Obstet Gynecol. 2019.
5. Maher C, Feiner B, Baessler K, Schmid C. Surgical management of pelvic organ prolapse in women. In: Maher C, editor. Cochrane database of systematic reviews. Chichester: John Wiley & Sons, Ltd; 2013. p. CD004014.
6. Meriwether KV, Antosh DD, Olivera CK, Kim-Fine S, Balk EM, Murphy M, et al. Uterine preservation vs hysterectomy in pelvic organ prolapse surgery: a systematic review with meta-analysis and clinical practice guidelines. Am J Obstet Gynecol. 2018;219(2):129–146.e2.
7. Park YJ, Kong MK, Lee J, Kim EH, Bai SW. Manchester operation: an effective treatment for uterine prolapse caused by true cervical elongation. Yonsei Med J. 2019;60(11):1074–80.
8. Singh P, Lim Wei Liang B, Han HC. A retrospective observational study on the outcomes and efficacy of the Manchester procedure as a uterine-sparing surgery for uterovaginal prolapse. J Gynecol Surg. 2018;34(6):275–8.
9. Oversand SH, Staff AC, Borstad E, Svenningsen R. The Manchester procedure: anatomical, subjective and sexual outcomes. Int Urogynecol J. 2018;29(8):1193–201.
10. Engelbredt K, Glavind K, Kjaergaard N. Development of cervical and uterine malignancies during follow-up after Manchester-Fothergill procedure. J Gynecol Surg. 2020;36(2):60–4.

19 Vaginal Hysterectomy and Pelvic Floor Repair with Local Anesthesia

Grigoriadis Themos, Zacharakis Dimitrios, Kalantzis Christos, Hatzilia Sophia, Pitsouni Elieni, Douskos Athanasios, Valsamidis Dimitris, and Athanasiou Stavros

19.1 Introduction

Vaginal hysterectomy (VH) is currently recommended by various medical societies through position statements and other commentary reports as the preferred approach for the surgical treatment of benign gynecological disease [1–4]. Moreover, the traditional surgical management for pelvic organ prolapse (POP) often includes VH with or without pelvic floor repair (PFR) [1]. Given the aging population and the higher prevalence of POP in the elderly, the number of women who will undergo VH for POP is estimated to grow dramatically over the next years [5].

Conventionally, VH is performed under either general or regional (spinal and/or epidural) anesthesia. It is known that both surgery and general anesthesia exert comparatively greater adverse effects on the elderly than on younger patients [6]. This is due to a progressive loss of the functional reserves that may render them more susceptible to anesthesia-mediated perioperative morbidity [6]. Furthermore, regional anesthesia also has known contraindications such as certain preexisting neurological disease, severe thrombocytopenia or coagulopathy, and severe mitral or aortic stenosis, pathologies that may have an increased incidence in elderly patients [7].

Local anesthesia has been utilized as an alternative anesthetic method for the surgical correction of POP [8–15]. The advantages of local anesthesia over both regional and general anesthesia techniques are well documented [16]. More specifically, local anesthesia has been shown to have minimal interference with homeostasis; a lower risk of postoperative nausea, vomiting, delirium, and cognitive dysfunction; need for postoperative analgesia; and an earlier fulfillment of discharge criteria [16]. To date, the use of local anesthesia for performing minor gynecological surgeries is becoming more popular aiming to improve patient recovery and to reduce institutional costs. In such cases, the combination of local anesthesia with conscious intravenous (iv) sedation has been shown to relieve patients' intraoperative distress and increase patients' comfort [8–13]. The available evidence on the use of local anesthesia is more extensive for relatively minor urogynecological procedures which do not require access to the peritoneum such as the placement of midurethral slings. However, only a few published studies report the feasibility of local anesthesia for more complex surgical procedures including VH [14, 15].

G. Themos (✉) · Z. Dimitrios · K. Christos · H. Sophia · P. Elieni · D. Athanasios · V. Dimitris · A. Stavros
Urogynecology Unit, National and Kapodistrian University, Athens, Greece
e-mail: dimivals@otenet.gr

F. Dökmeci, D. E. E. Rizk (eds.), *Insights Into Incontinence and the Pelvic Floor*,
https://doi.org/10.1007/978-3-030-94174-1_19

19.2 Literature Review

The use of local anesthesia for performing VH was firstly described by Sheth and Malpani [14] in 1992. This was a retrospective case series of 54 selected patients who underwent VH under local anesthesia within a period of 18 years (1970–1988). This study was mainly focused in the intraoperative technique of anesthesia and patient management and did not report any postoperative assessment data with the exception of a prolonged postoperative hospitalization (7 days or more).

In 1995 Miklos et al. [8] published a retrospective case series of 20 elderly patients undergoing minor vaginal reconstructive surgeries (anterior and posterior colporrhaphies, enterocele repair, and LeFort colpocleisis) under local anesthesia with sedation due to various medical contraindications for a general anesthesia. The authors commented that surgical correction of severe pelvic organ relaxation could be performed rapidly and safely using local anesthesia, although no cases of VH were included in this study.

In a recently published study, Axelson et al. [9] reported 80 cases of anterior repair under local anesthesia with i.v. sedation finding high rates (95.2%) of patient satisfaction. Moreover, Buchsbaum GM et al. [11] reported on 87 consecutive vaginal reconstructive procedures, including anterior and posterior colporrhapies, enterocele repairs, and colpocleises, performed under local anesthesia with i.v. sedation, with and without concomitant anti-incontinence procedures. Subsequently the same author [12] reported on more complex vaginal reconstructive surgery including either vaginal sacrospinous ligament suspension or vaginal paravaginal defect repair although all cases needing VH were excluded from this study. In this case series [12], all women (100%) reported being very satisfied from local anesthesia with sedation during their surgery.

The abovementioned studies evaluated the feasibility of local anesthesia for relatively minor vaginal reconstructive procedures. Athanasiou et al. [15] evaluated the feasibility of performing VH and pelvic floor repair (PFR) under local anesthesia and i.v. conscious sedation for women presenting with advanced POP. In this single center prospective case-control study, the "standard care" group consisted of 20 patients who underwent VH and PFR under a combined spinal-epidural (CSE) block, whereas the "local anesthesia" group consisted of 20 patients who underwent VH and PFR under local anesthesia and i.v. sedation. Primary outcomes included the intensity of postoperative pain (measured by a 10-cm visual analog scale [10 cm VAS, ranging from not at all, 0, to the most excruciating pain, 10]) and the percentage of patients with moderate/severe pain (defined as pain score ≥ 4 on the 10-cm VAS). Secondary outcomes included percentage of patients who used opioids, incidence of nausea/vomiting, level of sedation, and patient satisfaction rate. The study found that median pain intensity at rest was significantly lower in the local anesthesia group at 2 h, 4 h, and 8 h postoperatively. The percentage of women with moderate/severe pain was also significantly lower in the "local anesthesia" group compared to the "standard care" group (15% vs 61%, respectively, OR 0.11 (95% CI: 0.02–0.53)). The percentage of participants needing opioids in the postoperative period for additional pain control was statistically significant lower for the local anesthesia group (35% vs 95%, $p = 0.002$). Finally, patients of the "local anesthesia" group had statistically significant shorter time to first mobilization and shorter duration of postoperative hospitalization and reported higher levels of satisfaction.

Another study [16] evaluated the effect of local infiltration with ropivacaine for controlling postoperative pain in women undergoing VH and PFR for advanced POP under combined spinal-epidural (CSE) block. The abstract of this study was presented in the VI MIPS Annual Meeting in Barcelona, 25–27 April 2019, with the title **Intraoperative Local Infiltration with Ropivacaine 0.5%, in Women Undergoing Vaginal Hysterectomy and Pelvic Floor Repair: Randomized Double-Blind Placebo-Controlled Trial**, with authors Themos Grigoriadis, Christos Kalantzis, Dimitris Zacharakis, Sophia Hatzilia, Eleni Pitsouni, Athanasios Douskos, Dimitris Valsamidis, and Stavros Athanasiou.

19.3 Case Study

(a) **Aim and Scope**

Local infiltration with anesthetics at the surgical site blocks peripheral sensory nerves with low or absent systematic side effects. Nevertheless, it is unclear whether patients undergoing VH and pelvic floor repair for POP under CSE block may benefit from local infiltration with ropivacaine 0.5%. The aim of this study was to evaluate the effect of intraoperative local infiltration with ropivacaine 0.5% on postoperative pain in patients with symptomatic POP stage > II undergoing VH and pelvic floor repair. Specifically, women receiving local ropivacaine infiltration in the round ligaments (RL), the uterosacral ligaments (USL), and the perineal body (PB) were compared with women receiving placebo infiltration at the same sites.

(b) **Study Design and Material Methods**

This is a double-blind randomized 1:1 placebo-controlled trial included 59 women.

Eligible participants were allocated at random to the ropivacaine group or the placebo group by an independent anesthesiologist (HS) who was not involved in any other part of the study. The ropivacaine group received an infiltration of 30 mL ropivacaine 0.5% [5 mL in RL and 5 mL in USL (bilaterally), and 10 mL in PB], while the placebo group received an infiltration of 30 mL placebo solution (N/S 0.9%) [5 mL in RL and 5 mL in USL (bilaterally) and 10 mL in PB].

A patient-controlled analgesia (PCA) pump was placed in all participants, containing 40 mg morphine (0.5 mg/mL) plus 8 mg ondansetron (0.1 mg/mL). PCA was started after the end of surgery with a demand dose of morphine 1 mg i.v., a lockout period of 7 min after each bolus, and a maximum allowed dose of 16 mg/2 h. In addition, all participants received metoclopramide 10 mg/12 h i.v., ranitidine 100 mg/12 h i.v., paracetamol 1 g/8 h i.v., and diclofenac suppository 75 mg/12 h. Additionally, ondansetron 4 mg i.v. was used to treat nausea and vomiting whenever necessary.

The primary outcomes included pain intensity [measured by 10-cm visual analog scale (10-cm VAS)] and the number of patients with moderate/severe pain (pain ≥4 on 10-cm VAS). The evaluation of pain included assessment of static pain when the patients were at rest and assessment of dynamic pain after asking patients to produce a forceful cough. The secondary outcomes included cumulative morphine consumption (in mg), number of patients who used PCA, number of patients who reported the presence of nausea or vomiting (incidence of nausea or vomiting), and the level of sedation (measured by 10-cm VAS). All outcomes (primary and secondary) were collected and/or evaluated at 2, 4, 8, and 24 h postoperatively.

(c) **Results of the Study**

Overall, 82 patients were screened. Fifty-nine patients (29 and 30 in the ropivacaine and placebo groups, respectively) undergoing surgery were recruited, of which 50 (25 in each arm) were finally included in the study.

Median pain intensity at rest and during cough was significantly lower in the ropivacaine group compared with the placebo group up to 4 h postoperatively (Fig. 19.1). The effect of ropivacaine in reducing postoperative pain (at rest and during cough) was clinically meaningful up to 4 h (Cliff's delta 0.36–0.44) (Table 19.1). The number of women reporting moderate/severe pain was significantly lower in the ropivacaine group compared with the placebo group at rest and during cough up to 8 h postoperatively (Fig. 19.2). The odds of having moderate/severe pain in the ropivacaine group were 76–90% less than in the placebo group up to 8 h postoperatively.

Patients in the ropivacaine group consumed significantly less morphine compared with those in the placebo group up to 24 h postoperatively ($p = 0.02$). The odds of mor-

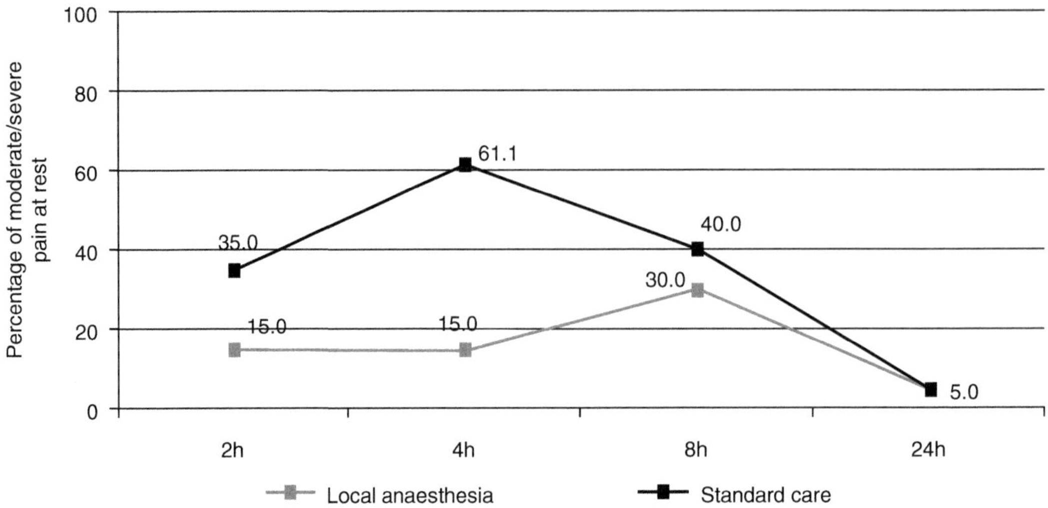

Fig. 19.1 Patients reporting moderate/severe pain at rest (16)

phine administration in the ropivacaine group at 4–24 h were 24–62% less than in the placebo group. Although nausea and/or vomiting and/or sedation did not differ between the groups, the odds of having nausea and/or vomiting (2–8 h postoperatively) were 28–78% less in the ropivacaine group compared with the placebo group. The findings of this study suggest that patients undergoing VH and PFR for POP could benefit from local infiltration with ropivacaine 0.5%.

19.4 Discussion

The use of local anesthesia in combination with i.v. sedation seems to be a feasible option in most women undergoing VH and PFR for the treatment of advanced uterovaginal prolapse. Current literature [14, 15] does not report any local anesthesia-related complications, whereas most of the patients reported being satisfied from this type of anesthesia.

Immediate postoperative pain seems to be significantly reduced in women undergoing surgery under local anesthesia although pain scores at and after 24 h do not differ among the various types of anesthesia. The mechanisms underlying the onset and persistence of pain caused by the tissue damage and nerve injury at VH are linked to the existence of complex circuits, which involve peripheral neural pathways, the spinal cord, and brain areas [17]. It is hypothesized that local anesthetics applied to the site of surgical injury may be more effective on blocking the acute postoperative pain arising from the surgical site compared to local anesthetics applied close to the nerves in the subarachnoid and epidural space (CSE block). In fact, the local anesthetics at the surgical site are binding to specific receptors located at the nerve membrane (on the sodium channel) leading to interruption of nerve conduction blocks and thus preventing the central sensitization in the spinal cord [17]. It is therefore important to emphasize the fact that the administration of a local anesthetic infiltration follows the concepts of a preemptive or a multimodal analgesia to improve the postoperative management of pain [18].

The percentage of patients consuming opioids for pain control during the first 24 h seems to be lower for patients undergoing surgery under LA [15]. Moreover, intraoperative local infiltration with ropivacaine during VH leads to reduction of postoperative pain, which is accompanied by significantly lower consumption of morphine up to 24 h postoperatively [16]. This is particularly important, as the widespread use of opioid analgesics has recently been called into question. In fact, there is an epidemic of opioid use, abuse, and mis-

Table 19.1 Primary outcomes at 2 h, 4 h, 8 h, and 24 h postoperatively

	Active group ($n = 25$)	Placebo group ($n = 25$)	Effect size	p-value
Pain at rest				
2 h				
Median (min-max)	0.5 (0.1–7.2)	1.1 (0.2–9.3)	−0.44 (95% CI -0.12, −0.68)	**0.007**
Moderate/severe intensity	1 (4%)	8 (32%)	OR 0.1 (95% CI 0.004, 0.65)	**0.03**
4 h				
Median (min-max)	1.3 (0.1–5.1)	3.1 (0.1–9.8)	−0.37 (95% CI -0.05, −0.63)	**0.02**
Moderate/severe intensity	4 (16%)	11 (44%)	OR 0.24 (95% CI 0.05, 0.87)	**0.03**
8 h				
Median (min-max)	1.3 (0.2–8.4)	2.6 (0.1–9.1)	−0.3 (95% CI 0.03, −0.57)	0.08
Moderate/severe intensity	3 (12%)	10 (40%)	OR 0.2 (95% CI 0.05, 0.87)	**0.02**
24 h				
Median (min-max)	0.5 (0–7)	0.6 (0–5.5)	−0.03 (95% CI 0.3, −0.34)	0.9
Moderate/severe intensity	2 (8%)	1 (4%)	OR 2 (95% CI 0.18, 24.6)	1
Pain during coughing				
2 h				
Median (min-max)	0.9 (0.1–8.9)	1.9 (0.1–10)	−0.36 (95% CI −0.03, −0.62)	**0.03**
Moderate/severe intensity	2 (8%)	10 (40%)	OR 0.13 (95% CI 0.03, 0.68)	**0.008**
4 h				
Median (min-max)	1.6 (0.1–4.7)	3.2 (0.3–9.6)	−0.4 (95% CI −0.11, −0.67)	**0.009**
Moderate/severe intensity	4 (16%)	13 (52%)	OR 0.18 (95% CI 0.05, 0.66)	**0.007**
8 h				
Median (min-max)	1.7 (0.2–8.5)	4 (0.1–9.5)	−0.31 (95% CI 0.02, −0.58)	0.06
Moderate/severe intensity	5 (20%)	13 (52%)	OR 0.23 (95% CI 0.07, 0.8)	**0.02**
24 h				
Median (min-max)	0.5 (0.1–5.8)	1 (0–6.4)	−0.13 (95% CI 0.2, −0.43)	0.4
Moderate/severe intensity	3 (12%)	1 (4%)	OR 3.27 (95% CI 0.32, 33.84)	0.6

Statistical significance was set at 5% ($p < 0.05$)

use, which results in significant postoperative morbidity [19, 20]. It is now firmly established that poorly controlled acute postoperative pain is among the strongest predictors for the development of chronic postsurgical pain and using escalating doses of opioids might only worsen the problem [19–21]. The use of local anesthesia could reduce the need for potent opioid analgesia after surgery.

The ability of a prompt postoperative mobilization with the use of LA is also considered of paramount importance. In particular, early mobilization could lower the risk of postoperative venous thrombosis while it simultaneously facilitates earlier restoration of the function of the bladder and bowel and thus quicker return to daily routine [22]. The aforementioned parameters are compatible with the "Enhanced Recovery After Surgery" (ERAS) protocols that have been recently adopted by many institutions, which have been related with favorable outcomes regarding patients' recovery [23, 24]. A critical point for those protocols is the intention for the reduction of opioid consumption, which is achieved with the use of local anesthetics and nerve blocks [23, 24].

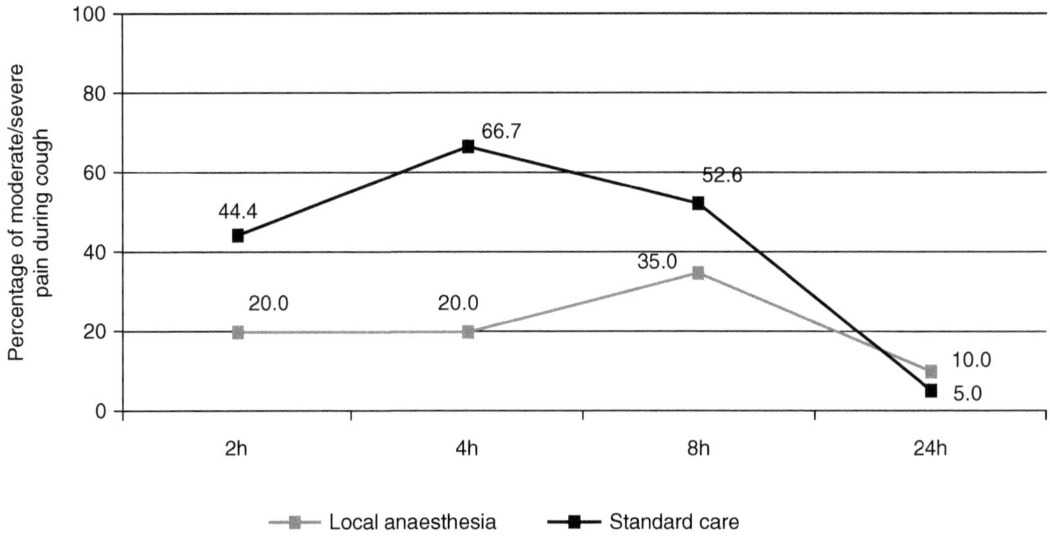

Fig. 19.2 Patients reporting moderate/severe pain during cough (16)

19.5 Conclusion

In conclusion local anesthesia has been shown to be a viable alternative to regional anesthesia in women undergoing VH for pelvic floor reconstruction offering reduced postoperative pain in the early postoperative period, less opioid use, and high patient satisfaction rate. This is particularly important for geriatric patients or patients with comorbidities having contraindications for general or regional anesthesia and for patients requiring an opioid-free anesthesia-analgesia or an enhanced recovery. In addition if regional anesthesia is the preferred anesthetic technique, local infiltration with ropivacaine may reduce postoperative pain and morphine consumption in women undergoing VH and PFR for pelvic floor reconstructive surgery.

Acknowledgments Grigoriadis Themos: Writing of chapter and case series; Zacharakis Dimitrios: Writing of chapter and case series; Kalantzis Christos: Writing of case series; Hatzilia Sophia: Writing of case series; Pitsouni Elieni: Writing of case series; Douskos Athanasios: Writing of case series; Valsamidis Dimitris: Writing of case series; Athanasiou Stavros: Writing of chapter and case series

References

1. Aarts JW, Nieboer TE, Johnson N, Tavender E, Garry R, Mol B et al. Surgical approach to hysterectomy for benign gynaecological disease. Cochrane Database Syst Rev. 2015;(8):CD003677. https://doi.org/10.1002/14651858.CD003677.pub5.
2. ACOG Committee Opinion No. 444. Choosing the route of hysterectomy for benign disease. American College of Obstetricians and Gynecologists. Obstet Gynecol. 2009;114:1156–1158.
3. AAGL Advancing Mininally Invasive Gynecology Worldwide. AAGL position statement: route of hysterectomy to treat benign uterine disease. J Minim Invasive Gynecol. 2011;18:1–3.
4. Moen M, Walter A, Harmanli O, Cornella J, Nihira M, Gala R, et al. Considerations to improve the evidence-based use of vaginal hysterectomy in benign gynecology. Obstet Gynecol. 2014;124:585–8.
5. Pelvic organ prolapse: ACOG Practice Bulletin, Number 214. Obstet Gynecol. 2019;134(5):e126–e142. https://doi.org/10.1097/AOG.0000000000003519.
6. Strøm C, Rasmussen LS, Sieber FE. Should general anaesthesia be avoided in the elderly? Anaesthesia. 2014;69(Suppl 1):35–44. https://doi.org/10.1111/anae.12493.
7. Olawin AM, Das J. Spinal anesthesia. [Updated 2020 Oct 13]. In: StatPearls [Internet]. Treasure Island: StatPearls Publishing; 2020. https://www.ncbi.nlm.nih.gov/books/NBK537299/.
8. Miklos JR, Sze EH, Karram MM. Vaginal correction of pelvic organ relaxation using local anesthesia. Obstet Gynecol. 1995;86:922–4.

9. Axelsen SM, Bek KM. Anterior vaginal wall repair using local anaesthesia. Eur J Obstet Gynecol Reprod Biol. 2004;112:214–6.
10. Flam F. Sedation and local anaesthesia for vaginal pelvic floor repair of genital prolapse using mesh. Int Urogynecol J Pelvic Floor Dysfunct. 2007;18:1471–5.
11. Buchsbaum GM, Albushies DT, Schoenecker E, Duecy EE, Glantz JC. Local anesthesia with sedation for vaginal reconstructive surgery. Int Urogynecol J Pelvic Floor Dysfunct. 2006;17:211–4.
12. Buchsbaum GM, Duecy EE. Local anesthesia with sedation for transvaginal correction of advanced genital prolapse. Am J Obstet Gynecol. 2005;193:2173–6.
13. Narayansingh GV, Kissoon W, Ramsewak SS. Local anaesthesia for vaginal hysterectomy in a patient with second degree utero-vaginal prolapse. J Obstet Gynaecol. 1993;13:73–4.
14. Sheth S, Malpani A. Vaginal hysterectomy for high risk patients under local anesthesia. J Gynecol Surg. 1992;8:65.
15. Athanasiou S, Zacharakis D, Grigoriadis T, Papalios T, Pitsouni E, Valsamidis D, et al. Vaginal hysterectomy with anterior and posterior repair for pelvic organ prolapse under local anesthesia: results of a pilot study. Int Urogynecol J. 2020;31:2109–16.
16. Athanasiou S, Hadzillia S, Pitsouni E, Kastanias S, Douskos A, Valsamidis D, et al. Intraoperative local infiltration with ropivacaine 0.5% in women undergoing vaginal hysterectomy and pelvic floor repair: randomized double-blind placebo-controlled trial. Eur J Obstet Gynecol Reprod Biol. 2019;236:154–9.
17. Levene JL, Weinstein EJ, Cohen MS, Andreae DA, Chao JY, Johnson M, et al. Local anesthetics and regional anesthesia versus conventional analgesia for preventing persistent postoperative pain in adults and children: a cochrane systematic review and meta-analysis update. J Clin Anesth. 2019;55:116–27. https://doi.org/10.1016/j.jclinane.2018.12.043.
18. Rosero EB, Joshi GP. Preemptive, preventive, multimodal analgesia. Plast Reconstr Surg. 2014;134:85S–93S. https://doi.org/10.1097/prs.0000000000000671.
19. Hollmann MW, Rathmell JP, Lirk P. Optimal postoperative pain management: redefining the role for opioids. Lancet. 2019;393(10180):1483–5. https://doi.org/10.1016/S0140-6736(19)30854-2.
20. Kumar K, Kirksey MA, Duong S, Wu CL. A review of opioid-sparing modalities in perioperative pain management: methods to decrease opioid use postoperatively. Anesth Analg. 2017;125(5):1749–60. https://doi.org/10.1213/ANE.0000000000002497.
21. Schuchat A, Houry D, Guy GP. New data on opioid use and prescribing in the United States. JAMA. 2017;318:425–6.
22. Flam F. Local anesthesia for hysterectomy in prolapse repair. Acta Obstet Gynecol Scand. 2007;86(4):502–3.
23. Kaye AD, Renschler J, Cramer K, Klein K, Granier A, Hart B, et al. The role of clinical pharmacology in enhanced recovery after surgery protocols: a comprehensive review. Anaesthesiol Intensive Ther. 2020;52(2):154–64. https://doi.org/10.5114/ait.2020.95020. PMID: 32419436.
24. Carter-Brooks CM, Du AL, Ruppert KM, Romanova AL, Zyczynski HM. Implementation of a urogynecology-specific enhanced recovery after surgery (ERAS) pathway. Am J Obstet Gynecol. 2018;219(5):495.e1–495.e10. https://doi.org/10.1016/j.ajog.2018.06.009.

Laparoscopic Surgery for Pelvic Organ Prolapse and Urinary Incontinence

20

Luis López-Fando, Marta Santiago, Javier Lorca, Martin Costal, Vanessa Viegas, Javier Gonzalvez, Mercedes Ruiz, Alvaro Sánchez, and Miguel Jiménez

The laparoscopic approach has become a revolution in surgery since George Kelling presented in 1901 the results of his research introducing the cystoscope described by Nitze through an orifice in the abdominal wall of a dog [1], until the later development of the automatic insufflator by Kurt Semm in 1966, among other many surgical instruments adapted to this approach, which led him to be considered the father of the laparoscopic technique [2]. Numerous studies have proven the laparoscopic approach to have a better complication rate and a shorter convalescence period, as it avoids many of the complicated incisions that are required for open surgery.

The retropubic vesical approach was used for the first time by Sánchez de Badajoz in 1988 [3] in order to perform a laparoscopic colposuspension, at first with intra- or extracavitary stitches; Ou in 1993 used a polypropylene mesh attached to the vaginal spoilers and the Cooper ligament [4].

L. López-Fando (✉) · M. Costal · V. Viegas · J. Gonzalvez
Urology Department, Hospital La Princesa, Madrid, Spain
e-mail: luis@urolf.com

M. Santiago · J. Lorca · M. Ruiz · A. Sánchez · M. Jiménez
Urology Department, Hospital Ramón y Cajal, Madrid, Spain
e-mail: msantiago.1@alumni.unav.es

The laparoscopic approach has granted a better understanding of the anatomical structures of the pelvis and a reduced complication rate compared to the open and vaginal surgical approaches. This chapter focuses in the two surgical techniques in which the laparoscopic is more relevant: the laparoscopic colposacropexy and the implantation of the artificial urinary sphincter, performing a review of the current literature and our own surgical experiences.

20.1 Laparoscopic Surgery for Pelvic Organ Prolapse: Colposacropexy

Pelvic organ prolapse (POP) is an increasingly relevant condition due to the aging of the population. Age, as well as obesity, gravida, and previous hysterectomy, is a risk factor for this entity.

Age is particularly relevant taking into account the figures obtained from the Spanish National Statistical Institute in January 2013, which estimate that 7,956,122 people over 65 years were registered in the general Spanish population, with women accounting for the 57% of the population over 65 years old (4,568,541). The population is experiencing a progressive increase in the life expectancy, which is again more common in the female population. Elderly patients are increasingly common, and not all of them must be considered as patients with limitations in their

F. Dökmeci, D. E. E. Rizk (eds.), *Insights Into Incontinence and the Pelvic Floor*,
https://doi.org/10.1007/978-3-030-94174-1_20

capacities. According to the European health survey, the percentages of women over 65 years old with a limitation in their daily activities in the last 6 months due to a health problem were 6.39% for great limitation, 22.15% for mild limitation, and 71.46% for no limitation.

The estimation of the probability of having any intervention for POP at 80 years old is 11.1%, and the risk of re-intervention is 30%. Wu et al. [5] calculate that the number of women with POP will increase of 46%, rising from 3.3 to 4.9 million cases between 2010 and 2050. Additionally, in that interval of time, Wu et al. [5] predict an increase of 47% in the patients undergoing a POP surgery.

The treatment of POP aims to restore the vesical, intestinal, and sexual functionality, as well as to correct the anatomy of the pelvis. Guidelines recommend surgery for the treatment of POP when conservative treatment has failed [6].

Traditionally a vaginal approach has been preferred in elderly patients, because of the shorter operating time and the reduced complication rate. The main inconvenient related to classical vaginal surgery performed with native tissue is POP relapse, requiring then a second intervention. Previous longitudinal studies have reported re-intervention rates that range from 0.7 to 5.4% [7]. Vaginal surgery with mesh arises due to the need to solve this problem. However, even if it has a better relapse rate, the complications are more frequent. In 2002, the FDA approved the first mesh for the treatment of POP, leading to an exponential increase of the use of transvaginal mesh for the treatment of pelvic floor conditions [8]. This same organism issued in October 2008 a Public Health Notification in response to the complications derivated from the urogynecological use of surgical mesh [9]. Currently the FDA places in class III (devices with high complication risk) transvaginal mesh, while it places in class I (low complication risk) the mesh used for abdominal colposacropexy.

Mesh colposacropexy is the gold standard technique because of its anatomical and functional long-term results, with a major complication rate inferior to 6% [10]. The laparoscopic approach offers a minimally invasive surgery with a better postoperative recovery compared to open surgery. There is scarce literature about the long-term complications in elderly patients undergoing this technique. In our unit laparoscopic colposacropexy was started in 2012 as the gold standard surgical technique after the failure of conservative treatment for POP, abandoning then the use of transvaginal mesh.

20.2 Case Study Laparoscopic Colposacropexy: A Safe Approach in Elderly Patients

Surgical Technique

- ***Patient position:*** the patient is placed in 30° Trendelenburg, with lower limbs in 45° abduction and flexed at the knees. A 14 Fr urethral catheter is placed (Fig. 20.1a).
- ***Trocar colocation:*** transperitoneal, through four trocars: two of 12 mm in the midline (one for the Hasson insertion, the other one between the pubis symphysis and the umbilicus) and two auxiliary trocars of 5 mm (Fig. 20.1a).
- ***Sigma and uterus mobilization:*** sigma and uterus are mobilized and fixated to the abdominal wall (Fig. 20.1b).
- ***Dissection and preparation of the sacrum:*** location of the anterior aspect of the sacrum and marking of the surface in which the mesh will be attached at the end of the surgery. It is crucial to carefully preserve the middle sacral artery in this step of the surgery.
- ***Rectovaginal space:*** a vaginal valve is of cardinal importance in order to achieve a correct tension that enables the visualization of the dissection planes. Opening of the peritoneum and dissection of the rectovaginal space, identifying the rectum. Careful dissection of the levator ani muscle on each side of the rectum (Fig. 20.2b and c).
- ***Attachment of the posterior mesh:*** stitches to each levator ani muscle. An additional stitch to extend the mesh in each uterosacral ligament and at the cervix level (Fig. 20.2d).
- ***Vesicovaginal space:*** the dissection starts with the opening of the peritoneum, and it extends distally until the posterior aspect of

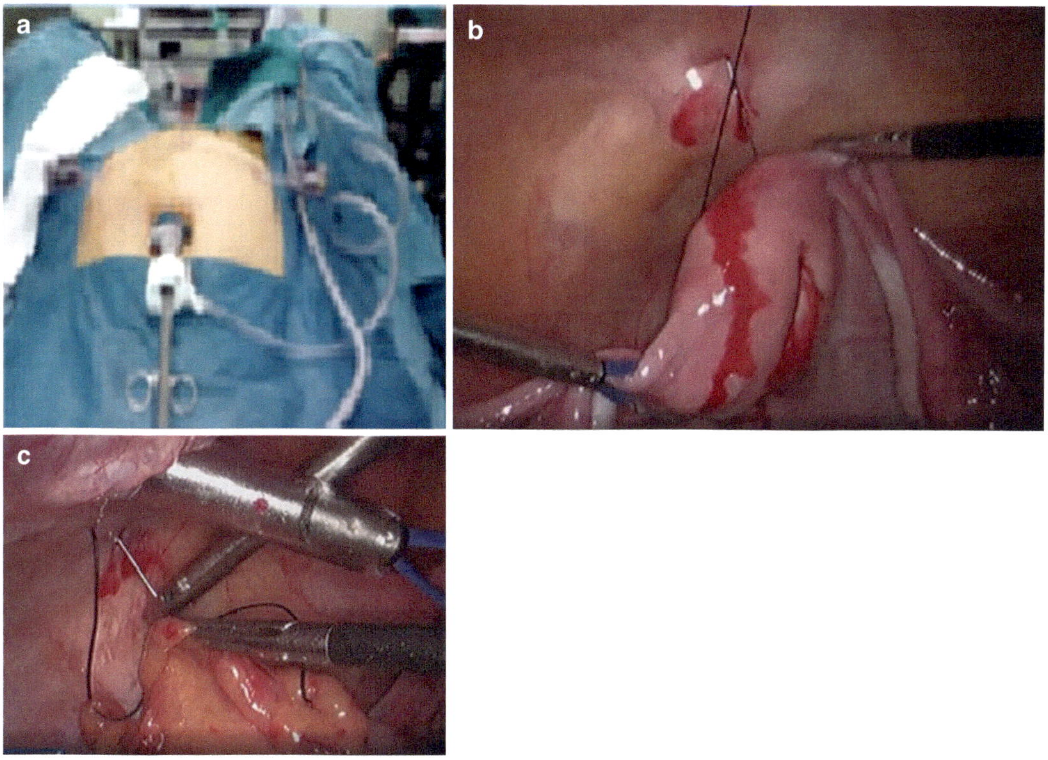

Fig. 20.1 (**a**) Patient position and trocar situation. (**b**) Uteros fixation. (**c**) Sigmoidopexy

the bladder neck is identified. The anterior mesh is attached to the anterior vaginal wall with a stitch and two additional lateral stitches in the lateral aspects of the vagina in order to extend the mesh (Fig. 20.3).

- ***Attachment of the mesh to the sacrum:*** both meshes are attached to the sacrum with an extracorporeal stitch of non-absorbable multifilament suture.
- ***Final maneuvers:*** reperitonization of meshes with absorbable suture.

When performing a review of the currently available literature about POP surgery, there are few studies that truly reflect the complications and long-term results in elderly patients. In the scarce available studies, the age threshold used to define the patients as elderly is 65 years old, which we believe is not an appropriate definition of the demographic reality in developed countries [7]. As a response to the population aging, in the last years, there has been a rapid expansion of the recognition and knowledge of the concept of fragility. The elderly patients have a vulnerable functional capacity; any intercurrent event can present as a decline in the functional status. There are several tools available to evaluate these patients at the time of a major surgical intervention or a medical treatment for their conditions, and these tools must be used by a multidisciplinary health supplier team in order to optimize the treatment results. An example of this is the participation of the International Society of Geriatric Oncology (SIOG) in the elaboration of the European Guidelines for the treatment of the different genitourinary malignancies. Such collaborations should be progressively assimilated when planning the treatment of genitourinary functional conditions. In the European Guidelines, the patients with a score over 14 in the G8 scale, or vulnerable patients with conditions that are susceptible of being reversed after an intervention, should receive the same treatment as younger patients [11]. The patients

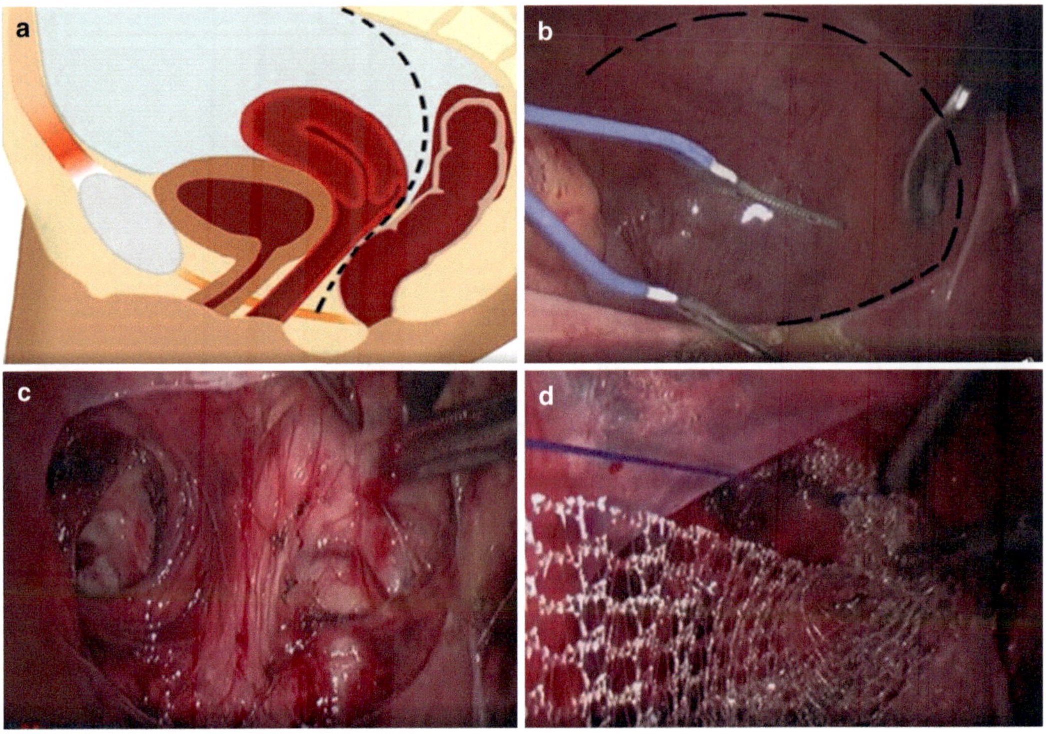

Fig. 20.2 Posterior dissection and mesh attachment

undergoing surgery in our series were over 14 points in the G8 scale.

With the progressive aging and increase of obesity in the population, it is to be expected a significant increase in the POP prevalence. In the United States, the number of women with symptomatic POP between 2010 and 2050 is estimated to increase in 46% in the best case scenario (from 3.3 to 4.9 millions of women) and in up to 200% in the worst case scenario (from 3.3 to 9.2 millions of women) [12]. These circumstances will lead to an increase in the demand for treatment and to the use of economic resources, as well as a need for a greater number of experienced health professionals in the diagnosis, assessment, and treatment of POP.

Traditionally, the vaginal approach has been the preferred one for elderly patients, as it was believed to have shorter operating times, a lower complication rate, and shorter hospital stay, all of these factors leading to reduced cost. After the emission of the alarm by the FDA, this approach has been widely questioned.

In the study by Skoczylas et al., 1385 surgical procedures for the treatment of POP in a single center from 2008 to 2011 are analyzed, with the objective of assessing the tendency in the surgical treatment of POP and the influence of the FDA notifications. A significant decrease in the use of vaginal mesh procedures was observed. In 2008 transvaginal mesh accounted for 27% of the procedures, being reduced to 15% after the first FDA alarm and to 5% after the second notification. They were finally limited to 2% of the interventions at the end of the year 2011. Following the same tendency, a significant increase of the number of procedures using native tissue for apical suspension was observed, as well as minimally invasive procedures such as laparoscopic and robot-assisted colposacropexy, so that at the end of the study the later was established as the most frequently performed intervention for the treatment of POP in that center [13]. In our center, laparoscopic colposacropexy was initiated in 2012, becoming then the gold standard intervention and abolishing the use of vaginal mesh for

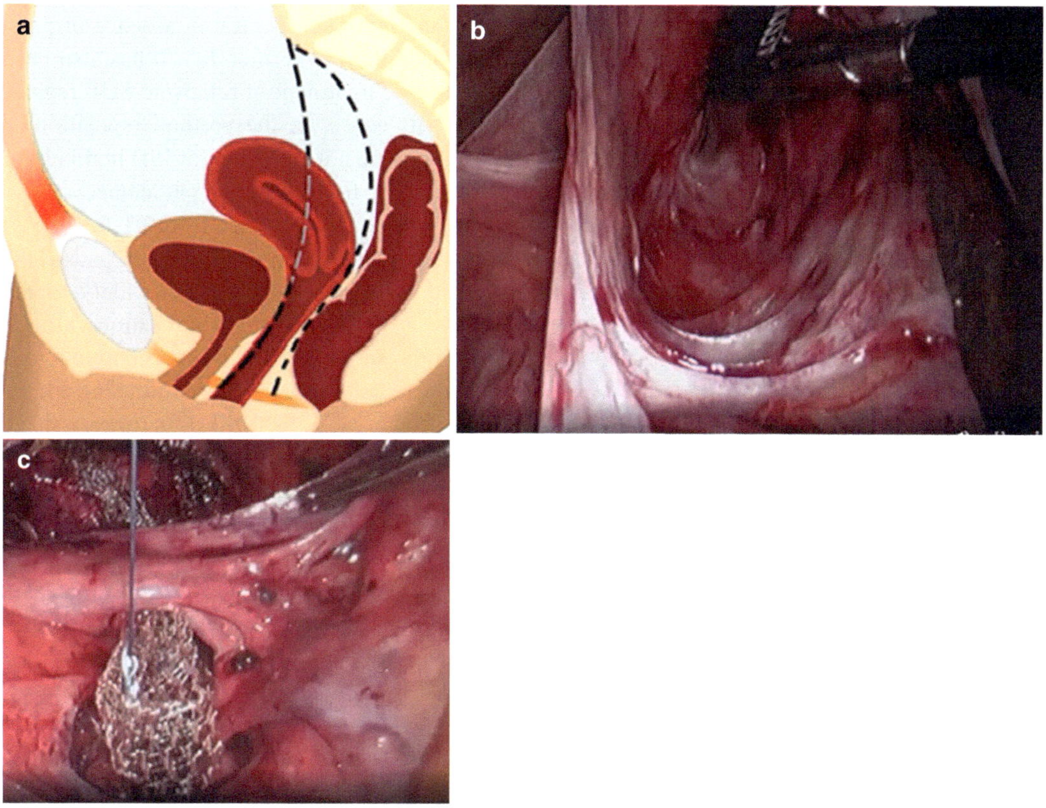

Fig. 20.3 Vesicovaginal space and sacrum fixation

the POP correction following the FDA indications.

When analyzing the complications between different approaches, according to the Prospere study results, for the correction of grade over 2 POP, the incidence of complications is lower in colposacropexy compared to vaginal surgery using native tissues; however, the difference was not statistically significant. In contrast, for over grade 3 POP, complications following colposacropexy are significantly less frequent compared to vaginal surgery. This study observed that there were no differences in symptoms, quality of life, and overall improvement between both techniques but there were differences in anatomical results in apical POP, favoring colposacropexy [14]. In our series, there were no significant differences in the incidence of complications in the different age groups. The relapse rate, defined as the presence of grade ≥2 POP in one or several compartments, was globally 4.4%, with no difference between age groups. The risk factors for relapse are not well defined, but there might be a positive correlation between advanced grade of POP and the repetition of classic surgical techniques with native tissue after a first surgical failure. This is the main problem of the classic vaginal approach. The relapse and re-intervention rates published in the literature are very variable, which complicates results comparison. In longitudinal studies re-intervention rates range from 0.7 to 5.4% [15].

As far as the economic aspect is concerned, the economical evaluation studies for transvaginal surgery have proven that the use of mesh is not cost-effective [16]. According to a comparative study of the direct cost of POP correction through different approaches, POP correction using laparoscopic colposacropexy shows reduced cost compared to transvaginal mesh, with no statistically significant differences. POP correction through laparoscopic colposacropexy presented a greater spend because of a longer surgical time, operating room occupation, and anesthesia; however, the transvaginal mesh group presented higher cost as a result of a more prolonged hospital stay and more expensive prosthetic material [6]. Laparoscopy offers the possibility of performing POP correction with an abdominal and minimally invasive approach, allowing with sufficient safety a hospital stay of 24 h, with a mean saving of 607.91 euros per procedure in hospital stay [17].

20.3 Laparoscopic Surgery for Urinary Incontinence in Female: Urinary Artificial Sphincter

Stress urinary incontinence (SUI) frequently affects the female population over 18 years old, with a prevalence ranging from 14 to 55% [18]. Surgical treatment is indicated when SUI is severe and impairs the patient's quality of life, after the failure of conservative treatment [19]. There are multiple surgical techniques for SUI correction. Currently, the more widely used are sub-urethral slings implanted through a retropubic (TVT®) or transobturator (TOT®) approach. A recent systematic review has observed lower efficacy of the TVT-Secur® mini-sling compared to TVT® and TOT®, leading to the withdrawal of the device from the market. Additionally, there is not sufficient scientific evidence to recommend any other mini-sling [20]. No statistically significant differences have been found between the prevalence of SUI resolution between the different sling techniques, and neither compared to colposuspension [21]. The long-term effectivity of sub-urethral slings is 43–91% for TOT® and 51–88% for TVT®. The risk factors for the failure of these techniques are relapsing SUI, intrinsic sphincter deficiency (ISD), concomitant vaginal hysterectomy, and the presence of associated apical compartment prolapse [22–24].

The indications for the implant of an artificial urinary sphincter (AUS) are not clearly defined. Many authors have demonstrated its utility in the treatment of SUI secondary to ISD (neurogenic and non-neurogenic), in absence or presence of urethral hypermobility. It has also been used for the treatment of relapsing SUI, regardless of its cause, as the urethral repositioning techniques are not validated for ISD in relapsing SUI [25–27]. Even if a high percentage of successes has been described, from 61 to 90% of completely continence (no use of pads), the implant of feminine AUS is not widely spread because of the frequent complications associated to the surgery [28, 29]. The complications risk is generally lower in the series using a laparoscopic approach [26, 30, 31]. In robot-assisted series, a high frequency of intra- and postoperative complications has also been described [32]. The risk of intraoperative erosion and postoperative extrusion of the sphincter (mainly caused by the wrong placement of the AUS) increases with the number of previous anti-incontinence interventions [30, 33].

20.3.1 Surgical Technique

- ***Patient position and trocars:*** similar to laparoscopic colposacropexy.
- ***Vesicovaginal space dissection:*** after gaining access to the peritoneal cavity, the first step consists in the dissection of the vesicovaginal space, similar to the laparoscopic colposacropexy technique (Fig. 20.4b). The dissection is distally extended until the posterior aspect of the bladder neck is identified. At this level the ureters are lateral and intramural, reducing the likelihood of intraoperative lesion. The use of a vaginal valve is crucial to enable a safe identification of the dissection planes (vesicovaginal and latero-vesical).
- ***Dissection of the latero-vesical spaces:*** the antero-lateral peritoneum is incised in one side, and the latero-vesical space is created. The dissection is extended lateral to the bladder until the endopelvic fascia is identified (Fig. 20.4d). The process is repeated in the contralateral side.
- ***Communication between the vesicovaginal and both latero-vesical spaces:*** with a dissector a communication is created between the

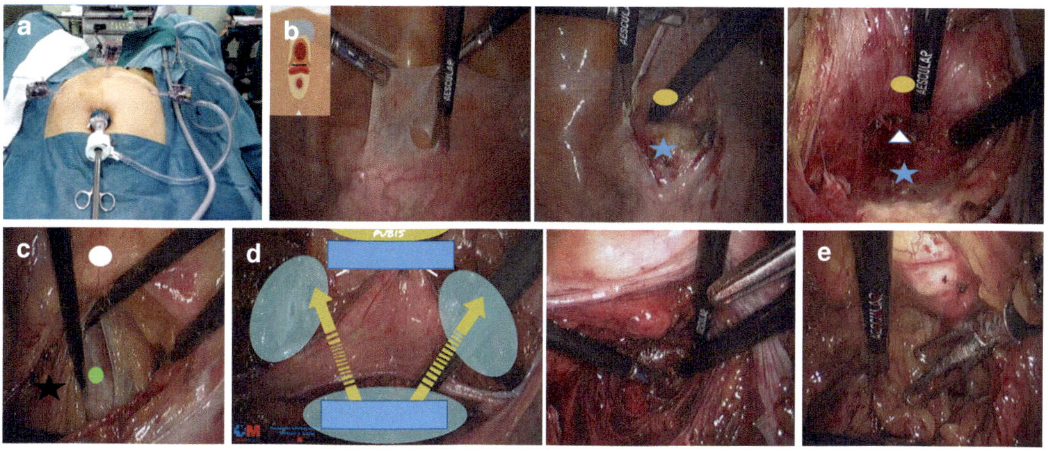

Fig. 20.4 Laparoscopic posterior approach to female urinary sphincter

vesicovaginal space and both latero-vesical spaces (Fig. 20.4d).

- ***Dissection of the anterior aspect of the bladder neck:*** the maximum possible length of the pubovesical ligament is preserved (Fig. 20.4e).
- ***Measurement of the bladder neck diameter and verification of bladder and vagina integrity:*** a meter is introduced through the infraumbilical 12 mm trocar. The diameter was 7.5 cm in the first patient and 6.5 cm in the second (Fig. 20.5a). The integrity of the bladder wall is verified through a cystoscopy and the vaginal wall through digital examination.
- ***Placement of the cuff and reservoir:*** the sphincter components are prepared. After voiding and purging them, a metallic tip is placed at the end of cuff and reservoir to keep them empty and free of air. For the activation pump, a protected hemostatic clamp is place in its end. The cuff is introduced through the 12 mm trocar and tied to a suture placed at the end of the meter (this step facilitates the placement of the cuff surrounding the bladder neck) (Fig. 20.5b). The reservoir is introduced through the same trocar, placing it in the left latero-vesical space (Fig. 20.5c).
- ***Externalization of the connections:*** a left suprapubic incision of approximately 2 cm is performed. Through this incision a 5 mm trocar is placed, in order to externalize the connections of the cuff and reservoir (Fig. 20.5d).
- ***Placement of the activation pump:*** a subcutaneous tunnel is created from the suprapubic incision, connecting the incision with the ipsilateral labia majora. The activation pump is placed through this tunnel (Fig. 20.5d).
- ***Connection of the components and verification of the correct functioning:*** the reservoir is filled with 23 cc of saline, and the components are connected using the habitual technique (Fig. 20.5e). The components are introduced in the peritoneal cavity, and the correct functioning of the sphincter is verified: with laparoscopic vision, after the pump is activated, the cuff is filled and in the cystoscopy the coaptation of the bladder neck is observed. Additionally, the correct location of the cuff distal to the ureteral meatus is verified through cystoscopy. After checking the correct functioning of the system, the AUS is deactivated, and it will be activated 6 weeks after the surgery.
- ***Closing of the peritoneum and abdominal incisions:*** hemostasia revision and closure of the three peritoneal incisions (Fig. 20.2f). No drainage is needed.

AUS is not widely spread for the treatment of female SUI, and its indications are not fully stablished. The consensus document of the European Association of Urology (EAU) and Urogynecology of 2017 claims that the AUS can improve SUI in women with ISD (level of evi-

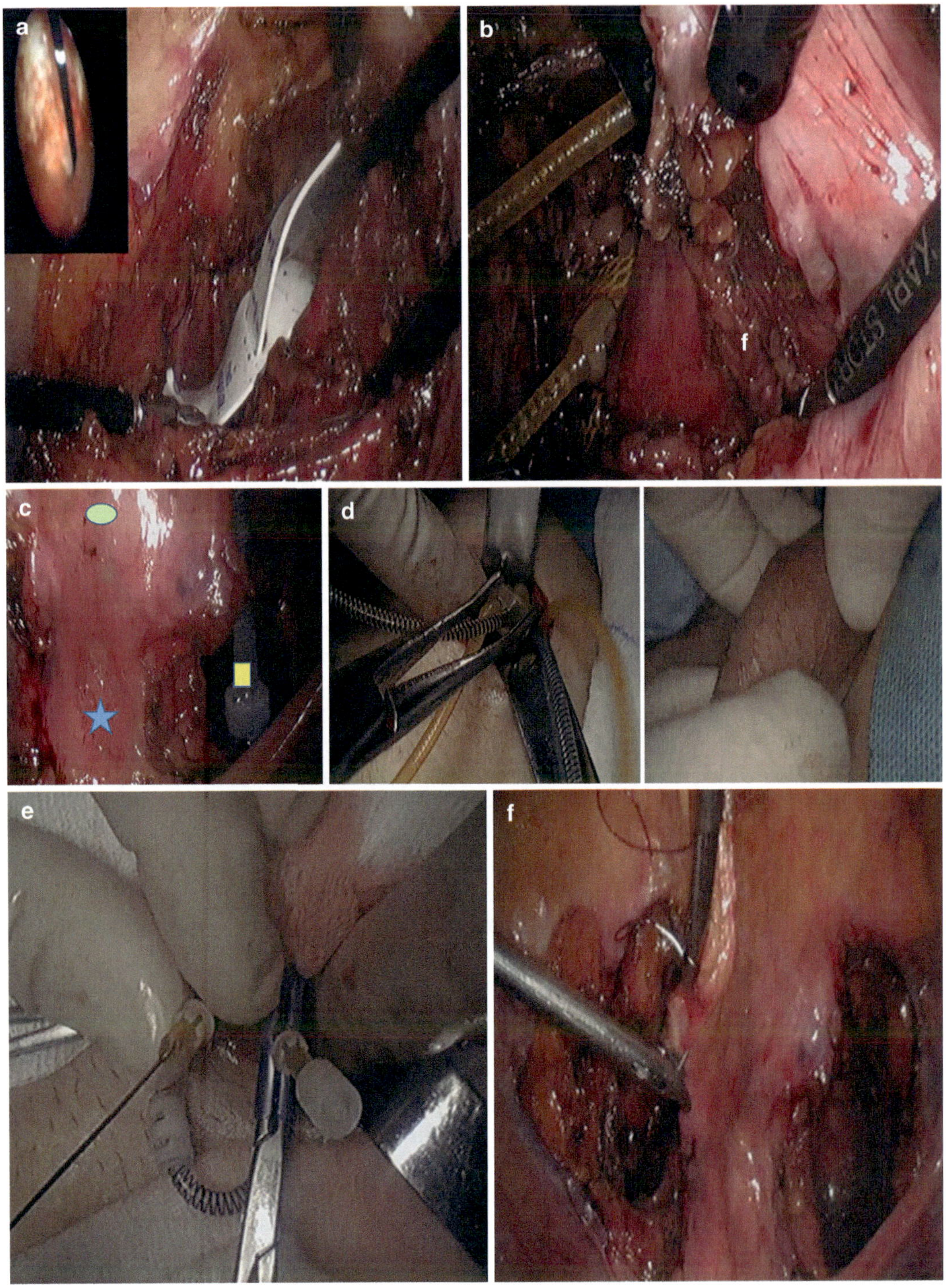

Fig. 20.5 Laparoscopic female urinary sphincter placement

dence 3). However, there are no available clinical trials that prove its efficacy, and it is consequently not recommended as a first-line treatment [19]. The American Urological Association (AUA) Guidelines on SUI of 2017 do not establish any recommendation on AUS [34]. The International Continence Society (ICS) recommends its use only in selected cases of relapsing SUI because of the need of further follow-up of the cases and the scarce data about the long-term efficacy of the treatment (grade C) [35].

The main current indication for AUS in the available literature is ISD, neurogenic and non-neurogenic [25–27]. ISD is characterized by a fixed urethra, absence of urethral hypermobility during Valsalva maneuvers, and low abdominal leak point pressure (ALPP) in urodynamic study [36]. The treatment options for ISD include bulking agents, pubovaginal mesh implant, or external compressive agents such as AUS [19]. The adjustable mesh (Reemex®) has demonstrated a high SUI resolution rate (89%). However, for patients with hypocontractile detrusor, there is a high obstruction risk, and achieving the right tension for the sling can be challenging [37]. On the other hand, the experience of POP correction using a laparoscopic approach, where the dissection of the vesicovaginal space is a mandatory step for the mesh placement, has allowed a reproduction of such dissection of the laparoscopic implant of AUS [6].

The optimal time for the AUS implant is controversial. Many authors consider it the first option treatment if ISD is demonstrated. Other authors prefer less invasive surgical techniques, such as slings, independently of the cause of SUI. Taking into account that the risk of intraoperative complications and posterior explant are higher if previous anti-incontinence procedures and pelvis surgeries are present [25], AUS should be considered after the failure of maximum one or two anti-incontinence surgical interventions [26, 29, 35].

The main contraindications for the implant of AUS are the absence of manual skills to manipulate the pump, urogynecological malformations, previous radiation, cutaneous infections in the external genitalia, vaginal or urethral conditions (p.e. urethral traumatism), overactive detrusor, or low bladder accommodation during the filling phase [28].

Regarding the surgical approaches used until the present day, the good results observed by some authors, in open surgery as well as in laparoscopic and robot-assisted interventions, have been poorly reproductible. In some robot series, a rate 36.4% of intraoperative complications and 27.3% explant have been described [32]. In open surgery, the vaginal approach has been associated with higher infection rates, erosion, and shorter survival of the AUS device, with an explant risk of 56% in 10 years [29]. Using a retropubic approach, Costa et al. report a 85% continence rate in the long term. After 3, 5, and 10 years, 92.0, 88.6, and 69.2% of the AUS were still in place, respectively [25]. The main limitation of this approach is the difficulty to place the cuff around the bladder neck because of the complicated access and identification of the dissection plane, especially in obese patients or women with previous pelvic surgeries. In laparoscopic and robot-assisted surgery, despite the magnified bladder neck vision that might ease the urethrovaginal dissection, the placement of the cuff around the posterior aspect of the bladder neck is performed blindly. Once the anterior aspect of the bladder neck is identified, the dissection of the posterior aspect is performed with a blunt dissector, but the space is never directly visualized [30, 31, 38, 39] (Fig. 20.3a). Vesical and vaginal perforations, especially vaginal at this level, which could go unnoticed, are potential causes of infection and cuff extrusion. Fournier et al. perform an incision of the anterior vesical wall, in order to be able to identify potential posterior perforations when using the blunt dissector [40]. However, this does not permit the diagnosis of vaginal perforations, and it adds potential complications derived from the vesical opening. By dissecting the vesicovaginal space, a blind access to the posterior aspect of the bladder neck is avoided, allowing greater security, better vision, and control [41].

In addition, using the laparoscopic approach permits to preserve the maximum length of the pubovesical ligament, due to its potential role in continence (vesical opening and closure) and as a support element [42, 43]. The presence of this ligament would limit the posterior displacement of the bladder and bladder neck. Consequently, the risk of erosion would also be decreased, particularly late erosion. Until the present day, all the groups that perform laparoscopic AUS completely section this ligament. On the other hand, a dissection of the pubovesical ligament fibers at the bladder neck would not imply changes in the diameter of the cuff.

Acute urinary retention is frequent in the immediate postoperative period due to urethral edema, with reported rates up to 45%, higher than in open surgery [30, 33]. There is no consensus on how long the patient should maintain the urethral catheter. The duration of the urethral catheter varies among the different series, varying from 2 to 7 days. Those authors in favor of maintaining the urethral catheter longer justify their decision with the intention of decreasing the risk of acute urinary retention. However, the longer urethral catheterization periods are associated with higher risk of urethral erosion. In our series, the catheter is maintained for 48 h. In cases of elevated post-void residual urine, depending on the symptoms and severity, the options would be conservative management or placing a new urethral catheter for another 48 h.

Lastly, the patient must also be informed of the risk of mechanic failure, with an incidence of 29% in 10 years, similar to the male AUS series. The main survival of the device is 11.2 years [44]. The laparoscopic approach allows a safe implant of the AUS with the advantage of tactile sensation and feedback.

20.4 Conclusion

Laparoscopic colposacropexy is a safe technique which offers the best anatomical and functional results in the long term for POP correction. The patients' age must not be an exclusion factor for this approach, and a holistic and individualized assessment must be performed, taking into account the patients' desires and expectations, in order to offer the best treatment option. The dissection of the vesicovaginal space similar to the laparoscopic colposacropexy technique allows to implant under direct vision the cuff surrounding the posterior aspect of the bladder neck. Preserving the pubovesical ligament can play a role in the achievement of continence and in limiting the posterior displacement of the bladder neck. Both technical details might reduce the risk of complications and allow the AUS implant to be a more reproductible intervention.

Acknowledgments Case study authors: Javier Lorca Álvaro - Marta Santiago González Clara Sánchez Guerrero - Francisco Javier Burgos Revilla.

References

1. Kelling G. Verhandlungen II Teil; 2 Hälfe, Versammlung deutscher Natur-forscher und Aertze. Hamburg; 1901. p. 119.
2. Semm K. Endoscopic intraabdominal surgery. In: Semm K, editor. Kiel; 1984.
3. Sánchez De Badajoz E, Chamorro F, Díaz Ramírez F, Marín Martín J. Anclaje cervical endoscópico. Nuevo tratamiento para la incontinencia de esfuerzo. Arch Esp Urol. 1988;41(2):127–30.
4. Ou CS, Presthus J, Beadle E. Laparoscopic bladder neck suspension using hernia mesh and surgical stapler. J Laparoendosc Surg. 1993;13:563.
5. Wu JM, Matthews CA, Conover MM, Pate V, Jonsson Funk M. Life-time risk of stress urinary incontinence or pelvic organ prolapsesurgery. Obstet Gynecol. 2014;123:1201–6.
6. Carracedo D, López-Fando L, Sánchez MD, et al. Cost analysis of surgical treatment for pelvic organ prolapse by laparoscopic sacrocolpopexy or transvaginal mesh. Análisis de costes del tratamiento del prolapso de órganos pélvicos mediante colposacropexia laparoscópica o malla transvaginal. Actas Urol Esp. 2017;41(2):117–22. https://doi.org/10.1016/j.acuro.2016.08.001.
7. Moreno-Mira R, García-Montes F, Lizarbe-Iranzo R, Martín-Jiménez Á. Influencia de la edad en el rendimiento de la colposacropexia laparoscópica [Influence of age on laparoscopic colposacropexy]. Ginecol Obstet Mex. 2015;83(7):447–453.
8. Tijdink M, Vierhout ME, Heesakkers JP, Withagen MI. Surgical management of mesh-related complications after prior pelvic floor reconstructive surgery with mesh. Int Urogynecol J. 2011;22:1395–404.
9. FDA public health notification: serious complications associated with transvaginal placement of surgical mesh in repair of pelvic organ prolapse and stress urinary incontinence. 2008. http://www.

fda.gov/MedicalDevices/Safety/AlertsandNotices/PublicHealthNotifications/ucm061976.htm.
10. Nygaard IE, McCreery R, Brubaker L, Connolly A, Cundiff G, Weber AM, Zyczynski H. Abdominal sacrocolpopexy: a comprehensive review. Obstet Gynecol. 2004;104:805–23.
11. Mottet N, et al. EAU-ESTRO-SIOG guidelines on prostate cancer. Part 1: screening, diagnosis, and local treatment with curative intent. Eur Urol. 2017;71:618.
12. Abrams P et al Members of the Committees. Recommendation of the International Scientific Committee: evaluation and treatment of urinary incontinence, pelvic organ prolapse and fecal incontinence. In: Abrams P, Cardozo L, Wagg A, Wein A, editors. Incontinence. International Consultation on Incontinence. 6th edn. Tokyo. 2016; pp. 2549–2605. isbn:978-0-9569607-3-3.2017
13. Skoczylas LC, Turner LC, Wang L, et al. Changes in prolapse surgery trends relative to FDA notifications regarding vaginal mesh. Int Urogynecol J. 2014;25:471–7.
14. Lucot JP, Fritel X, Debodinance P, Bader G, Cosson M, Giraudet G, Collinet P, Rubod C, Fernandez H, Fournet S, Lesavre M, Deffieux X, Faivre E, Trichot C, Demoulin G, Jacquetin B, Savary D, Botchorichvili R, Campagne Loiseau S, Salet-Lizee D, Villet R, Gadonneix P, Delporte P, Ferry P, Aucouturier JS, Thirouard Y, de Tayrac R, Fatton B, Wagner L, Nadeau C, Wattiez A, Garbin O, Youssef Azer Akladios C, Thoma V, Baulon Thaveau E, Saussine C, Hermieu JF, Delmas V, Blanc S, Tardif D, Fauconnier A, GROG (groupe de recherche en gynécologie et obstétrique). PROSPERE randomized controlled trial: laparoscopic sacropexy versus vaginal mesh for cystocele POP repair. J Gynecol Obstet Biol Reprod (Paris). 2013;42(4):334–41. https://doi.org/10.1016/j.jgyn.2013.03.012. Epub 2013 Apr 22.
15. Friedman T, Eslick GD, Dietz HP. Risk factors for prolapse recurrence: systematic review and meta-analysis. Int Urogynecol J. 2018;29:13–21.
16. Paz Valiñas L, Macía Cortiñas M, López-García M. Mallas transvaginales en la reparación del prolapso de órganos pélvicos. Red Española de Agencias de Evaluación de Tecnologías y Prestaciones del SNS. Axencia de Avaliación de Tecnoloxías Sanitarias de Galicia. Informes de evaluación de tecnologías sanitarias; 2014.
17. Moscatiello P, Carracedo D, Sánchez MD, et al. Analysis of minimally invasive sacrocolpopexy with 24-hour hospital stay for the treatment of pelvic organ prolapse. Análisis del tratamiento del prolapso de órganos pélvicos mediante colposacropexia mínimamente invasiva con 24horas de ingreso. Actas Urol Esp. 2019;43(9):509–14. https://doi.org/10.1016/j.acuro.2019.05.002.
18. Espuña Pons M. Incontinencia de orina en la mujer. Med Clin (Barc). 2003;120:464–72.
19. Chapple CR, Cruz F, Deffieux X, Milani AL, Arlandis S, Arti-bani W, et al. Consensus statement of the European Urology Association and the European Urogynaecological Association on the use of implanted materials for treating pelvic organ prolapse and stress urinary incontinence. Eur Urol. 2017;72:424–31.
20. Nambiar A, Cody JD, Jeffery ST, Aluko P. Single-incision sling operations for urinary incontinence in women. Cochrane Database Syst Rev. 2017. CD008709 [consultado 29Ene 2018]. http://onlinelibrary.wiley.com/doi/10.1002/14651858.CD008709.pub3/full.
21. Lapitan MCM, Cody JD, Mashayekhi A. Open retropubic colposuspension for urinary incontinence in women. Cochrane Database Syst Rev. 2017;CD002912 [consultado 29Ene 2018]. http://onlinelibrary.wiley.com/doi/10.1002/14651858.CD002912.pub7/full.
22. Ford AA, Rogerson L, Cody JD, Aluko P, Ogah JA. Mid-urethral sling operations for stress urinary incontinence in women. Cochrane Database Syst Rev. 2017;CD006375. [consul-tado 29 Ene 2018]. http://onlinelibrary.wiley.com/doi/10.1002/14651858.CD006375.pub4/full.
23. Smith AL, Karp DR, Aguilar VC, Davila GW. Repeat versus primary slings in patients with intrinsic sphincter deficiency. Int Urogynecol J. 2013;24:963–8.
24. Athanasiou S, Grigoriadis T, Zacharakis D, Skampardonis N, Lourantou D, Antsaklis A. Seven years of objective and subjective outcomes of transobturator (TVT-O) vaginal tape: why do tapes fail? Int Urogynecol J. 2014;25:219–25.
25. Costa P, Mottet N, Rabut B, Thuret R, Ben Naoum K, Wagner L. The use of an artificial urinary sphincter in women with type III incontinence and a negative Marshall test. J Urol. 2001;165:1172–6.
26. Chartier-Kastler E, van Kerrebroeck P, Olianas R, Cosson M, Mandron E, Delorme E, et al. Artificial urinary sphincter (AMS800) implantation for women with intrinsic sphincter deficiency: a technique for insiders? BJU Int. 2011;107:1618–26.
27. Phé V, Léon P, Granger B, Denys P, Bitker M-O, Mozer P, et al. Stress urinary incontinence in female neurological patients: long-term functional outcomes after artificial urinary sphincter (AMS 800TM) implantation. Neurourol Urodyn. 2017;36:764–9.
28. Hussain M, Greenwell TJ, Venn SN, Mundy AR. The current role of the artificial urinary sphincter for the treatment of urinary incontinence. J Urol. 2005;174:418–24.
29. Venn SN, Greenwell TJ, Mundy AR. The long-term outcome of artificial urinary sphincters. J Urol. 2000;164(3 Pt 1):702–6; discussion 706–707.
30. Mandron E, Bryckaert P-E, Papatsoris AG. Laparoscopic artificial urinary sphincter implantation for female genuine stress urinary in continence: technique and 4-year experience in 25 patients. BJU Int. 2010;106:1194–8; discussion 1198.
31. Ferreira C, Brychaert P-E, Menard J, Mandron E. Laparoscopic implantation of artificial urinary sphincter in women with intrinsic sphincter deficiency: mid-term outcomes. Int J Urol. 2017;24:308–13.

32. Biardeau X, Rizk J, Marcelli F, Flamand V. Robot-assisted laparoscopic approach for artificial urinary sphincter implantation in 11 women with urinary stress incontinence: surgical technique and initial experience. Eur Urol. 2015;67:937–42.
33. Rouprêt M, Misraï V, Vaessen C, Cardot V, Cour F, Richard F, et al. Laparoscopic approach for artificial urinary sphincter implantation in women with intrinsic sphincter deficiency incontinence: a single-centre preliminary experience. Eur Urol. 2010;57:499–504.
34. American Urological Association. Surgical treatment of female stress urinary incontinence (SUI): AUA/SUFU Guideline [Internet] [consultado 7 Dic 2017]. http://www.auanet.org/guidelines/stress-urinary-incontinence-(sui)-new-(aua/sufu-guideline-2017).
35. Rovner E, Athanasiou S, Choo MS, Cosson M, Dmochowski R, Golmesky A, et al. Surgery for urinary incontinence in women. En: Abrams P, Cardozo L, Wagg A, Wein A, editors. Incontinence. 6th edn. Tokyo: ICS; 2016. p. 1741---1854.
36. Murphy M, Culligan PJ, Graham CA, Kubik KM, Heit MH. Is the leak point pressure alone an accurate indicator of intrinsic sphincteric deficiency? Int Urogynecol J Pelvic Floor Dysfunct. 2004;15:294–7.
37. Park BH, Kim JC, Kim HW, Kim YH, Choi JB, Lee DH. Mid-term efficacy and complications of readjustable mid urethralsling (Remeex system) in female stress urinary incontinence with recurrence or intrinsic sphincter deficiency. Urology. 2015;85:79–84.
38. Phé V, Benadiba S, Rouprêt M, Granger B, Richard F, Chartier-Kastler E. Long-term functional outcomes after artificial urinary sphincter implantation in women with stress urinary incontinence. BJU Int. 2014;113:961–7.
39. Baldissera-Aradas JV, Rodríguez-Villamil L, González-Rodríguez I, Gil-Ugarteburu R, Fernández-Pello-Montes S, Mosquera-Madera J. Laparoscopic implantation of artificial urinary sphincter: an option for treating recurrent female urinary incontinence. Actas Urol Esp. 2016;40:406–11.
40. Fournier G, Callerot P, Thoulouzan M, Valeri A, Perrouin-Verbe MA. Robotic-assisted laparoscopic implantation of artificial urinary sphincter in women with intrinsic sphincter deficiency incontinence: initial results. Urology. 2014;84:1094–8.
41. Ercoli A, Campagna G, Delmas V, Ferrari S, Morciano A, Scambia G, et al. Anatomical insights into sacrocolpopexy for multicompartment pelvic organ prolapse. Neurourol Urodyn. 2016;35:813–8.
42. DeLancey JOL. Pubovesical ligament: a separate structure from the urethral supports ("pubo-urethral ligaments"). Neurourol Urodyn. 1989;8:53–61.
43. Ulmsten U. Some reflections and hypotheses on the pathophysiology of female urinary incontinence. Acta Obstet Gynecol Scand Suppl. 1997;166:3–8.
44. Petero VG, Diokno AC. Comparison of the long-term outcomes between incontinent men and women treated with artificial urinary sphincter. J Urol. 2006;175:605–9.

21 Laparoscopic Pectopexy

Pablo Doménech López, Vanessa Talavera Cobo, Cristina Gutiérrez Castañé, Santiago Chiva San Román, Ángel García Cortés, Francisco Javier Ancizu Marckert, Jose Enrique Robles García, Mateo Hevia Suárez, Jose María Velis Campillo, Maria Luisa Bayo Delgado, Fernando Ramón De Fata Chillón, Fernando Diez-Caballero Alonso, Marcos Torres Roca, Felipe Villacampa Aubá, David Rosell Costa, Bernardino Miñana López, and Juan Ignacio Pascual Piédrola

21.1 Introduction

Pelvic organ prolapse (POP) is defined as the descend of one or more organs through the anterior or posterior vaginal wall, or vaginal apex [1].

The main predisposing factors for the development of this pathology are vaginal labor, age, and obesity. In addition, there are some secondary factors such as abnormalities in the connective tissue or genetic variations on the pelvic architecture. All this adds up to make this pathology more frequent in Caucasian women [2].

The progressive aging of the population and the increasing of obesity rate prevalence are causing the incidence of this pathology to rise up. POP is not exempt from associate symptoms such as stress urinary incontinence (SUE) or urgency urinary incontinence (UUI) from mechanical causes.

According to the integral theory developed by Dr. Peter Papa Petros, nearly all women's pelvic floor symptoms can be explained by the variation of the anatomical position or descent of pelvic organs. The restitution of the organs to their correct place should suffice to solve all of the related pathologies.

The prevalence of POP is very variable. It is based on questionnaires whose main question is the presence of a vaginal lump, which underestimates slight or incipient prolapses [3].

Clinical history is characterized by the weigh sensation or the presence of a vaginal lump, urinary incontinence (which is actually five times more frequent than in normal population), fecal incontinence, and sexual function disorders or pain [4].

P. D. López (✉) · C. G. Castañé · S. C. S. Román · Á. G. Cortés · F. J. A. Marckert · J. E. R. García · M. H. Suárez · J. M. V. Campillo · F. D.-C. Alonso · M. T. Roca · D. R. Costa · J. I. P. Piédrola
Clínica Universidad de Navarra, Pamplona, Spain
e-mail: pdomenech@unav.es; cgutierrezc@unav.es; schiva@unav.es; agarcia.11@unav.es; fancizu@unav.es; jerobles@unav.es; fdcaballero@unav.es; mtroca@unav.es; drosell@unav.es; ipascualp@unav.es

V. T. Cobo · M. L. B. Delgado
Universidad de Navarra, Pamplona, Spain
e-mail: mbayo.1@alumni.unav.es

Fernando Ramón De Fata Chillón · F. V. Aubá · B. M. López
Clínica Universidad de Navarra, Madrid, Spain
e-mail: frchillon@unav.es; fvauba@unav.es; bminana@unav.es

F. Dökmeci, D. E. E. Rizk (eds.), *Insights Into Incontinence and the Pelvic Floor*,
https://doi.org/10.1007/978-3-030-94174-1_21

On the case of UUI, it should be noted that it is a pathology whose prevalence increases with age, rising from 20% in young women to over 50% in older or institutionalized women [5]. This pathology alone implies a significant decrease on the patient's quality of life, reducing their autonomy and their self-esteem which, in turn, affects their health directly [6].

Nowadays it is estimated that 11% of Western women may undergo pelvic floor reconstruction surgery at some point in their lifetime.

POP-Q classification is the most used system for measuring prolapse [7]. It uses anatomical references that consider the hymen as the 0 point: the sites above being negative and the ones below positive. It requires measuring 6 points to recreate the vaginal profile, establishing the different categories [8]. The treatment of POP and its associated symptoms is staggered, starting with hygienic-dietary measures and techniques of behavior modification or urination habit, escalating to pharmacological treatment or conservative anatomical restitution therapies such as the use of pessaries. Corrective surgery is considered as the final step.

21.2 Literature Review

21.2.1 Material and Methods

A systematic search was carried out using PubMed database. Searching was done in two stages with MESH tool. The first search was made with MESH terms "pelvic organ prolapse surgery" and "pectopexy"; ten articles were selected.

The second search was carried out using the terms "laparoscopy/therapeutic use" or "laparoscopy therapy" and "pelvic organ prolapse surgery" and "sacropexy or sacrocolpopexy" rendering 54 articles.

Inclusion criteria employed was defined as publication date after 2010, written in English with enough pectopexy content or relevant information. Articles about other procedures aside from POP surgical techniques have been excluded. Articles without full text availability were excluded.

Eight articles from the first search and ten from the second were selected.

The search was completed with widely recognized theoretical manuals about female pelvic organs and anatomy, including different theories about the functioning of female pelvic floor and the anatomical reconstruction.

21.2.2 About Female Pelvic Floor Anatomy

Based on integral theory, the female pelvis can be categorized in three different levels, each one related to different anatomical structures. They are categorized from inside to outside in level one, two and three [9].

On the first level, or level 1, the bladder and the uterus can be found. This level is located on top of the imaginary line that runs from the middle height of the pubic bone to the sacrum, leaving these two organs above it. The main ligaments contained in this compartment are the uterosacral ligament (USL) and the pubocervical fascia (PCF).

The second level goes from below the line of level 1 to immediately below the pubic bone, parallel to the previous line. It contains the cardinal ligaments (CL), the pubourethral ligaments (PUL), and the rectovaginal fascia (RVF) also known as Denonvilliers' fascia.

The last level contains the perineal membrane, external urethral ligaments (EUL), and perineal body.

The central point for the pelvic floor anchorage is known as the cervical ring (CR). On this point, the USL, CL, PCF, and RVF join. According to the bridge model [10], the descent of this structure can be the result of the loss of strength of the USLs, causing a vaginal prolapse, uterine descent, and urinary symptoms such as urgency or incontinence. USL anchor on the sides of S2–S4 level [11].

The rupture of the PCF would cause a severe cystocele or an anterior enterocele.

The pubovesical ligament (PVL) is the main support structure of the bladder. It is a rigid fibromuscular structure. During urination, due to its more rigid nature, the PVL remains firm while the longitudinal muscles of the anus (LMA) and the lifting plate (LP) contract, causing a force in a posterior-inferior direction that provoke the rotation of the bladder favoring the opening of the urethra [9]. The union of the LMA with the anterior bladder wall forms the Gilvernet precervical arch.

At the medial level, the PUL and EUL attach to the urethra outside the pelvis, beyond the perineal membrane on its medial area, supporting it [9].

The tendinous arch of the pelvic fascia (TAPF) is built by horizontal ligaments, which go from the pubis symphysis, above the PUL, to the ischial spine.

TAPF has lateral branches that join the PCF above and the RVF below, being the anchorage of the vagina.

The lifting muscles maintain the tension of the ligaments so that this structure simulates a hammock where the urethra is supported [12].

Dysfunction of the TAPF would cause a lateral defect and the descent of the urethra that would lead to stress urinary incontinence [13].

Finally, VFR, also called Denonvilliers' fascia, extends from the perineal body below the levator muscle to the lateral pillars of the rectum [14].

It is considered that continence and normal position of the pelvic organs are achieved by the interrelated functioning of the muscles, ligaments, and fascias. Deterioration or unbalance in any of the ligaments described above could favor the appearance of urinary or rectal pathology, as well as prolapses of the pelvic organs [10].

21.2.3 Colposacropexy Development

As it has been explained, anatomical position of the bladder, rectum, and vagina depends directly on the forces generated by ligaments, muscles, and fascias, as they have neither form nor structure in themselves. The relaxation and contraction of the muscles from the wall of these organs allow the continence and evacuation when they have enough support because, in all three cases, they are mostly container organs [9].

Risk factors induce an excessive laxity in the connective tissue of any of the pelvic compartments. The prolapse is named depending on the structure that protrudes. Even at rest, a certain amount of tension is required in the vaginal membrane to keep all the structures balanced [15].

Most of the pelvic floor ligaments are related to the vagina and/or uterus due to the position of the vagina. It is medial between the bladder and the rectum, so any damage to those ligaments will alter the entire pelvic axis.

Uterus value is often underestimated because of the hysterectomy usually carried out in POP surgery. However, this organ has an important role on the anchoring of the ligaments such as USL or CL, as well as providing blood flow to them [10].

The closure and opening of the urethra depend largely on the integrity of the pubococcygeal muscle (PCM). The correct anchoring of the PCM in the urethra will allow the activity of the lifting plate (LP) and longitudinal anus muscle (AML), whose contraction closes the proximal urethra in a "C" shape and whose relaxation opens it in an "O" shape for urination. In addition, the PCM requires an "H"-shaped contraction to help to closure the urethra [9]. Dysfunction of the ligaments leads to a loss of strength which results in prolapse due to excessive laxity. It is essential to repair the laxity of the suspensory ligaments in order to regain their previous length and tension. If they are restored, the pelvis gains again its anatomical shape and thus its function.

First-line treatment for symptomatic POP consists on the use of pessary. However, only 14% continue with this option in long term [16].

Most cases are treated with a surgical procedure, being colposacropexy the current gold standard.

The open approach POP correction surgery was described by Lane in 1962. He demonstrated its superior results when compared to sacrospinous ligament fixation [17].

The resolution of the prolapse is achieved in 91% of cases, and 96% of patients show clear satisfaction after the operation. The results are more favorable in women who have had a previous hysterectomy or if a supracervical hysterectomy is performed, because a greater distance is achieved between the mesh and the ureter, minimizing the risk of incontinence and the risk of re-intervention due to any possible cause [18]. The main reason for re-intervention "de novo" emergency incontinence and the second in frequency is the recurrence of MOP (with a prevalence of 5.1%). There is a 40% decrease in re-operation risk for every 10 years that pass since the patient had the surgery. At this point, the possibility of assessment bias must be taken into account for two reasons: first, because older women are less likely to undergo reoperation and choose more conservative measures and, second, because the doctor himself limits surgery in older women [19].

Forty percent of women have a POP greater than or equal to grade two. The unstoppable aging of the population is increasing this problem, so it is important to know the quality of life (QoL) and sexual function of patients after undergoing this intervention. Two questionnaires have been used for this purpose: the FSFI for female sexual function and the P-QOL for quality of life, being evaluated both before and after surgery. The scores of these questionnaires improved significantly after pectopexy surgery, with an undeniable relationship between the absence of a vaginal lump and the feeling of general improvement after surgery [20].

Laparoscopic and robotic surgeries have less morbidity but are associated with a higher economic cost. Both require a longer learning curve than open abdominal surgery [18]. In the Kenton et al. study [21], the total number of patients expressed an improvement in their symptoms, with no significant differences between the group that received laparoscopy and those that received robotic surgery. There were also no significant differences in postoperative quality of life. Sexual activity was improved in both groups [21].

80% of colposacropexies are currently performed using minimally invasive methods, a fact that demonstrates generalization of these techniques in the last decade, although it has not yet been possible to obtain evidence of their superiority to open abdominal surgery [18]. However, it is true that the use of these techniques favors the correction of SUI, which usually appears simultaneously with POP and whose presence must be evaluated before surgery [22].

In the comparative studies of laparoscopic and robot-assisted surgery, the assessment of quality of life was evaluated with the ICIQ-VS (International Consultation on Incontinence Questionnaire-Vaginal Symptoms) questionnaire, which was sent between 6 and 36 months to all patients undergoing surgery. Satisfaction was 86%, with a decrease in scores in all domains of the questionnaire. This improvement proved to be statistically significant as well as clinically relevant [16].

Robotic colposacropexy is currently indicated in anterior and/or apical vaginal prolapses and in posterior asymptomatic defects that could not be resolved in a first surgery. The advantages of robotics over laparoscopy are greater freedom of movement and improved optical systems, which result in better visualization of the protrusion and greater precision and speed in locating the sutures. Furthermore, in robotics, the main surgeon is not that dependent on the quality of his assistants [23]. In the long term, robotics has shown that 95% of patients do not require re-intervention for the same problem in the following 5 years, in contrast to 17% of re-interventions required in the open abdominal surgery group.

21.2.4 Pectopexy, the Beginning

However, it is still curious how all pathologies of descent of pelvic organs are resolved with a single surgical technique, colposacropexy, which generates a new ligament between the cervix and cervical stump with the sacral promontory. The placement of a mesh at this level has side effects that may be relevant in patients undergoing the operation, with rates of constipation of more than 30% and the appearance of symptoms related to sexual activity due to the displacement of the vaginal axis [11].

In addition, increasing of obesity rates and intestinal adhesions due to prior abdominal interventions is an obstacle to colposacropexy in the access to the promontory.

As a solution to these problems G. Noé and C. Banarjee proposed in 2007 [24] laparoscopic pectopexy, a surgical technique initially intended for obese women with BMI >30. For this purpose, the use of the lateral part of the right and left iliopectineal ligaments is proposed for the fixation of the mesh, which are stronger than sacrospinous ligament and TAPF [11].

This location is associated with a reduced incidence of lateral defects.

This technique maintains the indications for traditional colposacropexy [11]: the existence of a greater prolapse of grade 1 according to the POP-Q system, in seating and supine position. It is also recommended for women in whom it's difficult to access the anterior longitudinal ligament.

When compared with colposacropexy, pectopexy has better surgical time, faster recovery rate, less cost, and less morbidity [25], but these advantages are not significant due to the small number of patients nowadays [26].

21.3 Case Study: The Laparoscopic Pectopexy Surgical Technique as a Treatment of Apical and Anterior Compartment Defects of the Female Pelvic Floor

(a) **Aim and Scope**

Colposacropexy is the gold standard treatment for apical defects of the female pelvic floor, attaching the mesh to the sacrum or promontorium, being the most employed technique with success rates near 90%.

However, this procedure is not exempt of secondary effects, especially the newly appearance of constipation which can affect up to 37% of the patients [24].

Currently, we face an elderly population with higher obesity rates, which difficult the access to the sacrum for the attachment of the mesh, even more if they have suffered from previous abdominal surgery.

The technique that we show today was developed in 2011, due to these sociodemographic conditions.

Laparoscopic pectopexy allows a physiological repositioning of the pelvic floor organs which avoids constipation and allows a correct vaginal dynamic.

(b) **Material and Methods**

Here we present the case of a 59-year-old woman with a grade 3 cystocele and a grade 1 descending uterus.

Before the surgery we performed an urodynamic study where we did not identify positive leak points asking the patient to cough or perform Valsalva maneuver.

We performed the operation using standard endoscopic equipment (a 10-mm optical device inserted via a 12-mm trocar and 5-mm instruments) and polyvinylidene fluoride (PVDF) monofilament mesh (DynaMesh® PVDF, 3 × 15 cm).

We performed the surgery following the steps described in Karl Günter Noé's article. "Laparoscopic Pectopexy: A New Technique of Prolapse Surgery for Obese Patients."

(c) **Study Results**

The surgery could be performed satisfactorily. No adverse events turned up during surgery nor in the recovering time. The operating time for this procedure was 96 min.

21.4 Discussion

The main objective of any reconstructive surgery should be to achieve the anatomical restitution of the affected organ. The balance of forces in the female pelvic floor is affected by multiple ligaments and muscles. If surgical technique is able to obtain an anatomical anchor for the ligaments, it will be able to obtain patient's well-being too. Anatomical and functional points of view should be at the same level, because the anatomical restitution is followed by functional restitution.

All works analyzed about laparoscopic pectopexy on different databases coincide on the great advantage of this technique. This surgery enables an easier access in obese women and in those who have been through others abdominal surgeries.

Pectopexy is not inferior when it is compared with gold standard. Without adding any risk, laparoscopic pectopexy allows the surgeon to get a more physiological reconstruction of female pelvis, and it avoids some of the most frequent secondary effects of colposacropexy, like constipation.

Pectopexy is not a common surgery. The generalization of this technique is difficult due to the high requirements needed to perform it. Surgeon experience and laparoscopic skills are the cornerstones in the learning of this procedure, which has a larger learning curve compared with open surgery.

These factors condition the spread of this new technique, which is relegated to the second line. Colposacropexy is supported by greater evidence, and more years to measure the results, but the potential that pectopexy seems to have, force us to have an open mind and think that maybe not every level of female pelvic floor can be treated successfully with the same technique.

21.5 Conclusions

Laparoscopic pectopexy is a safe and feasible technique that allows a physiological recovery of the female pelvic floor. No additional secondary effects appeared with this procedure.

Further studies are recommended for long-term results against the gold standard laparoscopic sacropexy.

References

1. International Continence Society [Internet]. ICS. 2019. https://www.ics.org/.
2. Maher C, Barber MD, Jelovsek JE. Pelvic organ prolapse. Lancet. 2007;369:1027–38.
3. Olsen A, Smith V, Bergstrom J, Collin J. Epidemiology of surgically managed pelvic organ prolapse and urinary incontinence. Obstet Gynecol. 1997;89:501–6.
4. Rogers RG, Fashokun TB. Pelvic organ prolapse in women: Epidemiology, risk factors, clinical manifestations, and management. [Internet]. 2019. https://www.uptodate.com/contents/pelvic-organ-prolapse-in-women-epidemiology-risk-factors-clinical-manifestations-andmanagement?search=pelvic%20organ%20prolapse%20clinica%20manifestation&source=search_result&selectedTitle=1~106&usage_type=default&display_rank=1#H17
5. Lucas MG, Bosch RJ, Burkhard FC, Cruz F, Madden TB, Nambiar AK, et al. EAU guidelines on surgical treatment of urinary incontinence. Eur Urol. 2012;62(6):1118–29.
6. Li J, Yang L, Pu C, Tang Y, Yun H, Han P. The role of duloxetine in stress urinary incontinence: a systematic review and meta-analysis. Int Urol Nephrol. 2013;45(3):679686.
7. Boyd S, O'Sullivan D, Tulikangas P. Use of the pelvic organ quantification system (POPQ) in published articles of peer-reviewed journals. Int Urogynecol J. 2017;28:1719–23.
8. Bump R, Norton P. Epidemiology and natural history of pelvic floor dysfunction. Obstet Gynecol Clin N Am. 1998;25:723–46.
9. Petros P. The International Continence Society and Integral Theory systems for management of the incontinent female-a comparative analysis. Pelviperineology. 2007;26:25–9.
10. Petros P. The integral system. Central Eur J Urol. 2011;64(3):110.
11. Banerjee C, Noé K. Laparoscopic pectopexy: a new technique of prolapse surgery for obese patients. Arch Gynecol Obstet. 2010;284:631–5.
12. Petros PEP. The female pelvic floor: function, dysfunction and management according to the integral theory. Springer; 2011.
13. Petros P, Papadimitriou J. Evolution of midurethral and other mesh slings—a critical analysis. Neurourol Urodyn. 2013;32(4):399–406.
14. DeLancey JO. Structural support of the urethra as it relates to stress urinary incontinence: the hammock hypothesis. Am J Obstet Gynecol. 1994;170(6):171320; discussion 1720–3.
15. Petros P. The female pelvic floor. 2nd ed. Berlin Heidelberg: Springer; 2010. p. 14–50. The anatomy and dynamics of pelvic floor function and dysfunction.
16. Price N, Slack A, Jackson S. Laparoscopic sacrocolpopexy: an observational study of functional and anatomical outcomes. Int Urogynecol J. 2010;22:77–82.
17. Campbell P, Cloney L, Jha S. Abdominal versus laparoscopica sacrocolpopexy: a systematic review and meta-analysis. CME. 2016;71:435–42.
18. Lee R, Mottrie A, Payne C, Waltregny D. A review of the current status of laparoscopic and robot assisted

sacrocolpopexy for pelvic organ prolapse. Eur Urol. 2014;65:1128–37.
19. Vandendriessche D, Sussfeld J, Giraudet G, Lucot J. Complications and reoperations after laparoscopic sacrocolpopexy with a mean follow-up of 4 years. Int Urogynecol J. 2016;28:231–9.
20. Tahaoglu A, Bakir M, Peker N, Bagli İ, Tayyar A. Modified laparoscopic pectopexy: short-term follow-up and its effects on sexual function and quality of life. Int Urogynecol J. 2018;29:1155–60.
21. Kenton K, Mueller E, Tarney C, Bresee C. One-year outcomes after minimally invasive sacrocolpopexy. Female Pelvic Med Reconstr Surg. 2016;22:382–4.
22. Heesakkers J, Vierhout M. Prolapse surgery: which technique and when? Curr Opin Urol. 2011;21:281–5.
23. Hudson C, Northington G, Lyles R, Karp D. Outcomes of robotic sacrocolpopexy. Female Pelvic Med Reconstr Surg. 2014;20:252–60.
24. Noé K, Spüntrup C, Anapolski M. Laparoscopic pectopexy: a randomised comparative clinical trial of standard laparoscopic sacral colpo-cervicopexy to the new laparoscopic pectopexy. Short-term postoperative results. Arch Gynecol Obstet. 2012;287:275–80.
25. Noé K, Schiermeier S, Alkatout I, Anapolski M. Laparoscopic pectopexy: a prospective, randomized, comparative clinical trial of standard laparoscopic sacral colpocervicopexy with the new laparoscopic pectopexy—postoperative results and intermediate-term follow-up in a pilot study. J Endourol. 2015;29:210215.
26. Biler A, Ertas I, Tosun G, Hortu I, et al. Perioperative complications and short-term outcomes of abdominal sacrocolpopexy, laparoscopic sacrocolpopexy, and laparoscopic pectopexy for apical prolapse. Int Braz J Urol. 2018;44:9961004.

Part IV

Chronic Bladder Disorders

22 Bladder Pain Syndrome and Interstitial Cystitis in Women

Mehmet Murat Seval, Bulut Varlı, Kazibe Koyuncu, Şerife Esra Çetinkaya, and Fulya Dökmeci

22.1 Introduction

Bladder pain syndrome/interstitial cystitis is a chronic condition characterized by pelvic pain, pressure, or discomfort accompanied by lower urinary tract symptoms, such as urgency and frequency. Several different nomenclatures regarding this clinical condition are used in the literature interchangeably, including hypersensitive bladder, bladder pain syndrome (BPS), painful bladder syndrome (PBS), interstitial cystitis (IC), and combinations of these terms (IC/PBS, BPS/IC, and IC/BPS). However, BPS is increasingly preferred to be referred to as IC, and the term IC, defined by the presence of Hunner's lesions, is referred to represent a different disease process with different diagnostic and therapeutic features [1].

In addition to the nomenclature, the definition of the clinical condition also varies between international societies. The definition of the International Society for the Study of BPS (ESSIC) requires symptoms to be present for longer than 6 months: "Chronic pelvic pain, pressure or discomfort of >6 months' duration, perceived to be related to the urinary bladder, accompanied by at least one other urinary symptom such as persistent urge to void or urinary frequency. Confusable diseases as the cause of the symptoms must be excluded" [2]. This definition has used the term "persistent urge to void" for the sensation of pressure or discomfort that many patients describe rather than pain. The American Urological Association decided to use the nomenclature "interstitial cystitis/bladder pain syndrome" (IC/BPS) and described this condition as "an unpleasant sensation (pain, pressure, discomfort) perceived to be related to the urinary bladder, associated with lower urinary tract symptoms of more than six weeks duration, in the absence of infection or other identifiable causes" [3]. In this definition, suffering from the abovementioned symptoms for more than 6 weeks was found to be sufficient for a diagnosis.

The incidence of IC/BPS varies in different populations worldwide. An estimated prevalence of 100–200 per 100,000 has been reported, with a 5:1 female-to-male dominance and a mean average age of 51 years [4]. The prevalence of BPS/IC has also been shown to be higher in first-degree relatives than the general population [5].

Although the pathogenesis of the disease remains unclear, it is generally accepted that an unknown mutual effect triggers immune and neu-

M. M. Seval (✉) · B. Varlı · Ş. E. Çetinkaya · F. Dökmeci
Department of Obstetrics and Gynecology, Ankara University School of Medicine, Cebeci Hospital, Ankara, Turkey
e-mail: seval@ankara.edu.tr

K. Koyuncu
Department of Obstetrics and Gynecology, Istanbul Kartal Dr. Lütfi Kırdar City Hospital, Istanbul, Turkey

F. Dökmeci, D. E. E. Rizk (eds.), *Insights Into Incontinence and the Pelvic Floor*,
https://doi.org/10.1007/978-3-030-94174-1_22

roendocrine factors, which induce a vicious cycle provoking an inflammatory response in the urothelium [6]. All etiological factors presented in the literature lead to urothelial dysfunction and increased permeability and can be listed as urinary toxic substances, infections, immune cell activation (especially the mast cells), autoimmune mechanisms, autonomic nerve changes, inhibition of bladder urothelial cell proliferation, and decreased microvascular density resulting in hypoxia and genetic predisposition. The urothelium plays an important role as a barrier to irritants in urine by providing a protective dense inner layer consisting of glycosaminoglycans, chondroitin sulfate, and sodium hyaluronate on the luminal surface and by the intercellular junctions between urothelial cells. Damage of the protective inner layer of the bladder appears to be the key factor triggering inflammation, irritation, neurogenic responses, and numerous other reactions resulting in the clinical presentation of bladder pain syndrome [7, 8]. Although the exact etiology of the defect in this protective layer is currently unknown, strategies targeting to put the main consisting substances back have been investigated extensively and have given promising results in providing symptom relief.

Many studies have been conducted to reveal objective diagnostic criteria for the diagnosis of BPS/IC. However, neither any objective tool nor a pathognomonic finding could be obtained from the investigations. In fact, diagnostic criteria differ among the international societies [1]. Generally, a clinical diagnosis is established mainly on the basis of a comprehensive medical history, including questions about suprapubic pain related to bladder filling, increased urinary frequency and urinary urgency, and the exclusion of urinary tract infections or other diseases causing chronic pelvic pain. Voiding diaries and validated questionnaires may be preferred to standardize the symptoms and quality of life in the diagnosis [9]. A detailed physical examination should be performed, including abdominal examination for bladder fullness and tenderness, pelvic examination for pain mapping of the genital and pelvic regions, neurological examination, and pelvic muscle strength assessment. Urinary dipstick and urine culture are recommended to rule out hematuria or infection. Even though it is not recommended in routine practice, urodynamic monitoring may allow observing detrusor overactivity or reduced bladder capacity, suggestive of BPS/IC [10]. In cases of clinical suspicion, diagnostic cystoscopy should be performed not only to exclude malign conditions but also to demonstrate Hunner's lesions, which have been described by Guy L. Hunner as patches of red mucosa exhibiting small vessels radiating to a central pale scar [11]. A bladder biopsy should be considered to exclude malignancies and eosinophilic or tuberculotic cystitis. Counting tryptase-positive bladder mast cells histopathologically may be helpful to define detrusor mastocytosis, which is considered diagnostic for BPS/IC [12]. Hydrodistention of the bladder is not widely used as it can cause serious complications, such as rupture and necrosis, and may provide little useful information beyond history and physical examination findings. However, it might be performed in some cases, keeping in mind that it must be performed always before bladder wall biopsy to prevent rupture of the bladder.

Since the pathophysiology of BPS/IC is not understood clearly, treatment options have focused on the repair of the potential disease mechanisms that cause the vicious cycle, thereby relieving symptoms and increasing quality of life. Thus, the realistic goals of the preferred treatment option should be discussed carefully with patients, giving clear information that BPS/IC is a chronic disease and explaining that it has no curative treatment and may require long-term processes followed by remissions and exacerbations.

The management of BPS/IC occurs in a stepwise manner, from conservative to more invasive treatment approaches. Behavioral modifications, physical therapy, stress reduction, and dietary manipulations outline conservative management, which is recommended as first-line therapy 4). Medical treatments can be evaluated in two groups as systemic or intravesical, according to the method of application. Apart from these treatment options, hydrodistention and fulguration of Hunner's ulcers, intravesical botulinum toxin A injections, sacral neuromodulation, and surgical options including substation cystoplasty or urinary diversion are considered as the more advanced treatment steps in the management of BPS/IC.

Non-steroidal anti-inflammatory drugs, analgesics, antidepressants (amitriptyline), antihistamines (cimetidine, hydroxyzine), immunosuppressants (cyclosporine), and sodium pentosan polysulfate are the medical agents available to use per orally. Intravesical treatment agents include dimethyl sulfoxide, hyaluronic acid (HA), chondroitin sulfate, lidocaine, and their combinations, which will be reviewed and discussed below together with a case study.

22.2 Literature Review

Hyaluronic acid is a mucopolysaccharide that is present in the GAG layer of the urothelium [4]. Intravesical application of HA may theoretically repair the damaged GAG layer, which is considered to play a key role in the pathogenesis of BPS/IC. It has also been proposed that HA has an inhibitory action on mast cell degranulation, which is crucial in the pathogenesis of the disease [13].

Several studies in the literature have investigated the efficacy of HA in BPS/IC patients. Hung et al. have demonstrated significant improvements in the pain visual analogue scale (VAS) and the Interstitial Cystitis Symptom and Problem Index (ICSI and ICPI) scores in a prospective, multicenter study evaluating 103 women with refractory BPS/IC who underwent intravesical HA therapy. In this study, a significant improvement of the bladder pain symptoms was noted in 73.3% of patients, while bladder storage symptoms were improved in only less than half (47.2%) of the patients. Thus, they have concluded that HA treatment was more efficient in improving bladder pain than storage symptoms of BPS/IC [14].

Similarly, Akbay et al. have found significant improvements in VAS, ICSI, and ICPI scores in the 75.9–94.4% range in short-term follow-up after intravesical instillation of HA in 54 women with BPS/IC [15]. In another study, significant improvements in urinary bladder pain, urgency, nocturia, and quality of life have been demonstrated with intravesical HA at 15 months of follow-up [16].

Liang et al. have investigated psychological and urinary symptoms in 30 patients with newly diagnosed BPS/IC after intravesical HA treatment. In contrast to the improvements in bladder pain and lower urinary tract symptoms in patients, they reported that no significant changes were observed in psychological and sexual functional scores [17].

Engelhardt et al. demonstrated that 50% of patients reported complete remission of bladder symptoms at a mean 4.9 years follow-up without any additional therapy to the intravesical HA treatment and concluded that intravesical hyaluronan provides a high rate of symptom remission, both acutely and in the long term, in a considerable number of patients [18].

The effects of the presence of Hunner's ulcers and previous treatment modalities on the therapeutic outcome of intravesical HA have also been investigated. In a study that included 33 BPS/IC patients, intravesical HA instillation was reported to be an effective and safe treatment for BPS/IC, whereas previous treatment modalities and the presence of Hunner's ulcers did not affect the efficacy of HA instillation [19].

Shao et al. evaluated the efficacy of intravesical HA instillation after hydrodistention for the treatment of patients with IC and small bladder capacities in a prospective open-label controlled trial. In a total of 47 patients, they reported that intravesical HA treatment prolonged the effect of bladder hydrodistention [20].

In a prospective randomized study comparing the clinical efficacies of intravesical chondroitin sulfate (CS) and HA in patients with BPS/IC, both CS and HA have been shown to be effective treatment methods. However, CS was found to be superior to HA in terms of 24 h frequency, nocturia, and the interstitial cystitis problem index (ICPI) in short-term follow-up [21].

There are also a number of studies investigating the efficacies of combinations of HA with other intravesical therapies. Cervigni et al. evaluated the efficacy of the combination of intravesical HA and CS in BPS/IC patients refractory to previous treatments. They assessed symptoms and quality of life using a visual analogue scale and 3-day voiding diaries and validated questionnaires over a period of 3 years. They concluded that this treatment combination produced a sustained improvement in symptoms up to 3 years [7]. In a study comparing the efficacy of intravesical CS with combined HA/CS treatment in women, the intravesical HA/CS combination was found to be superior to CS alone in terms of ICSI, ICPI, and daytime and nighttime frequency [22].

In another randomized, open-label, multicenter study, Cervigni et al. compared the efficacy, safety, and costs of an intravesical HA/CS combination with dimethyl sulfoxide (DMSO) alone in 110 women with BPS/IC. They demonstrated that treatment with HA/CS appears to be as effective as DMSO with potentially more favorable and acceptable safety and cost-effectiveness profile [8].

Lv et al. compared the efficacy of HA combined with alkalinized lidocaine to two control groups provided with lidocaine or HA monotherapy. Among the 45 participants, the combination group demonstrated significant improvement at 2 weeks that continued until the completion of the trial at 48 weeks. Monotherapy with alkalinized lidocaine demonstrated an improvement at 2 weeks, but the therapeutic benefit ceased at week 24, while monotherapy with HA had a later onset of improvement at 4 weeks but remained beneficial throughout the study [23].

A web-based survey analysis has evaluated perceptions of success or failure of all previous BPS/IC treatment modalities in 1628 women. The most effective treatments were found to be oral drugs in a range of 35.1–65.5%. However, only 31.9% of the patients reported improvement in their clinical situations with intravesical HA therapy, while the other intravesical agents demonstrated an improvement rate of 33.3–56.2%. It has been emphasized that the available data were still insufficient to demonstrate the effectiveness of the intravesical HA treatment [24].

Meta-analyses and systematic reviews have been conducted analyzing the efficacy of various intravesical treatment agents in BPS/IC [25–27]. Pyo et al. have analyzed intravesical HA and combined HA/CS treatment in 10 studies including 390 women at a follow-up of 6 months. Changes in VAS, ICSI, ICPI, bladder, and voided volumes were used as outcome measures, and significant improvements in these measures were found with both HA and the combination of HA/CS [25].

Barua et al. analyzed 19 trials involving dimethyl sulfoxide (DMSO), pentosan polysulfate (PPS), and low and high molecular weight HA and CS, including 801 patients. Four trials included both male and female patients. The most commonly used tools were VAS, ICSI, ICPI, and the Pain, Urgency, and Frequency (PUF) score. Follow-up varied mostly between 6 weeks and 4.9 years. The highest improvement in symptoms and response rate was found for high molecular weight HA [26].

A very recent meta-analysis by Liu et al. included 11 randomized controlled trials with 902 patients and evaluated 8 intravesical agents for the treatment of BPS/IC, DMSO, HA, CS, combined HA/CS, onabotulinumtoxinA (ONBA), lidocaine, and resiniferatoxin (0.05 μm and 0.1 μm). VAS, ICSI, and ICPI were used as primary outcome measures. 0.1 μm resiniferatoxin was found to be more effective according to ICPI and ICSI. Combined HA/CS was found to be more effective according to VAS and ranked second in ICSI and third in ICPI [27].

22.3 Case Report: Intravesical Hyaluronic Acid Instillation for Interstitial Cystitis/Bladder Pain Syndrome—Case Series

(a) **Aim and Scope**
As reviewed above, intravesical instillation of hyaluronic acid may repair and replenish the protective bladder barrier against infiltration of urinary ingredients in patients with BPS/IC. The objective of this report was to demonstrate the experience of single center with intravesical hyaluronic acid installation

for women with *refractory* BPS/IC to medical treatments.

(b) **Study Design and Method**

A total of seven patients were followed in a university hospital urogynecology department between March 2016 and October 2018. Women with urinary tract infection or malignancy, urolithiasis, and neurological pathologies were excluded. The women were diagnosed as BPS/IC according to the American Urology Association Guideline [3]. All the patients presented with Hunner's lesions at cystoscopy and were refractory to conservative and oral treatments (analgesics, anticholinergics, and antidepressants). Intravesical hyaluronic acid was administered at a dose of 50 mL/120 mg sterile sodium HA (HYACYST®—Molecular weight: 152 kDa) using 12F hydrophilic Foley catheters. The intravesical instillations were performed weekly in the first month and monthly through the second to fourth months, with a total of eight intravesical doses. Treatment success was evaluated using the change in visual analogue scale (VAS) pain scoring and the Patients Global Impression of Improvement (PGI-I) after completion of therapy.

(c) **Results**

The mean age of the women was 59.7 years (42–88 years) and the mean body mass index was 31.4 kg/m^2 (24.9–40 kg/m^2). The mean VAS score decreased from 8.1 (range: 6–10) to 6.1 (range: 4–8) after treatment. However, this decrease was not statistically significant ($p = 0.140$). The overall characteristics of the patients are summarized in Table 22.1. The mean PGI-I score was 4.1 for all patients at the end of the treatment. With regard to the PGI-I scores, two patients (28.5%) reported an improvement, three patients (43.0%) reported no change, and two patients (28.5%) reported worsening in their clinical conditions. One of the two cases who showed improvement in the PGI-I score (#2) had severe detrusor overactivity during ambulatory urodynamic monitoring before the treatment (Fig. 22.1) and demonstrated a dramatic decrease in detrusor overactivity after intravesical hyaluronic acid treatment. As a result, the effectiveness of intravesical HA treatment in refractory BPS/IC patients was found to be limited.

22.4 Discussion

Intravesical instillation agents appear to be promising in the treatment of BPS/IC, but the quest for higher efficacy therapies that improve outcomes continues and proves that a fully satisfactory suc-

Table 22.1 Characteristics of the study population

Case #	Age (years)	BMI (kg/m^2)	Previous pelvic surgery	Previous vaginal delivery	Menopause status	VAS (before treatment)	VAS (after treatment)	PGI-I
1	45	32.1	Colporrhaphy anterior-posterior	2	Pre-menopausal	7	6	6
2	88	24.9	–	4	Post-menopausal	6	6	4
3	62	40	–	0	Post-menopausal	10	7	4
4	58	29.2	–	3	Post-menopausal	10	4	2
5	60	28.3	–	3	Post-menopausal	10	4	3
6	63	35.6	Burch	3	Post-menopausal	8	8	4
7	42	30	Mini-sling	2	Pre-menopausal	6	8	6

BMI body mass index, *VAS* visual analogue scale, *PGI-I* Patients Global Impression of Improvement

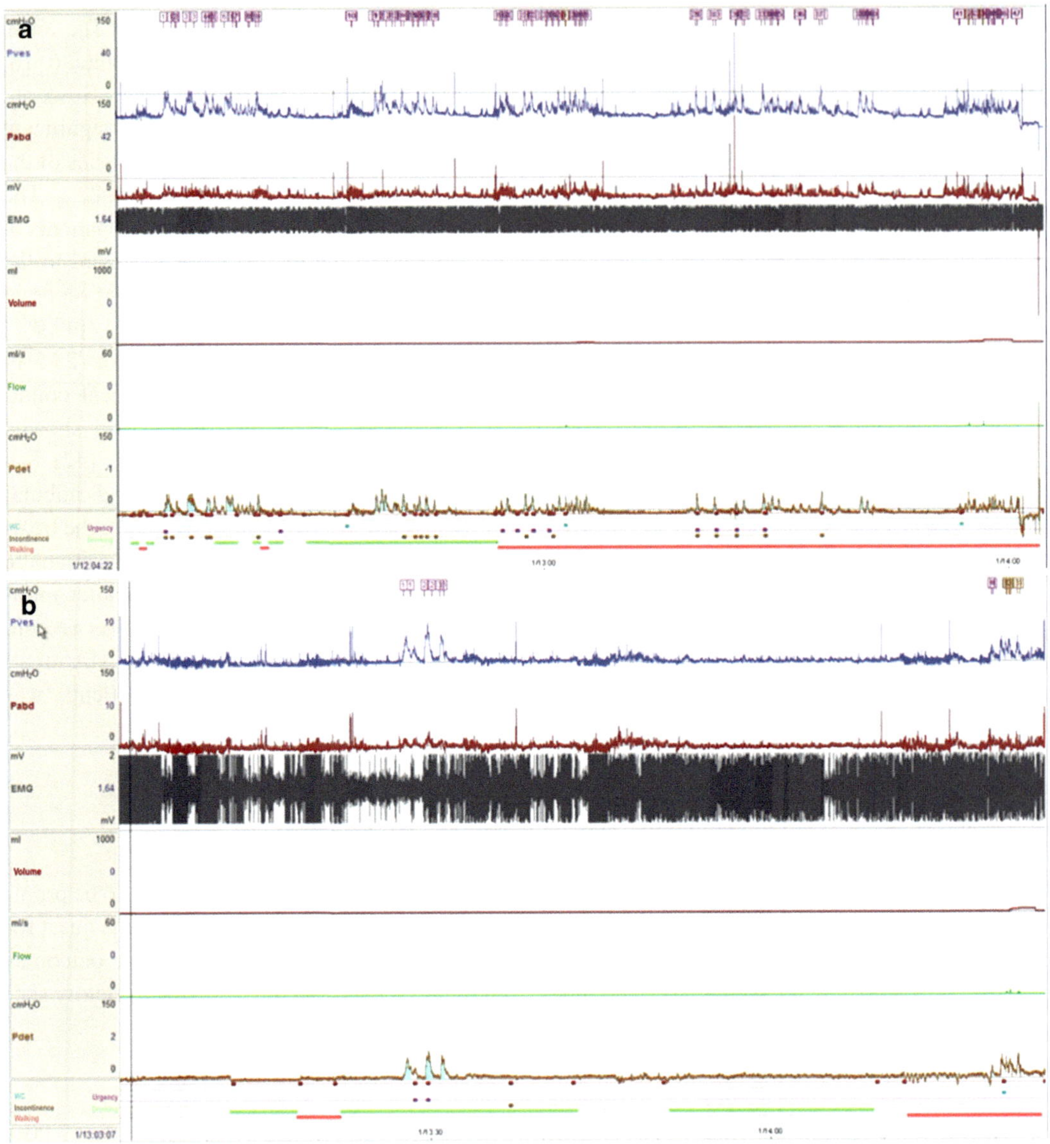

Fig. 22.1 (**a**) Initial ambulatory urodynamic monitoring of Case #2 presenting severe detrusor overactivity. *(Cystometry duration, 112 min; number of urgency, 11; number of incontinence, 18; number of urgency incontinence, 18; number of detrusor overactivity, 47)*. (**b**) Control ambulatory urodynamic monitoring after intravesical hyaluronic acid treatment. *(Cystometry duration, 81 min; number of urgency, 2; number of incontinence, 1; number of urgency incontinence, 1; number of detrusor overactivity, 4)*

cess rate has not yet been clearly achieved. The main reason for the lack of successful management is the unsolved etiopathogenesis of BPS/IC. Moreover, different definitions and various diagnostic criteria used for this disorder resulting in heterogeneous study populations, heterogeneity in the previous treatments of women, numerous agents with different administration schemes and periods, and varying outcome measures make the interpretation of the results of the studies difficult.

As mentioned previously, the cystoscopic observation of Hunner's lesions is suggested to provide the diagnosis of a different disease process which may require different treatment options. Such patients might be considered to be a more difficult group with whom to achieve success. All of the women in the case study had Hunner's lesions at cystoscopy and were all refractory to many previous medical treatment agents. Despite the number of patients being too small, it was interesting to observe that the detrusor overactivity diminished significantly after eight intravesical HA instillations at 4 months.

22.5 Conclusion

BPS/IC is a complicated chronic condition caused by multiple etiologies and pathophysiology that is not yet clearly understood. Since the bladder urothelium plays a unique role in being a barrier protecting bladder interstitium from the irritants of the urine, the strategies targeting to repair this protective layer may be promising for better treatment outcomes of the disorder. New treatment modalities should be investigated in well-designed future studies with long-term follow-up.

References

1. Malde S, Palmisani S, Al-Kaisy A, Sahai A. Guideline of guidelines: bladder pain syndrome. BJU Int. 2018;122(5):729–43.
2. van de Merwe JP, Nordling J, Bouchelouche P, Bouchelouche K, Cervigni M, Daha L, et al. Diagnostic criteria, classification, and nomenclature for painful bladder syndrome/interstitial cystitis: an ESSIC proposal. Eur Urol. 2008;53(1):60–7.
3. Hanno PM, Burks DA, Clemens JQ, Dmochowski RR, Erickson D, Fitzgerald MP, et al. AUA guideline for the diagnosis and treatment of interstitial cystitis/bladder pain syndrome. J Urol. 2011;185(6):2162–70.
4. Hanno P, Dinis P, Lin A, Nickel C, Nordling J, et al. Bladder Pain Syndrome. In: Abrams P, Cardozo L, Adrian Wagg, Wein A, editors. Incontinence. 6th edn. International Continence Society; 2017. p. 2203–302.
5. Warren JW, Jackson TL, Langenberg P, Meyers DJ, Xu J. Prevalence of interstitial cystitis in first-degree relatives of patients with interstitial cystitis. Urology. 2004;63(1):17–21.
6. Cervigni M, Morciano A, Campagna G. Bladder pain syndromes/interstitial cystitis and the overactive pelvic floor. In: Padoa A, Rosenbaum T, editors. The overactive pelvic floor. 2016. p. 57–71.
7. Cervigni M, Natale F, Nasta L, Mako A. Intravesical hyaluronic acid and chondroitin sulphate for bladder pain syndrome/interstitial cystitis: long-term treatment results. Int Urogynecol J. 2012;23(9):1187–92.
8. Cervigni M, Sommariva M, Tenaglia R, Porru D, Ostardo E, Giammò A, et al. A randomized, open-label, multicenter study of the efficacy and safety of intravesical hyaluronic acid and chondroitin sulfate versus dimethyl sulfoxide in women with bladder pain syndrome/interstitial cystitis. Neurourol Urodynam. 2016;36(4):1178–86.
9. Parsons CL, Dell J, Stanford EJ, Bullen M, Kahn BS, Waxell T, et al. Increased prevalence of interstitial cystitis: previously unrecognized urologic and gynecologic cases identified using a new symptom questionnaire and intravesical potassium sensitivity. Urology. 2002;60(4):573–8.
10. Nordling J, Anjum FH, Bade JJ, Bouchelouche K, Bouchelouche P, Cervigni M, et al. Primary evaluation of patients suspected of having interstitial cystitis (IC). Eur Urol. 2004;45(5):662–9.
11. Hunner GL. A rare type of bladder ulcer in women. Southern Med J. 1915;8(5):410.
12. Gamper M, Regauer S, Welter J, Eberhard J, Viereck V. Are mast cells still good biomarkers for bladder pain syndrome/interstitial cystitis? J Urol. 2015;193(6):1994–2000.
13. Boucher WS, Letourneau R, Huang M, Kempuraj D, Green M, Sant GR, et al. Intravesical sodium hyaluronate inhibits the rat urinary mast cell mediator increase triggered by acute immobilization stress. J Urol. 2002;167(1):380–4.
14. Hung M-J, Tsai C-P, Lin Y-H, Huang W-C, Chen G-D, Shen P-S. Hyaluronic acid improves pain symptoms more than bladder storage symptoms in women with interstitial cystitis. Taiwan J Obstet Gynecol. 2019;58(3):417–22.
15. Akbay E, Cayan S, Kilinc C, Bozlu M, Tek M, Efesoy O. The short-term efficacy of intravesical instillation of hyaluronic acid treatment for bladder pain syndrome/interstitial cystitis. Turk J Urol. 2018;45(2):129–34.
16. Scarneciu I, Bungau S, Lupu A-M, Scarneciu CC, Bratu OG, Martha O, et al. Efficacy of instillation treatment with hyaluronic acid in relieving symptoms in patients with BPS/IC and uncomplicated recurrent urinary tract infections—long-term results of a multicenter study. Eur J Pharm Sci. 2019;139:105067.
17. Liang C-C, Lin Y-H, Hsieh W-C, Huang L. Urinary and psychological outcomes in women with interstitial cystitis/bladder pain syndrome following hyaluronic acid treatment. Taiwan J Obstet Gynecol. 2018;57(3):360–3.
18. Engelhardt PF, Morakis N, Daha LK, Esterbauer B, Riedl CR. Long-term results of intravesical hyaluronan therapy in bladder pain syndrome/interstitial cystitis. Int Urogynecol J. 2011;22(4):401–5.

19. Kim A, Lim B, Song M, Choo M-S. Pretreatment features to influence effectiveness of intravesical hyaluronic acid instillation in refractory interstitial cystitis/painful bladder syndrome. Int Neurourol J. 2014;18(3):163–7.
20. Shao Y, Shen Z-J, Rui W-B, Zhou W-L. Intravesical instillation of hyaluronic acid prolonged the effect of bladder hydrodistention in patients with severe interstitial cystitis. Urology. 2010;75(3):547–50.
21. Gülpınar Ö, Esen B, Kayış A, Gökçe Mİ, Süer E. Clinical comparison of intravesical hyaluronic acid and chondroitin sulfate therapies in the treatment of bladder pain syndrome/interstitial cystitis. Neurourol Urodynam. 2017;37(1):257–62.
22. Arslan B, Gönültaş S, Gökmen E, Özman O, Avci MA, Özdemir E. Outcomes of intravesical chondroitin-sulfate and combined hyaluronic-acid/chondroitin-sulfate therapy on female sexual function in bladder pain syndrome. Int Urogynecol J. 2019;30(11):1857–62.
23. Lv Y-S, Zhou H-L, Mao H-P, Gao R, Wang Y-D, Xue X-Y. Intravesical hyaluronic acid and alkalinized lidocaine for the treatment of severe painful bladder syndrome/interstitial cystitis. Int Urogynecol J. 2012;23(12):1715–20.
24. Lusty AJ, Kavaler E, Zakariasen K, Tolls V, Nickel JC. Treatment effectiveness in interstitial cystitis/bladder pain syndrome: do patient perceptions align with efficacy based guidelines? Can Urological Assoc J. 2017;12(1):E1–5.
25. Pyo J-S, Cho WJ. Systematic review and meta-analysis of intravesical hyaluronic acid and hyaluronic acid/chondroitin sulfate instillation for interstitial cystitis/painful bladder syndrome. Cell Physiol Biochem. 2016;39(4):1618–25.
26. Barua JM, Arance I, Angulo JC, Riedl CR. A systematic review and meta-analysis on the efficacy of intravesical therapy for bladder pain syndrome/interstitial cystitis. Int Urogynecol J. 2015;27(8):1137–47.
27. Liu S, Zhang C, Peng L, Lu Y, Luo D. Comparative effectiveness and safety of intravesical instillation treatment of interstitial cystitis/bladder pain syndrome: a systematic review and network meta-analysis of randomized controlled trials. Int Urogynecol J. 2020:1–11.

23 Treatment of Interstitial Cystitis/Bladder Pain Syndrome with Palmitoylethanolamide/Polydatin

Marilena Gubbiotti, Stefano Rosadi, and Antonella Giannantoni

The problem with inflammation is not how often it starts, but how often it fails to subside.
(Nathan and Ding, Nonresolving Inflammation, 2010)

The new concept underlying the neuropathic pain which provides the link between neurons and non-neuronal immunocompetent cells (mast cells and microglia) with a cascade of pro- and anti-inflammatory cytokines introduces the innovative pain management with Palmitoylethanolamide (PEA). PEA was identified in the 1950s as being an active anti-inflammatory agent in chicken egg yolk [1] and is currently used in a wide range of therapeutic areas.

PEA (N-(2-hydroxyethyl) hexadecanamide) is a member of the N-acylethanolamine family composed of a fatty acid and ethanolamine and collectively named as "fatty acid ethanolamines" (FAEs), with antiallodynic and antihyperalgesic properties. They are endogenous molecules activated in the body due to tissue damage or stimulation of inflammatory responses and nociceptive fibers [2]. The mechanism of action of PEA with the strongest evidence is for an action upon the nuclear receptor peroxisome proliferator-activated receptor α (PPARα), receptor proteins that function as transcription factors regulating the expression of genes (especially, the α- and γ-isoforms of PPAR are associated with pro-inflammatory effects [3]. Other mechanisms of action of PEA involve effects on mast cells [4], CB_2-like cannabinoid receptors [5], ATP-sensitive K^+-channels [6], TRP channels [7], and NFkB [8].

M. Gubbiotti (✉) · S. Rosadi
Department of Urology, Pelvic Unit, San Donato Hospital, Arezzo, Italy

A. Giannantoni
Functional and Surgical Urology Unit, Department of Medical and Surgical Sciences and Neurosciences, University of Siena, Siena, Italy
e-mail: antonella.giannantoni@unisi.it

23.1 Microglia, Mast Cells, and Their Role in Neuropathic Pain

Although the pathogenesis of Interstitial Cystitis/Bladder Pain Syndrome (IC/BPS) remains in part unknown, bladder, perineal, lower abdominal pain, and bleeding of the urothelium could be suggestive of bladder inflammation.

The high prevalence in IC/BPS patients of comorbid functional somatic syndromes, characterized by chronic pain in the absence of clearly identifiable peripheral pathology [9], suggest that the altered central pain processing could be a contributory factor to the chronic pain in IC [10].

An increase in mast cell density in the urothelium and sub-urothelium areas of patients with IC/BPS has been demonstrated [11].

F. Dökmeci, D. E. E. Rizk (eds.), *Insights Into Incontinence and the Pelvic Floor*,
https://doi.org/10.1007/978-3-030-94174-1_23

Glia provides a link between neuroinflammation and neuropathic pain, and microglia, in particular, shows increased activity in multiple pain-processing pathways in response to peripheral injury [12]. Systemic inflammation gives rise to signals that communicate with the brain and leads to changes in metabolism and behavior, including the expression of a pro-inflammatory phenotype by microglia.

The activation of microglia leads to the transformation of an adaptive central nervous system (CNS) inflammatory response to systemic inflammation, with deleterious consequences [13].

Microglia and astrocytes also respond to proinflammatory signals released from other cells of immune origin: mast cells represent an important peripheral immune signaling link to the brain in an inflammatory setting [14]. Mast cells participate in disease development, in nociceptive pain by sensitization of peripheral nerve fibers, and in persistent stimulation of afferent somatosensory fibers to promote onset of central sensitization and to shift to chronic and neuropathic pain [15]. Upon degranulation, mast cells release algogenic substances which activate or sensitize nociceptors, thereby contributing directly to neuropathic pain. Nerve resident peripheral nerve mast cells represent the first line of activation at the point of damage and facilitate recruitment of neutrophils and macrophages [16]. Rapid release of nerve growth factor from mast cells also produces sensitization of nociceptors via the latter's high-affinity nerve growth factor-trkA receptors (and indirectly via other peripheral cell types; [17]).

23.2 Endogenous Mechanisms as a Therapeutic Approach

Chronic inflammatory processes such as those sustaining neuropathic pain may be counteracted by the production of lipid mediators able to switch off inflammation. Chronic inflammatory conditions may lower the levels or actions of these molecules. The administration of such lipid mediators might provide an avenue "to commandeer nature's own anti-inflammatory mechanisms and induce a 'dominant' program of resolution" [18].

Among these natural mediators are the FAEs and therefore also PEA. PEA is formed from N-acylated phosphatidylethanolamine (NAPE) by several enzymatic pathways, the principal one involving a membrane-associated NAPE phospholipase D which generates the respective NAE and phosphatidic acid [19]. This enzyme converts N-palmitoyl-phosphatidyl-ethanolamine into PEA. In the mammalian brain, NAEs are hydrolyzed by (1) fatty acid amide hydrolase in the endoplasmic reticulum, which breaks down NAEs into the corresponding fatty acid and ethanolamine; (2) lysosomal NAE-hydrolyzing acid amidase (NAAA) is found mainly in macrophages, where it hydrolyzes NAEs with less than 18 carbon atoms, i.e., PEA, but not N-oleoylethanolamine and N-stearoylethanolamine. In contrast, fatty acid amide hydrolase hydrolyzes all three NAEs [15].

PEA is produced/hydrolyzed by microglia and mast cells; it downmodulates mast cell activation and controls microglial cell behaviors. Tissue levels of PEA are elevated in brain areas involved in nociception and in spinal cord following neuropathic pain induction, as well as conditions associated with pain development [16]. Its ability to modulate inflammation and pain in animal studies has led to the proposal of this endogenous fatty acid amide as a component of a complex homeostatic system that controls the baseline threshold for both inflammation and pain.

23.3 Pharmacological Effects of PEA in IC/BPS

Current approaches to pain management involve inflammation target enzymes, ion channels, RNAs, and epigenetics. An alternative strategy to inhibiting inflammation would be "to commandeer nature's own anti-inflammatory mechanisms to induce a dominant program of resolution" [18].

Pharmacological effects of PEA are improved by phenols such as polydatin (PLD), a molecule with antioxidant and anti-inflammatory properties. PEA plus PLD acts by inhibiting edema and hyperalgesia, associated with a significant inhibition of the pro-inflammatory and pro-nociceptive cytokines IL-1B, TNF-alfa, and IL-6.

Preclinical studies about the management of chronic pain with the association of PEA and PLD showed a significant reduction in the inflammatory process and pain associated with an experimental rat model of surgically induced endometriosis [20].

Esposito et al. demonstrated that a co-micronized PEA/PLD, given orally, is protective and anti-nociceptive, with overall inhibition of the effects of reactive oxygen species exerted peripherally and centrally [21].

The IC/BPS etiology, and consequently its treatment, is still an "enigma." Recently, it has been recognized that IC/BPS is not an organ-specific syndrome but an urogenital manifestation of regional or systemic abnormalities characterized by neuropathic pain presenting with burning, jabbing, or searing sensations and is often associated with allodynia, hyperalgesia, and hyperesthesia. The site of the causative injury in neuropathic pain can be at peripheral or central level.

Treatment modalities vary largely, with many behavioral, pharmacological, mini-invasive, and invasive surgical procedures.

The aim of treatment is to achieve symptom control by addressing the underlying pathophysiological process. Few well-designed, randomized controlled trials have been conducted until now on different treatment modalities, and this still precludes the development of evidence-based management strategies.

It is now clear that no single treatment is curative and that symptom control may require combination therapy. To date, there is general agreement on the use of some agents, orally or intravesically administered, as indicated by the EAU guidelines on chronic pelvic pain [22] and the AUA Guidelines for the Diagnosis and Treatment of Interstitial Cystitis/Bladder Pain Syndrome [23].

The IC/BPS treatment is based on maximizing symptomatic control and minimizing possible adverse effects.

In the last years, PEA was introduced as an innovative approach. Few clinical studies are available about the use of PEA in the treatment of IC/BPS. Cervigni et al. have shown the potential benefit of PEA/PLD in controlling urologic symptoms (particularly urinary frequency) and reducing pain intensity in patients affected by IC/BPS. The efficacy and safety of PEA in the long-term follow-up have also been confirmed [24].

23.4 Case Study

Gubbiotti et al. provide preliminary evidences on the efficacy and safety of PEA/PLD in IC/BPS patients, as an add-on therapy to conventional pharmacological regimens, in the management of pain-resistant patients. The study included 23 patients (10 males and 13 females, mean age: 60.7 ± 14.2 years) poorly responsive to conventional pharmacological agents, who were analyzed by medical history, physical examination, 3-day bladder diary, and pain intensity evaluation on the Visual Analogue Scale (VAS). Patients received PEA/PLD 100 mg tablets, once daily (sublingually administered), while continuing their previous pharmacological treatments and were evaluated again at 3 and 6 months follow-up. All patients were under different poly-pharmacotherapies for IC/BPS (i.e., amitriptyline, nimesulide, pregabalin, tapentadol, skeletal muscle relaxants), and at baseline 34.7% of patients had bladder pain/burning (P/B) sensation, 30.4% had urethral P/B, 17.6% had dyspareunia, 13% had anal P/B, and 4.3% had prostate P/B. Twelve cases also presented with urgency and five with urgency urinary incontinence (UUI). After 3 months of therapy with PEA/PLD, 20 patients showed a significant reduction in pain (mean ± SD VAS score increased from 3.6 ± 1.3 to 6.8 ± 1.3); urgency persisted in six patients and UUI in three. At 6-month follow-up, pain completely disappeared in 5% of patients while substantially decreasing in the remaining cases. Only three patients stopped assuming PEA/PLD at 3-month follow-up due to lack of efficacy, and no side effects have been recorded during PEA/PLD administration. With this study it is possible to conclude that the significant pain intensity reduction could be attributed to the downregulation of must cell degranulation via an "autacoid local inflammation antagonism." This observational study provides preliminary evidence suggesting that PEA/PLD as add-on treatment to conventional pharmacological regimens in patients suffering from IC/BPS contributes to a significant pain intensity reduction. Worth of noting, relief in pain was obtained in the included patients without any consistent side effect [25].

Confirmation of these initial findings will require randomized, double-blind, placebo-controlled clinical trials to evaluate rates of respondents in subgroups of patients, in order to understand the efficacy of micronized PEA/PLD combination as a therapy for IC/BPS.

As an endogenous compound, PEA has no adverse effects at pharmacological doses while possessing a double therapeutic effect (anti-inflammatory and antinociceptive, [26]).

Acknowledgments
Authors of Chapter: Marilena Gubbiotti, Stefano Rosadi, Antonella Giannantoni.

Authors of Case study: Marilena Gubbiotti, Jacopo Adolfo Rossi de Vermandois*, Daniele Maglia§, Roberta Cagini*, Antonella Giannantoni.

* Urology Clinic, Department of Medicine and Surgery, University of Perugia, Perugia, Italy.

§ ASL 9 Macerata, Department of Urology, Italy.

References

1. Coburn A, Graham C, Haninger J. The effect of egg yolk in diets on anaphylactic arthritis (passive arthus phenomenon) in the guinea pig. J Exp Med. 1954;100:425–35.
2. Gubbiotti M, Giannantoni M. Chapter 6. Suprapontine lesions and bladder and bowel dysfunctions: assessment, treatment and rehabilitation. Management of the central nervous system chronic pelvic pain. Springer Nature Switzerland AG; 2020.
3. Baker D, Pryce G, Croxford JL, Brown P, Pertwee RG, Makriyannis A, et al. Endocannabinoids control spasticity in a multiple sclerosis model. FASEB J. 2001;15(2):300–2.
4. Hansen HS. Effects of diet on tissue levels of palmitoylethanolamide. CNS Neurol Disord Drug Targets. 2013;12:17–25.
5. Calignano A, La Rana G, Piomelli D. Antinociceptive activity of the endogenous fatty acid amide, palmitoylethanolamide. Eur J Pharmacol. 2001;419:191–8.
6. Romero TRL, Duarte IDG. N-Palmitoyl-ethanolamine (PEA) induces peripheral antinociceptive effect by ATP-sensitive K^+-channel activation. J Pharmacol Sci. 2012;118:156–60.
7. Lowin T, Apitz M, Anders S, Straub RH. Anti-inflammatory effects of N-acylethanolamines in rheumatoid arthritis synovial cells are mediated by TRPV1 and TRPA1 in a COX-2 dependent manner. Arthritis Res Ther. 2015;17:321.
8. D'Agostino G, La Rana G, Russo R, Sasso O, Iacono A, Esposito E, et al. Central administration of palmitoylethanolamide reduces hyperalgesia in mice via inhibition of NF-$_{\kappa}$B nuclear signalling in dorsal root ganglia. Eur J Pharmacol. 2009;613:54–9.
9. Clauw DJ, Schmidt M, Radulovic D, Singer A, Katz P, Bresette J. The relationship between fibromyalgia and interstitial cystitis. J Psychiatr Res. 1997;31:125–31.
10. Schrepf A, O'Donnell M, Luo Y, Bradley CS, Kreder K, Lutgendorf S. Inflammation and inflammatory control in interstitial cystitis/bladder pain syndrome: associations with painful symptoms. Pain. 2014;155(9):1755–61.
11. Liu HT, Shie JH, Chen SH, Wang YS, Kuo HC. Differences in mast cell infiltration, E-cadherin, and zonula occludens-1 expression between patients with overactive bladder and interstitial cystitis/bladder pain syndrome. Urology. 2012;80(1):225.e13–8.
12. Gao YJ, Ji RR. Chemokines, neuronal-glial interactions, and central processing of neuropathic pain. Pharmacol Ther. 2010;126:56–68.
13. Cunningham C. Microglia and neurodegeneration: the role of systemic inflammation. Glia. 2013;61(1):71–90.
14. Chen CC, Grimbaldeston MA, Tsai M, Weissman IL, Galli SJ. Identification of mast cell progenitors in adult mice. Proc Natl Acad Sci U S A. 2005;102(32):11408–13.
15. Skaper SD. Mast cell - glia dialogue in chronic pain and neuropathic pain: blood-brain barrier implications. CNS Neurol Disord Drug Targets. 2016;15(9):1072–8.
16. Zuo Y, Perkins NM, Tracey DJ, Geczy CL. Inflammation and hyperalgesia induced by nerve injury in the rat: a key role of mast cells. Pain. 2003;105(3):467–79.
17. Koda H, Mizumura K. Sensitization to mechanical stimulation by inflammatory mediators and by mild burn in canine visceral nociceptors in vitro. J Neurophysiol. 2002;87(4):2043–51.
18. Tabas I, Glass CK. Anti-inflammatory therapy in chronic disease: challenges and opportunities. Science. 2013;339(6116):166–72.

19. Facci L, Dal Toso R, Romanello S, Buriani A, Skaper SD, Leon A. Mast cells express a peripheral cannabinoid receptor with differential sensitivity to anandamide and palmitoylethanolamide. Proc Natl Acad Sci U S A. 1995;92(8):3376–80.
20. Di Paola R, Fusco R, Gugliandolo E, Crupi R, Evangelista M, Granese R, et al. Co-micronized Palmitoylethanolamide/Polydatin treatment causes endometriotic lesion regression in a rodent model of surgically induced endometriosis. Front Pharmacol. 2016;7:382.
21. Esposito E, Impellizzeri D, Bruschetta G, Cordaro M, Siracusa R, Gugliandolo E, Crupi R, Cuzzocrea S. A new co-micronized composite containing palmitoylethanolamide and polydatin shows superior oral efficacy compared to their association in a rat paw model of carrageenan-induced inflammation. Eur J Pharmacol. 2016;(782):107–18.
22. Engeler DS, Baranowski AP, Dinis-Oliveira P, Elneil S, Hughes J, Messelink EJ, van Ophoven A, Williams AC, European Association of Urology. The 2013 EAU guidelines on chronic pelvic pain: is management of chronic pelvic pain a habit, a philosophy, or a science? 10 years of development. Eur Urol. 2013;64:431–9.
23. Hanno PM, Burks DA, Clemens JQ, Dmochowski RR, Erickson D, Fitzgerald MP, Forrest JB, Gordon B, Gray M, Mayer RD, Newman D, Nyberg L Jr, Payne CK, Wesselmann U, Faraday MM, Interstitial Cystitis Guidelines Panel of the American Urological Association Education and Research, Inc. AUA guideline for the diagnosis and treatment of interstitial cystitis/bladder pain syndrome. J Urol. 2011;185:2162–70.
24. Cervigni M, Nasta L, Schievano C, Lampropoulou N, Ostardo E. Micronized palmitoylethanolamide-polydatin reduces the painful symptomatology in patients with interstitial cystitis/bladder pain syndrome. Biomed Res Int. 2019;2019:9828397.
25. Gubbiotti M, Giannantoni A. Interstitial cystitis/bladder painful syndrome: the use of palmitoylethanolamide/polydatin as add-on therapy in pain-resistant patients. J Urol Suppl. 2018;201(4):e692–3. MP47–13.
26. Petrosino S, Iuvone T, Di Marzo V. N-palmitoyl-ethanolamine: biochemistry and new therapeutic opportunities. Biochimie. 2010;92(6):724–7.

Overactive Bladder Syndrome in Women

24

Berna Haliloglu Peker, Ali Gursoy, Erdin Ilter, Aygen Celik, Erdal Yucel, Serpil Bozkurt, Umit Ozekici, and Hakan Peker

24.1 Introduction

Overactive bladder syndrome (OAB) is defined as urinary urgency, usually with urinary frequency and nocturia, with or without urgency urinary incontinence [1, 2]. A wide variety of therapeutic options are currently available for the treatment of OAB. Lifestyle changes (caffeine restriction, smoking cessation, timing of liquid food intake, physical exercise, weight loss), electrical stimulation, bladder training, and pelvic floor muscle training with or without biofeedback are first-line conservative treatment options in OAB. The next treatment options are pharmacological or neuromodulating treatment of the bladder. In addition to lifestyle changes, the first-line treatment method to be applied to women diagnosed with OAB is pelvic floor muscle training [3].

B. Haliloglu Peker (✉) · A. Gursoy · E. Ilter · A. Celik · U. Ozekici
Department of Obstetrics and Gynecology, Maltepe University Faculty of Medicine, Istanbul, Turkey
e-mail: umit.ozekici@maltepe.edu.tr

E. Yucel
Department of Obstetrics and Gynecology, Zeynep Kamil Women and Children Diseases Training and Research Hospital, Istanbul, Turkey

S. Bozkurt
Private Clinic, Istanbul, Turkey

H. Peker
Nisantasi Vocational School, Nisantasi University, Istanbul, Turkey

24.2 Literature Review

Functional electrical stimulation (FES), a method used to stimulate pelvic floor muscles, was first described by Caldwell in 1963. The mechanism of action of electrical stimulation in the treatment of urinary incontinence is thought to be to strengthen the structural support of the urethra and bladder neck, to ensure the resting and active closure of the proximal urethra, to strengthen the pelvic floor muscles, to prevent reflex bladder contractions, and to change the vascularity of the urethral and bladder neck tissues [4]. In a review, intravaginal stimulation was found to be effective in treatment of urge urinary incontinence, while there is no support for its use for stress urinary incontinence [5].

Anticholinergic agents are first option for pharmacological treatment in OAB cases. They block postganglionic muscarinic receptors with variable selectivity for different receptor subtypes. Therefore, they reduce bladder contraction, reduce intravesical pressure, and raise the volume threshold for micturition. Side effects of these drugs such as dry mouth, blurred vision, dry eyes, and constipation are the most important factors that prevent patients from continuing the treatment. Due to these side effects, only a minority of patients continue on anticholinergic drug therapy for more than 6 months [6]. Other medication options for OAB include mirabegron and botulinum toxin A. Tibial and sacral nerve stimu-

F. Dökmeci, D. E. E. Rizk (eds.), *Insights Into Incontinence and the Pelvic Floor*,
https://doi.org/10.1007/978-3-030-94174-1_24

lation have also been shown to improve symptoms of OAB [7].

24.3 Case Study: Does Functional Electrical Stimulation Increase Cure Rates in Patients Whom Not Exactly Satisfied with Anticholinergic Treatment?

(a) **Aim and Scope**
The role of FES in patients whom not exactly satisfied with anticholinergic treatment is unclear. For these patients, we aim to investigate whether FES plus anticholinergic treatment is efficient or not.

(b) **Study Design and Material Methods**
Eighty-five women with OAB were given anticholinergic treatment (fesoterodine, 8 mg Toviaz®) at outpatient clinic of Urogynecology Division, Maltepe University. After 3 months, satisfaction of treatment was assessed. Thirty women whom not satisfied with anticholinergic treatment were included in the study. For these women, FES treatment was added to anticholinergic treatment. After 3 months, patients were assessed. The difference between pre- and post-treatment IIQ scores, objective cure rates, subjective cure rates, digital vaginal palpation scores, and the procedure recommendation rate to another patient were assessed.

(c) **Results of the Study**
The mean age was 54.1 ± 15.6. The objective and subjective cure rates were significantly higher in anticholinergic plus FES treatment when compared with only anticholinergic treatment (53% vs 0% for objective cure, 70% vs 33.3% for subjective cure, $p < 0.0001$ and $p = 0.005$, respectively). The difference between pre- and post-treatment IIQ scores was significantly higher in anticholinergic plus FES treatment (1.80 ± 1.82 vs 6.43 ± 5.09, $p = 0.004$). The digital vaginal palpation scores were found to be increased after FES (1 point for 16.6%, 2 points for 46.9%, 3 points for 34.6%). The procedure recommendation rate to another patient was also significantly higher in anticholinergic plus FES treatment (73.3% vs 0%, $p < 0.0001$).

24.4 Discussion

Many studies comparing anticholinergic therapy and FES have shown that FES treatment is less costly and has fewer side effects [8, 9]. However, a study comparing trospium hydrochloride with intravaginal electrical stimulation in the treatment of OAB showed similar benefit in both treatment modalities. In addition, discontinuation of both treatments in overactive bladder syndrome leads to worsening of objective and subjective symptoms [10].

The use of anticholinergic drugs together with non-pharmacological treatments provides an additive effect in OAB treatment. In this study, addition of FES treatment in women whom not full satisfied with anticholinergic treatment increased cure rates.

24.5 Conclusion

Adding FES treatment to patients whom not full satisfied with anticholinergic treatment seems to increase cure rates.

Acknowledgments None.

References

1. Abrams P, Cardozo L, Fall M, Griffiths D, Rosier P, Ulmsten U, Van Kerrebroeck P, Victor A, Wein A, Standardisation Sub-committee of the International Continence Society. The standardisation of terminology in lower urinary tract function: report from the Standardisation Sub-committee of the International Continence Society. Urology. 2003;61(1):37–49. https://doi.org/10.1016/s0090-4295(02)02243-4. PMID: 12559262.
2. Haylen BT, de Ridder D, Freeman RM, Swift SE, Berghmans B, Lee J, Monga A, Petri E, Rizk DE,

Sand PK, Schaer GN, International Urogynecological Association; International Continence Society. An International Urogynecological Association (IUGA)/ International Continence Society (ICS) joint report on the terminology for female pelvic floor dysfunction. Neurourol Urodyn. 2010;29(1):4–20. https://doi.org/10.1002/nau.20798. PMID: 19941278.
3. Firinci S, Yildiz N, Alkan H, Aybek Z. Which combination is most effective in women with idiopathic overactive bladder, including bladder training, biofeedback, and electrical stimulation? A prospective randomized controlled trial. Neurourol Urodyn. 2020;39(8):2498–508. https://doi.org/10.1002/nau.24522. Epub 2020 Sep 22. PMID: 32960999.
4. Stewart F, Berghmans B, Bø K, Glazener CM. Electrical stimulation with non-implanted devices for stress urinary incontinence in women. Cochrane Database Syst Rev. 2017;12(12):CD012390. https://doi.org/10.1002/14651858.CD012390.pub2. PMID: 29271482; PMCID: PMC6486295.
5. Schreiner L, Santos TG, Souza AB, Nygaard CC, Silva Filho IG. Electrical stimulation for urinary incontinence in women: a systematic review. Int Braz J Urol. 2013;39(4):454–64. https://doi.org/10.1590/S1677-5538.IBJU.2013.04.02. PMID: 24054395.
6. Vozmediano-Chicharro R, Blasco Hernández P, Madurga-Patuel B. Insights into the management of overactive bladder with transdermal oxybutynin: a practical review. Res Rep Urol. 2020;12:321–30. https://doi.org/10.2147/RRU.S266400. PMID: 32884926; PMCID: PMC7434563.
7. Hersh L, Salzman B. Clinical management of urinary incontinence in women. Am Fam Phys. 2013;87(9):634–40. Erratum in: Am Fam Physician. 2013 Oct 1;88(7):427. PMID: 23668526.
8. Arruda RM, Castro RA, Sousa GC, Sartori MG, Baracat EC, Girão MJ. Prospective randomized comparison of oxybutynin, functional electrostimulation, and pelvic floor training for treatment of detrusor overactivity in women. Int Urogynecol J Pelvic Floor Dysfunct. 2008;19(8):1055–61. https://doi.org/10.1007/s00192-008-0586-y. Epub 2008 Mar 11. PMID: 18330483.
9. Amaro JL, Gameiro MO, Kawano PR, Padovani CR. Intravaginal electrical stimulation: a randomized, double-blind study on the treatment of mixed urinary incontinence. Acta Obstet Gynecol Scand. 2006;85(5):619–22. https://doi.org/10.1080/00016340500495058. PMID: 16752244.
10. Ozdedeli S, Karapolat H, Akkoc Y. Comparison of intravaginal electrical stimulation and trospium hydrochloride in women with overactive bladder syndrome: a randomized controlled study. Clin Rehabil. 2010;24(4):342–51. https://doi.org/10.1177/0269215509346092. Epub 2010 Mar 8. PMID: 20212061.

25 Overactive Bladder Syndrome in Men

Laura Mateu Arrom, Laia Sabiote Rubio, Cristina Gutierrez-Ruiz, Virginia Martinez, Joan Palou, and Carlos Errando

25.1 Introduction

Overactive bladder syndrome (OAB) is defined as the presence of urgency, with or without urgency incontinence and usually with increased daytime frequency and nocturia; moreover, it is often associated with the urodynamic finding of detrusor overactivity [1]. According to a large population-based survey [2], 10.8% of men older than 18 years present with symptoms of OAB, and this percentage increases significantly with age [2].

First-line treatment for idiopathic OAB consists in conservative measures as well as pharmacologic treatment. However, most patients discontinue their use for various reasons, such as inadequate efficacy or side effects [3]. Several randomized controlled trials have shown that treatment with intradetrusor onabotulinumtoxinA (BoNT-A) injections represents a safe and effective option for patients who fail pharmacologic treatment [4, 5], the most common adverse effects being urinary tract infection and urinary retention requiring clean intermittent catheterization (CIC), which occur in 20% and 9% of cases, respectively [4].

The vast majority of patients included in studies to date have, however, been females [6–9]. Few authors have assessed the results of this treatment in male patients [10, 11]. Thus, rates of treatment response, complications, and continuation on treatment in this population remain controversial. Moreover, predictive factors for efficacy or occurrence of complications are still unclear.

25.2 Literature Review

Current European Urology Guidelines on treatment of urinary incontinence state that 100U of onabotulinumtoxinA, dissolved in 10 mL of saline and injected in 20 points of the bladder wall excluding the trigone, can be used to treat OAB with refractory urge urinary incontinence in adults of both genders. They recommend this treatment in patients who have failed conservative therapy such as pelvic floor muscle training or drug treatment.

However, it is also stated that small numbers of males were included in the trials assessing the intradetrusor onabotulinumtoxinA injection treatment results [6, 12].

L. Mateu Arrom (✉) · L. Sabiote Rubio
C. Gutierrez-Ruiz · V. Martinez · J. Palou · C. Errando
Fundació Puigvert, Barcelona, Spain

F. Dökmeci, D. E. E. Rizk (eds.), *Insights Into Incontinence and the Pelvic Floor*,
https://doi.org/10.1007/978-3-030-94174-1_25

25.3 Case Study: Predictive Factors for Clinical Improvement, Treatment Continuation, and Complications After BoNT-A in Male Patients with Idiopathic Overactive Bladder Syndrome

(a) **Aim and Scope**

The aim of the study was to assess treatment response, complications, and the rate of continuation on treatment after midterm follow-up in male patients with idiopathic OAB as well as to define preoperative predictive factors for each of these.

(b) **Study Design and Material Methods**

A retrospective analysis was conducted of male patients older than 18 years who had been treated with a first intradetrusor injection of 100U BoNT-A for refractory idiopathic OAB since 2007 in a single department.

A revision was made of the patients' clinical charts regarding the age at onset of OAB symptoms, previous pharmacologic treatments or bladder outlet obstruction surgery, and comorbidities assessed by the Charlson Comorbidity Index, which is a validated index that was developed to predict mortality according to the load of comorbidity of each patient [13].

A urodynamic test was performed in all patients prior to treatment and was reported according to the International Urogynecological Association (IUGA)/International Continence Society (ICS) recommendations [1]. Patients without evidence of detrusor overactivity were also excluded from further analysis. In each patient we calculated the bladder outlet obstruction index (BOOI), the bladder contractility index (BCI), and the voiding efficiency [14]. Preoperative assessment also included an ultrasound scan with transabdominal prostate volume measurement and a PSA blood test.

Treatment consisted in the injection of 100U Botox® (Allergan, Inc., Irvine, CA) diluted in 10 mL saline and distributed in 20 dots in all bladder walls excluding the trigone (Fig. 25.1). Injection was performed with a 5-Fr 4-mm depth needle via a rigid cystoscope, with the patient under sedation or spinal anesthesia.

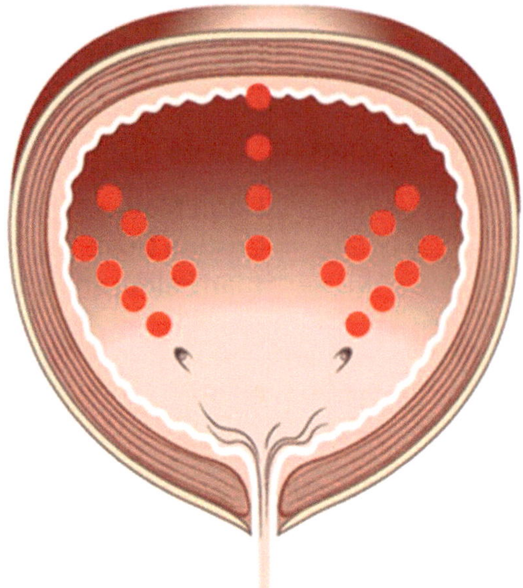

Fig. 25.1 Scheme of onabotulinumtoxinA intradetrusor injection

Follow-up consisted in uroflowmetry with post-void residual urine (PVR) measurement at 3 weeks and a clinical visit and urodynamic test at 3 months after the procedure. Efficacy was assessed using a Spanish validated single-item treatment benefit scale (TBS) [15, 16]: "My condition (urinary problems, urinary incontinence) has: 1—greatly improved, 2—improved, 3—not changed, 4—worsened after treatment." Answers 1 and 2 were considered to indicate that the patient had perceived a benefit from their treatment (treatment response), while answers 3 and 4 were interpreted as indicating no perceived benefit from treatment (non-response to treatment). Complications observed after treatment were classified according to the Clavien-Dindo (CD) classification [17]. CIC was indicated in patients with a PVR greater than 200 mL and symptoms such as difficulty voiding or urinary infection. The presence of PVR in the absence of symptoms was not considered a complication of treatment. In the absence of complications, further follow-up consisted in a clinical visit every 6 months.

Continuation on treatment was considered present if, at the last visit, patients had received a BoNT-A injection within the preceding 12 months. Patients who discontinued treatment were openly asked about their reasons for discontinuation.

A descriptive analysis of the series was performed, and the relationship between preoperative variables and treatment response, treatment continuation, and complications was assessed with the chi-square test for categorical variables and the Student's *t* test and Mann-Whitney U test for continuous variables when appropriate. Statistically significant relationships in the univariate study ($p < 0.05$) were evaluated in the multivariate study (logistic regression). To avoid overestimation of the treatment continuation rate, we excluded patients with a follow-up duration of <12 months from treatment continuation analysis. Ethical approval and written patient consent were obtained prior to enter the study.

(c) **Results of the Study**

One hundred and seventy-seven patients were included, with a mean age of 71.5 ± 11.2 years. Thirty-nine patients (22%) had underwent a radical prostatectomy and 15 patients (8.5%) pelvic radiotherapy, 39 patients (22%) had prior history of transurethral resection of the prostate, 32 patients (18.1%) suffered from diabetes, and mean Charlson Comorbidity Index punctuation was 4.1 ± 1.9.

All patients had undergone a urodynamic study prior to treatment demonstrating the presence of detrusor overactivity. Bladder contractility index was 103.8 ± 27.9, bladder outlet obstruction index was 19.5 ± 29.1, and voiding efficiency was 89.5 ± 17.4%. Twenty eight patients (15.8%) had a BOOI over 40.

One hundred and five patients (59.3%) reported response to treatment. Only a previous transurethral resection of the prostate was related with clinical improvement ($p = 0.015$).

After treatment, 23 (13%) complications were detected: 2 cases of mild hematuria (1.1%) (CD 1), 3 cases of urinary infections (1.6%) (CD2), and 18 cases of acute urinary retention (10.2%) (CD2). In the multivariate analysis, diabetes ($p = 0.043$) and a BOOI > 40 ($p = 0.016$) were predictive factors of complications.

Mean follow-up was 39.5 ± 20.4 months. One hundred and forty patients (79%) had a follow-up over 12 months. Among them, 101 patients (72.1%) discontinued BoNT-A treatment. Reasons for discontinuation were lack of efficacy in 27 patients (26.7%), adverse effects in 5 patients (5%), and lack of severe symptoms in 31 patients (30.6%), and 19 patients (18.8%) did not desire reinjection and 19 patients (18.8%) due to other reasons. A lower prostatic volume was related with the persistence on treatment in the multivariate analysis ($p = 0.025$).

25.4 Discussion

In this study the treatment response, occurrence of complications, and treatment continuation rate after BoNT-A injection in male patients with idiopathic OAB was assessed. The results suggested that most patients respond to treatment. However, the vast majority of them discontinue treatment for various reasons.

Previous randomized controlled trials assessing the efficacy of BoNT-A injection, in which almost 90% of patients were females, showed that a 61–63% rate of treatment response can be expected after treatment according to TBS results [6, 7]. While some authors report that subjective benefit is achieved after BoNT-A treatment in male patients [18], other authors have suggested that this benefit could be lower in male than in female patients [11].

In the present series, the majority of patients responded to treatment as assessed using the TBS.

Thus, these results suggest that the treatment efficacy of BoNT-A injection in males could be similar to that in the female population.

In this study, approximately 11% of patients required CIC during follow-up as compared with a rate of 8% in studies assessing both male and female patients but with a greater representation of females [4].

Regarding male patients, Rahnama'i et al. [10] reported a CIC rate of 24%, but that study included a heterogeneous group of patients of whom 28% were suffering from neurogenic detrusor overactivity. Recently, Faure Walker et al. [11] observed that 42% of male patients required CIC after treatment, a significantly higher rate than in female patients. However, they included patients treated with different doses of BoNT-A and started CIC in patients with symptomatic PVR >150 mL, a more conservative criterion than that employed in our study. Therefore, although the present results suggest that the need for CIC could be higher in male patients, more studies are needed to confirm the rate of this complication in this population.

Some authors have assessed long-term results after BoNT-A injection in terms of treatment continuation [19, 20], showing that the discontinuation rate can be as high as 70% after 8 years of follow-up [19], with no differences between men and women [19], and with most discontinuations being due to tolerability issues [19, 20]. The discontinuation rate observed in our series is similar to that reported previously, although the presence of complications explained only a low number of treatment discontinuations.

The present study has some limitations. First, it had a retrospective design, and there was not a control group. However, all patients in the study reported outcomes on a validated TBS, and all patients underwent urodynamic tests preoperatively. Second, the follow-up was only 3 years; thus we can report merely a midterm and not a long-term treatment continuation rate. The main strength of the present study is that the series analyzed herein comprises a homogeneous group of patients, excluding neurogenic patients and those receiving doses other than 100 U.

25.5 Conclusion

Although most male patients with idiopathic OAB present a treatment response after intradetrusor onabotulinumtoxinA injection, the vast majority will discontinue treatment. The prostatic volume could be related to persistence on treatment.

Complications after treatment with onabotulinumtoxinA in male with OAB are mild and infrequent. Diabetes and a bladder outlet obstruction index over 40 could predict their appearance.

References

1. Haylen BT, de Ridder D, Freeman RM, et al. An International Urogynecological Association (IUGA)/ International Continence Society (ICS) joint report on the terminology for female pelvic floor dysfunction. Neurourol Urodyn. 2010;29(1):4–20.
2. Irwin DE, Milsom I, Hunskaar S, et al. Population-based survey of urinary incontinence, overactive bladder, and other lower urinary tract symptoms in five countries: results of the EPIC study. Eur Urol. 2006;50(6):1306–14.
3. Chapple CR, Nazir J, Hakimi Z, et al. Persistence and adherence with mirabegron versus antimuscarinic agents in patients with overactive bladder: a retrospective observational study in UK clinical practice. Eur Urol. 2017;72(3):389–99.
4. Cui Y, Zhou X, Zong H, et al. The efficacy and safety of onabotulinumtoxin A in treating idiopathic OAB: a systematic review and meta-analysis. Neurourol Urodyn. 2015;34(5):413–9.
5. López Ramos H, Torres Castellanos L, Ponce Esparza I, et al. Management of overactive bladder with onabotulinumtoxin A: systematic review and meta-analysis. Urology. 2017;100:53 8.
6. Chapple C, Sievert KD, MacDiarmid S, et al. OnabotulinumtoxinA 100 U significantly improves all idiopathic overactive bladder symptoms and quality of life in patients with overactive bladder and urinary incontinence: a randomised, double-blind, placebo-controlled trial. Eur Urol. 2013;64(2):249–56.
7. Nitti VW, Dmochowski R, Herschorn S, et al. Onabotulinumtoxin A for the treatment of patients

with overactive bladder and urinary incontinence: results of a phase 3, randomized, placebo controlled trial. J Urol. 2017;197(2S):S216–23.
8. Fowler CJ, Auerbach S, Ginsberg D, et al. Onabotulinumtoxin A improves health-related quality of life in patients with urinary incontinence due to idiopathic overactive bladder: a 36-week, double-blind, placebo-controlled, randomized, dose-ranging trial. Eur Urol. 2012;62(1):148–57.
9. Denys P, Le Normand L, Ghout I, et al. Efficacy and safety of low doses of onabotulinumtoxin A for the treatment of refractory idiopathicoveractive bladder: a multicentre, double-blind, randomised, placebo-controlled dose-ranging study. Eur Urol. 2012;61(3):520–9.
10. Rahnama'i MS, Marcelissen TAT, Brierley B, et al. Long-term compliance and results of intravesical botulinum toxin A injections in male patients. Neurourol Urodyn. 2017;36(7):1855–9.
11. Faure Walker NA, Syed O, Malde S, et al. Onabotulinum toxin A injections in men with refractory idiopathic detrusor overactivity. Urology. 2019;123:242–6.
12. Mangera A, Andersson KE, Apostolidis A, Chapple C, Dasgupta P, Giannantoni A, et al. Contemporary management of lower urinary tract disease with botulinum toxin A: a systematic review of botox (onabotulinumtoxinA) and dysport (abobotulinumtoxinA). Eur Urol. 2011;60(4):784–95.
13. Charlson M, Szatrowski TP, Peterson J, et al. Validation of a combined comorbidity index. J Clin Epidemiol. 1994;47:1245–51.
14. Abrams P. Bladder outlet obstruction index, bladder contractility index and bladder voiding efficiency: three simple indices to define bladder voiding function. BJU Int. 1999;84(1):14–5.
15. Colman S, Chapple C, Nitti V, et al. Validation of treatment benefit scale for assessing subjective outcomes in treatment of overactive bladder. Urology. 2008;72(4):803–7.
16. Errando-Smet C, Ruiz MA, Villacampa-Aubá F, et al. [Spanish cultural adaptation and psychometrical validation of the treatment benefit scale (TBS) in the symptomatic treatment of overactive bladder]. Med Clin (Barc). 2013;140(1):6–13.
17. Dindo D, Demartines N, Clavien PA. Classification of surgical complications: a new proposal with evaluation in a cohort of 6336 patients and results of a survey. Ann Surg. 2004;240(2):205–13.
18. Habashy D, Losco G, Tse V, et al. Botulinum toxin (Onabotulinumtoxin A) in the male non-neurogenic overactive bladder: clinical and quality of life outcomes. BJU Int. 2015;116(Suppl 3):61–5.
19. Marcelissen TA, Rahnama'i MS, Snijkers A, et al. Long-term follow-up of intravesical botulinum toxin-A injections in women with idiopathic overactive bladder symptoms. World J Urol. 2017;35(2):307–11.
20. Mohee A, Khan A, Harris N, et al. Long-term outcome of the use of intravesical botulinum toxin for the treatment of overactive bladder (OAB). BJU Int. 2013;111(1):106–13.

Part V

Genitourinary Syndrome of Menopause and Recurrent Urinary Tract Infection

Effect of Laser Therapy on the Vaginal Epithelium

26

Svetlana Jankovic

Abbreviations

HE	Hematoxylin-eosin staining
HSP	Heat shock proteins
PAS	Periodic acid-Schiff
SMA	Smooth muscle actin antibodies
TGF-β	Transforming growth factor-β
VAS	Visual analog scale
VHI	Vaginal Health Index
VVA	Vulvovaginal atrophy

The average age of menopause is approximately 50 years worldwide. Nowadays more than 95% of women reach menopause with the life expectancy of nearly 30 years. Vulvovaginal atrophy (VVA), also known as genitourinary syndrome of menopause, is a public and social health problem involving more than 50% of menopausal women [1, 2]. A diagnosis of vaginal atrophy is made based on vaginal and genitourinary symptoms and a gynecological examination. In menopause, some women have different typical symptoms of VVA: vaginal dryness, itching, burning, dyspareunia, irritation or bleeding [3], and a variety of urinary disorders (urgency, increased frequency, nocturia, dysuria, incontinence, recurrent urinary tract infection, and bleeding) [4]. These symptoms may produce emotional distress and sexual dysfunctions.

However, many women hesitate to report vaginal-related symptoms, primarily because of embarrassment [4] and the belief that their symptoms are an inevitable part of aging [5]. In contrast to the vasomotor menopausal symptoms, which are usually transient, VVA is getting worst over the years with negative consequences on sexuality and quality of life aging [6]. However, only 25% of patients decide to seek medical attention [7].

Fractional CO_2 laser has shown skin tissue remodeling properties, with the effect of producing new collagen and elastic fibers [8]. In fact, the generated high temperature obtained with a CO_2 laser is able to induce a heat shock response, which can produce changes in cellular metabolism. These changes are rapid and transient and are characterized by the activation of a small family of proteins referred to as the heat shock proteins (HSP). HSP 70, which is overexpressed following laser irradiation, causes the stimulation of transforming growth factor-β (TGF-β), and it is known that TGF-β plays a crucial role in the inflammatory response and production of the new collagen and extracellular matrix. A few studies have shown the efficacy and safety of a fractional micro ablative CO_2 laser in the treatment of VVA [9–12].

S. Jankovic (✉)
Department of Obstetrics and Gynecology, "Narodni Front", Belgrade, Serbia

Belgrade University Medical School, Belgrade, Serbia

F. Dökmeci, D. E. E. Rizk (eds.), *Insights Into Incontinence and the Pelvic Floor*, https://doi.org/10.1007/978-3-030-94174-1_26

26.1 Case Study: Histopathological Findings of the Vaginal Epithelium After the Laser Therapy in Postmenopausal Women

The aim of this study was to evaluate the efficacy of fractional CO_2 laser therapy in sexually active menopausal patients who had dyspareunia related to vulvovaginal atrophy (VVA).

This prospective study was conducted between January and December 2015 and included sexually active postmenopausal women with symptoms related to VVA. Women entered the study after an informed written consent was obtained.

Thirty-two postmenopausal patients underwent laser treatment. Inclusion criteria were being sexually active last 4 weeks, symptoms of VVA, age $\geq$ 50 years, and absence of menstruation for $\geq$12 months. Exclusion criteria were use of any hormone replacement therapies (either systemic or local) within the 12 months prior to inclusion in the study; acute or recurrent urinary tract infections; active genital infections; pelvic organ prolapse staged $\geq$ II according to the pelvic organ prolapse quantification system; previous reconstructive pelvic surgery; and any serious disease or psychiatric disorders. VVA was confirmed by biopsy findings before the first treatment. Postmenopausal women were treated intravaginally with the fractional micro ablative CO_2 laser system (SmartXide^2 V^2 LR, Monalisa Touch; DEKA, Florence, Italy), using the following settings: dot power 35 W, dwell time 1000 μs, dot spacing 1000 μm, and the smart stack parameter from 1 to 3. The vaginal probe was inserted and rotated along the vaginal canal, to provide a complete treatment of the vaginal wall, using laser energy transmission. A treatment cycle included three laser applications, with the pause of 6–8 weeks. The procedure was performed in the outpatient clinic and did not require any specific preparation or anesthesia. Anamnestic data were collected. Before the study and 4 weeks after the third treatment, women were evaluated by using the Gloria Bachmann's Vaginal Health Index score (VHI) that consists of five characteristics of the vaginal wall: elasticity, fluid volume, pH, epithelial integrity, and moisture. Each parameter was graded from 1 to 5. If the total score is <15, the vagina is considered atrophic [13]. The severity of VVA symptoms (vaginal burning, vaginal itching, vaginal dryness, and dyspareunia) was measured using a 10 cm visual analog scale (VAS), where the left extreme of the scale, number 1, indicated "absence of symptom" and the right, number 10, indicated "symptom as bad as it could be."

Biopsies had been done after the third laser treatment to confirm the changes in the vaginal epithelium. Four weeks after the last treatment, the women rated the overall level of satisfaction with the treatment by answering the following question: "Taking into consideration the variations in VVA symptoms, in overall well-being and quality of life, as well as the adverse effects experienced, if any, how would you define your level of satisfaction with the laser treatment?" Answers were scored on a 5-point Likert scale (very satisfied, satisfied, uncertain, dissatisfied, and very dissatisfied). Satisfaction with the treatment was defined when the answers were "very satisfied" or "satisfied." The primary outcome of the study was to evaluate the change of the vaginal tissue between baseline and 4 weeks after the last treatment follow-up. Secondary outcomes of the study were to evaluate sexual function and patients' satisfaction after the laser procedure. Data presented in the text and tables are reported as means ± standard deviation, medians, or percentages (%). Evaluation whether continuous variable had normal distribution was done by Shapiro Wilks W Test. For defining statistical significance (p-value) of continuous indicators before/after the treatment, paired t-test was used for variables with normal distribution and Wilcoxon signed ranks test for variables that did not have normal distribution. Everything is statistically significant for $p < 0.05$. For defining statistical significance of category indicators prior/after the treatment, Fisher's exact test was used.

Thirty-two patients participated in this study. All of them have signed the written consent for the study. From a statistical and descriptive point of view, the patient group had an average age of

55.3 ± 4.7 years. The average duration of the menopause was 6.9 ± 3.8 years. Twenty-four women (75%) previously had only vaginal delivery, 6 women (18.75%) only had cesarean section delivery, and 2 women (6.25%) had both vaginal delivery and cesarean section delivery.

The VHI score before the first treatment was 11.6 ± 3.08 and after the third treatment was 19.2 ± 2.9. Four weeks after the third laser application, the VHI score improved significantly ($p < 0.001$), as we can see at Chart 26.1.

Every woman reported to have some of the symptoms related to vulvovaginal atrophy, such as itching, burning, dyspareunia, or dryness, with some intensity (1–10). We have shown statistically significant difference in values prior and after the treatment for all symptoms ($p < 0.001$), as it is shown at the Chart 26.2.

More than three quarters (78.1%) of patients were very satisfied with the treatment effects. Satisfied were the rest of seven patients (21.9%). It is presented at the Chart 26.3. There were neither neutral nor unsatisfied patients.

Each sample in our study taken before and after the therapy was examined histopathologically using standard hematoxylin-eosin staining (HE), immunohistochemically using CD 34 and smooth muscle actin (SMA) antibodies, and histochemically using Masson trichrome, periodic acid-Schiff (PAS), and Alcian blue staining.

Vaginal epithelium samples which were taken before therapy (Fig. 26.1) showed moderate orthokeratosis, while the cell glycogenization was minimal or absent (PAS reaction and Masson trichrome stain were used to detect glycogen). Thickness of epithelium was minimally to moderately reduced with the presence of the chronic inflammatory infiltrate. The collagen fibers are thin. The lamina propria has a chronic inflammatory infiltrate composed predominantly of lymphocyte. Plasma cells are less present. The deeper parts of the lamina propria have shown the signs of reduced collagen.

Samples taken after the therapy have shown decreased orthokeratosis of vaginal epithelium without perceptible changes of glycogenization, comparing to previous biopsy (PAS reaction and Masson trichrome stain). Stromal collagenization showed pronounced Alcian blue positivity (Fig. 26.2) and reduction of Masson trichrome staining intensity. These changes may indicate the increased synthesis of mucopolysaccharidoses (Fig. 26.3), which appears as a mark of tissue regeneration. Number of new blood vessels was mildly to moderately increased (CD34/alpha SMA) (Fig. 26.4), compared to the biopsy taken before the therapy. The formation of new papillae pervading the epithelium with newly formed and extended small vessels is presented at the Fig. 26.5. After the treatment, the epithelium shows signs of recovery; chronic infiltration is reduced, even lost completely; and collagen fibers are thicker, numerous, and more concentrated.

Chart 26.1 VHI score before and after treatment

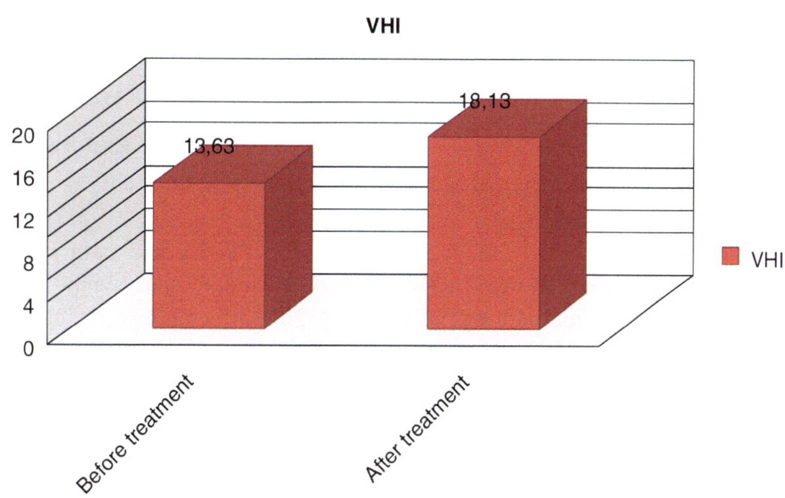

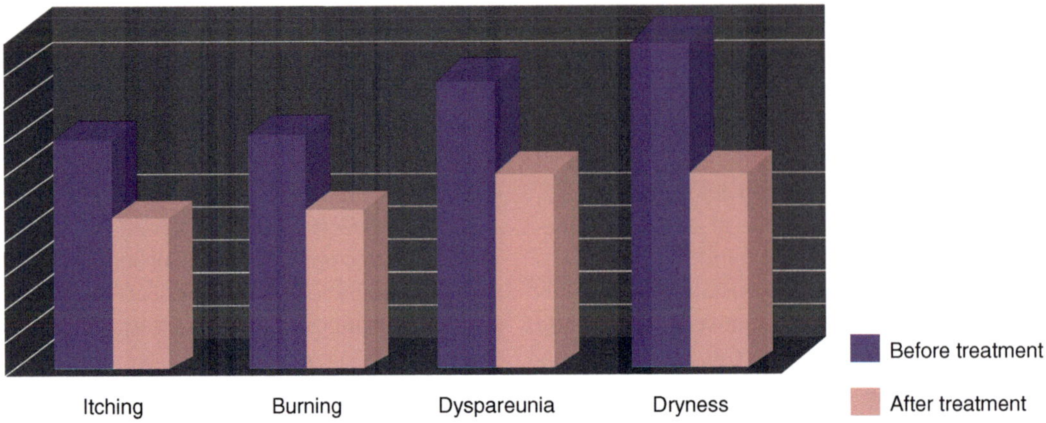

Chart 26.2 Vaginal symptoms before and after therapy

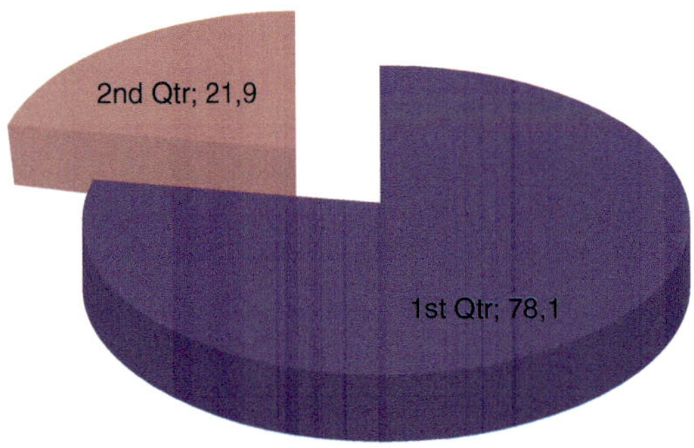

Chart 26.3 Patient satisfaction after the treatment

In Figs. 26.2, 26.3, 26.4, and 26.5, we can see thickening of the epithelium after the laser therapy with the epithelial cells maturation, desquamation of the epithelial surface, and formation of glycogen. We can also notice the formation of new thin fibrils and fibroblasts supporting a renewal of the extracellular matrix with functional restoration in the connective tissue underlying the vaginal epithelium.

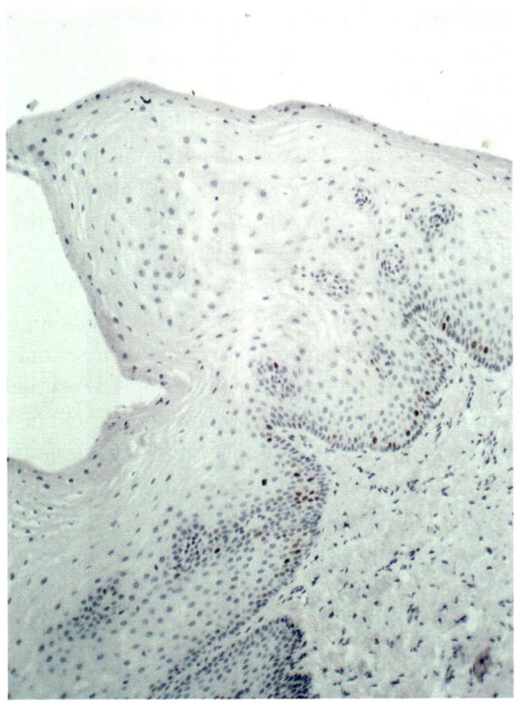

Fig. 26.1 Vaginal epithelium before therapy

26.2 Discussion

In the recent Vaginal Health: Insights, Views & Attitudes (VIVA) international survey of 3520 women, the 45% of postmenopausal women who reported vaginal discomfort experienced a range of symptoms, including dryness (83%), dyspareunia (42%), involuntary urination (30%), soreness (27%), itching (26%), burning (14%), and pain (11%) [2]. Despite all these unpleasant symptoms, less than one third of affected women seek for medical assistance [7], by the reason of embarrassment, shyness, and the belief that their symptoms are an inevitable part of aging [4].

Women in Serbia hesitate to report any symptoms of VVA and sexual dysfunction because of

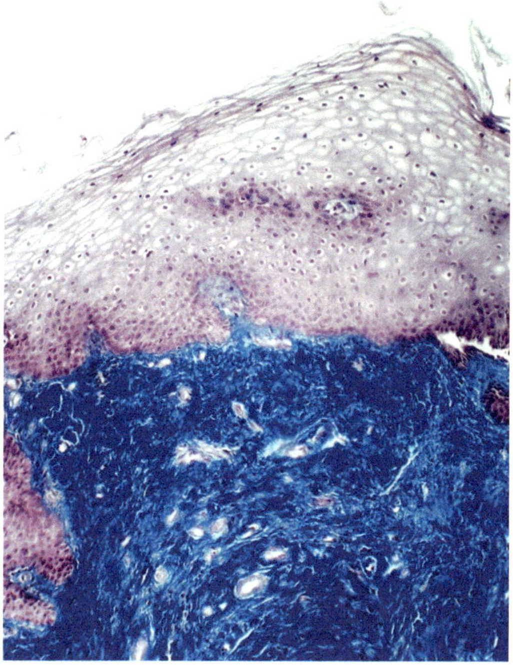

Fig. 26.2 Vaginal epithelium after therapy (stromal collagenization)

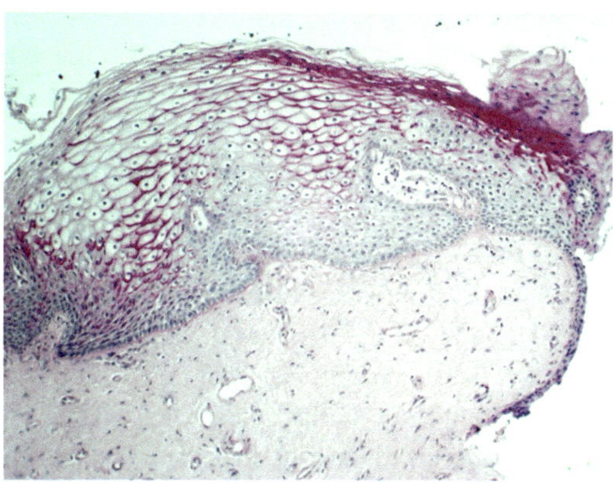

Fig. 26.3 Vaginal epithelial after therapy—increased synthesis of mucopolysaccharidoses

embarrassment. They think that nothing can be done. But it is promising that they fell comfortable to discuss with doctors if they start to talk about this.

CO_2 laser has been widely used in dermatology and plastic surgery. CO_2 laser generates heat and vaporizes the water content of the cells. The fractional CO_2 laser causes acute termoablative

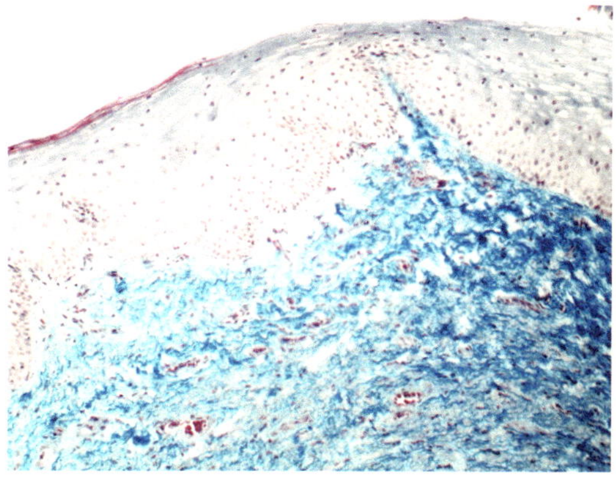

Fig. 26.4 Vaginal epithelial after therapy—increased number of new blood vessels

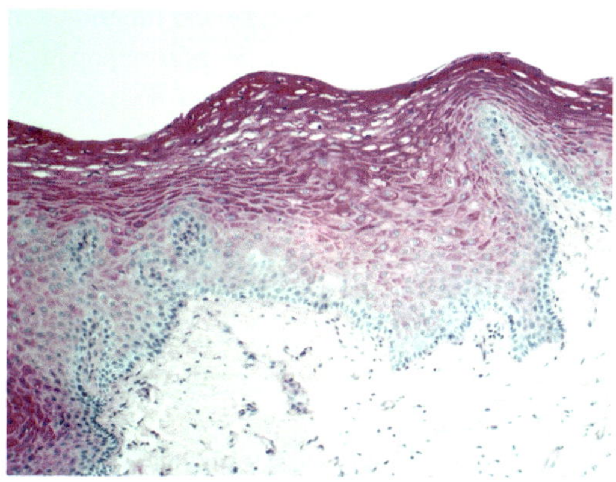

Fig. 26.5 Vaginal epithelial after therapy—increased number of papillae

damage, following the proliferation, and stimulates the synthesis of the new collagen and cellular matrix substances. This technology is used to improve elasticity and hydration of the vaginal walls, and it could relieve discomfort in menopausal women associated with the symptoms of vulvovaginal atrophy.

Gaspar et al. [14] reported significant histological improvement in the vaginal tissue; more than 50% increase in collagen fibers and fibroblastic activity respecting the biopsy before and after fractional CO_2 laser treatment in combination with platelet-rich plasma. Longo et al. [15] reported long-term effect on the tissue collagen remodeling of the skin was present 3 months after the laser treatment. Ex vivo data obtained from vaginal wall specimens have shown significant connective tissue remodeling, without showing any kind of damage to the surrounding tissues [16]. Zerbinati demonstrated the stimulation of collagen synthesis, increase of acidic mucopolysaccharides in the ground matrix, and increase of glycogen in the epithelial cells in the vaginal tissue of patients after fractional CO_2 laser treatment [17]. Salvatore et al. [9, 12] noticed that a treatment cycle of three laser applications significantly improved both most bothersome symptoms of VVA and scores of vaginal health at 12-week follow-up in women not responding or being unsatisfied with previous local estrogen therapies. In 2015, Salvatore demonstrated that fractional CO_2 laser treatment is associated with a significant improvement of sexual function and satisfaction with sexual life in postmenopausal women with VVA symptoms [11]. Perino published the study that indicates a significant improvement in VVA symptoms in women after three laser sessions with fractional CO_2 laser [10]. In fact, 91.7% of the patients was satisfied or very satisfied with the procedure.

Vaginal mucosa in reproductive age is well supplied with blood, and the epithelium consists of significantly larger number of cell layers, particularly rich in glycogen. Postmenopausal vaginal mucosa is atrophic (caused by decreased estrogen levels) with reduced presence of blood vessels and a significantly thinner epithelium with lack of glycogen.

Salvatore and Zerbinati described the following important histological changes after vaginal laser treatment protocol:

- A thickening of the epithelium, with the maturation of epithelial cells and desquamation at the epithelial surface as in premenopause.
- A new formation of papillae indenting the epithelium with newly formed and extended small vessels.
- In the connective tissue underlying the epithelium, the formation of new thin fibrils and morphological features of fibroblasts supporting a renewal of the extracellular matrix with functional restoration [12, 17].

These findings are similar to our research.

Samples taken after the therapy have shown decreased orthokeratosis of vaginal epithelium without perceptible changes of glycogenization, comparing to previous biopsy (PAS reaction and Masson trichrome stain). Stromal collagenization showed pronounced Alcian blue positivity and reduction of Masson trichrome staining intensity. These changes may indicate the increased synthesis of mucopolysaccharidoses, which appears as a mark of tissue regeneration. Number of new blood vessels was mildly to moderately increased (CD34/alpha SMA) compared to the biopsy taken before the therapy.

After the treatment, the epithelium shows signs of recovery; chronic infiltration is reduced, even lost completely; and collagen fibers are thicker, numerous, and more concentrated.

Salvatore et al. in 2015 have studied microscopic and ultrastructure aspects of the collagen and elastic components of the vaginal epithelium. They also approved the laser-induced activity of connective tissue proper cells, particularly fibroblasts. Treatment protocols were compared according to histological findings, particularly in maximal depth and connective changes achieved. This histological study shows that fractional CO2 laser can produce a remodeling of vaginal connective tissue without causing damage to surrounding tissue [18].

Salvatore et al. (2018) have investigated microscopic, ultrastructure, and biochemical modifications of the structural components of postmenopausal atrophic vaginal mucosa tissues 1 h following a single fractional laser CO_2 application. They are suggesting that the activation of regenerative mechanisms is expressed both in the connective tissue—with the formation of new vessels, new papillae, and new collagen—and in the epithelium with the associated thickening and desquamation of cells at the mucosal surface. Salvatore et al. proved effective early remodeling of the extracellular matrix. These early restoring modifications 1 h after the laser therapy could be enhanced and stabilized with a long-lasting effect by subsequent laser applications in an effective, experienced plan as a clinical treatment that ensures to vaginal mucosa of postmenopausal women a renewed healthy condition, according Salvatore et al. [19].

26.3 Conclusion

Laser treatments stimulate regeneration of the vaginal mucosa with new collagen fibers production that thickens and strengthens the vaginal structure. Samples taken after the therapy have shown signs of the recovery: increased stromal collagenization and increased synthesis of mucopolysaccharidoses, which appears as a mark of tissue regeneration. Number of new blood vessels was mildly to moderately increased compared to the biopsy taken before the therapy.

Number of papillae was significantly increased after the therapy. Significant reduction of vaginal atrophy symptoms is demonstrated in postmenopausal women after the laser therapy. Statistically significant improvement ($p < 0.001$) is shown for all symptoms of VVA and VHI score ($p < 0.001$). More than three quarters of patients were very satisfied after the treatment.

Treatment with fractional CO_2 laser appeared to be effective, achieving significant improvement of all symptoms related to VVA in menopausal women.

References

1. Santoro N, Komi J. Prevalence and impact of vaginal symptoms among postmenopausal women. J Sex Med. 2009;6(8):2133–42.
2. Nappi RE, Kokot-Kierepa M. Vaginal Health: Insights, Views & Attitudes (VIVA): results from an international survey. Climacteric. 2012;15(1):36–44.
3. Nappi RE, Kokot-Kierepa M. Women's voices in the menopause: results from an international survey on vaginal atrophy. Maturitas. 2010;67(3):233–8.
4. Goldstein I, Dicks B, Kim NN, et al. Multidisciplinary overview of vaginal atrophy and associated genitourinary symptoms in postmenopausal women. Sex Med. 2013;1(2):44–53.
5. Goldstein I. Recognizing and treating urogenital atrophy in postmenopausal women. J Women Health (Larchmt). 2010;19:425–32.
6. Leiblum S, Bachman G, Kemmann E, et al. Vaginal atrophy in the postmenopausal woman: the importance of sexual activity and hormones. J Am Med Assoc. 1983;249:2195–8.
7. Ibe C, Simon JA. Vulvovaginal atrophy: current and future therapies (CME). J Sex Med. 2010;7:1042–50.
8. Tierney EP, Hanke CW. Fractionated carbon dioxide laser treatment of photoaging: prospective study in 45 patients and review of the literature. Dermatol Surg. 2011;37(9):1279–90.
9. Salvatore S, Leone Roberto Maggiore U, Origoni M, et al. Microablative fractional CO2 laser improves dyspareunia related to vulvovaginal atrophy: a pilot study. J Endometriosis. 2014;6(3):150–6.
10. Perino A, Calligaro A, Forlani F, et al. Vulvo-vaginal atrophy: a new treatment modality using thermo-ablative fractional CO2 laser. Maturitas. 2015;80(3):296–301.
11. Salvatore S, Nappi RE, Parma MN, et al. Sexual function after fractional microablative CO2 laser in women with vulvovaginal atrophy. Climacteric. 2015;18:219–25.
12. Salvatore S, Nappi RE, Zerbinati N, et al. A 12-week treatment with fractional CO_2 laser for vulvovaginal atrophy: a pilot study. Climacteric. 2014;17:1–7.
13. Bachmann G. Urogenital ageing: an old problem newly recognized. Maturitas. 1995;22(Suppl):S1–5.
14. Gaspar A, Addamo G, Brandi H. Vaginal fractional CO2 laser: a minimally invasive option for vaginal rejuvenation. Am J Cosmet Surg. 2011;28:156–62.
15. Longo C, Galimberti M, De Pace B, et al. Laser skin rejuvenation: epidermal changes and collagen remodeling evaluated by in vivo confocal microscopy. Lasers Med Sci. 2013;28:76–9.
16. Tierney EP, Hanke CW. Ablative fractionated CO2, laser resurfacing for the neck: prospective study and review of the literature. J Drug Dermatol. 2009;8:723–31.
17. Zerbinati N, Serati M, Origoni M, et al. Microscopic and ultra- structural modifications of postmenopausal atrophic vaginal mucosa after fractional carbon dioxide laser treatment. Laser Med Sci. 2015;30: 429–36.
18. Salvatore S, Maggiore ULRM, Athanasiou S, et al. Histological study on the effects of microablative fractional CO2 laser on atrophic vaginal tissue: an ex vivo study. Menopause. 2015;22(8):845–9.
19. Salvatore S, França K, Lotti T, Parma M, et al. Early regenerative modifications of human postmenopausal atrophic vaginal mucosa following fractional CO_2 laser treatment open access maced. J Med Sci. 2018;6(1):6–14.

Recurrent Urinary Tract Infection

27

Cristóbal Ramírez Sevilla, Esther Gómez Lanza, Juan Llopis Manzanera, Juan Antonio Romero Martin, and Miguel Ángel Barranco Sanz

27.1 Introduction

Urinary tract infections (UTI) are the most common infections in humans with a prevalence of 150 million in the world in 2013 [1].

The World Health Organization report of April 2014 warns that common infections will again be life-threatening due to the increase in bacterial resistance [2–4].

We know that UTI have high prevalence and have a high economic impact and deteriorate the quality of life. It can be serious if cause pyelonephritis and urinary sepsis [4–6].

In this scenario, active immunoprophylaxis is presented as an effective and safe option to reduce the episodes and symptoms of recurrent UTI (rUTI), without increasing bacterial resistance and improving quality of life [7–12].

C. R. Sevilla (✉) · J. L. Manzanera · J. A. R. Martin · M. Á. B. Sanz
Urology Department, Hospital de Mataró, Barcelona, Spain
e-mail: jllopis@csdm.cat; jaromero@csdm.cat; mabarranco@csdm.cat

E. G. Lanza
Urology Department, Hospital Moisés Broggi de Sant Joan Despí, Barcelona, Spain

27.2 Literature Review

In prevention we have Uromune® since October 2010 in Spain.

From 2010 to the present, we can consult different publications on the results of Uromune® for prevention of rUTI. In 2013, a doctoral thesis from the University of Salamanca compared a group of 159 patients who received Uromune® along 3 months to 160 who received prophylaxis with antibiotics for 6 months and analyzed the results at 3, 9, and 15 months, demonstrating a great benefit in the group treated with uromune®. These results were published in International Urogynecology Journal in 2012 [13].

In 2015 the same group from the University of Salamanca published in Frontiers Journal a great difference of Uromune® with respect to antibiotics in a larger study with 360 vs 339 patients [14].

Moreover we can check the good results of Uromune® in a poster presented in the 2016 annual International Continence Society meeting with a short series of only 24 patients and a 12-month follow-up, obtaining 86% of the patients without recurrence.

The British Journal of Urology International in 2018 published a series of 75 women treated with Uromune® without recurrence in 78% after 1 year of follow-up [9].

The benefits of non-antibiotic measures such as active immunoprophylaxis in the prevention of

F. Dökmeci, D. E. E. Rizk (eds.), *Insights Into Incontinence and the Pelvic Floor*,
https://doi.org/10.1007/978-3-030-94174-1_27

recurrent UTI are explained in Nature Reviews Urology Journal also in 2018 [15].

We conclude with the European Association of Urology 2020 Guidelines that recommend the following [16, 17]:

- About the immunoactive prophylaxis for recurrent urinary tract infections (rUTI): OM-89 (Uro-Vaxom) is an oral vaccine that can be recommended for female patients with rUTI.
- About antimicrobials for preventing rUTI with continuous low-dose antimicrobial prophylaxis and post-coital prophylaxis: It is mandatory to offer both options when behavioral modifications and non-antimicrobial measures have been unsuccessful.

27.3 Case Study: Immunoprophylaxis with Autovaccine Uromune® Presents Better Effectiveness Against Prevention with Antibiotitcs or with Vaccine from the Collection Strain in Recurrent Urinary Tract Infections

(a) **Aim and Scope**

The objective of this study has been to analyze the efficacy of the Uromune® autovaccine in relation to Uromune® vaccine from the collection strain and the prophylaxis with antibiotics in the reduction of the UTI episodes at 3 and 6 months of follow-up.

Exclusion criteria (Table 27.1):

Table 27.1 Exclusion criteria

Neurogenic bladder
Symptomatic urinary lithiasis
Ureteral catheter, nephrostomy
Moderate-severe urinary incontinence (pad test, ICIQ-SF)
BPH with IPSS >15
Post-void residual urine >100 mL
Urinary diversion

(b) **Study Design** (Table 27.2)

Table 27.2 Study design

$n = 131$ patients from 2 urban hospitals
3 or more uncomplicated UTI in the previous 12 months
Prospective evaluation from 2016 to 2018
Uromune® sublingual with 2 pulsations on an empty stomach every 24 h for 3 months
Variables: number of UTI at the beginning, at 3 and 6 months after treatment, sex, and menopause
Effectiveness was defined in the presence of 0–1 UTI after treatment at 3 or 6 months
Menopause was defined as woman aged 50 or over

(c) **Material and Methods** (Table 27.3)

Table 27.3 Material and methods

$n = 131$
Group A (ATB): 42 (64.3% cefuroxime 125 mg daily, 35.7% fosfomycin 3 g weekly)
Group B (Uromune® autovaccine): 44
Group C (Uromune® from collection strain): 45

(d) **Results of the Study**

The mean age was 71 years with a range of 22–93 years. The female sex represented 76% and the male 24%. 89% of the women were menopausal and 11% premenopausal.

At the beginning of the treatment, 90.2% had between 3 and 6 UTI, with a maximum of 9 UTI.

3 months after the end of treatment the results were:

- Group A presented 0–1 UTI at 66% (0 UTI at 31% and 1 UTI at 35%)
- Group B presented 0–1 UTI at 86.4% (0 UTI at 27% and 1 UTI at 59%)
- Group C presented 0–1 UTI at 86.7% (0 UTI at 48% and 1 UTI at 37%)

At 6 months the results were:

- Group A had 0–1 UTI at 50% (0 UTI at 19% and 1 UTI at 31%)
- Group B had 0–1 UTI at 72.8% (0 UTI at 20% and 1 UTI at 52%)
- Group C had 0–1 UTI in 71.1% (0 UTI in 20% and 1 UTI in 51%)

27.4 Discussion

The 2020 EAU Guidelines recommend the use of continued or post-coital treatment with antibiotics after unsuccessful testing of the other alternatives, including active immunoprophylaxis, with a level of evidence 1a compared to 1b with antibiotics [16, 17].

Uromune® has been marketed in Spain since October 2010 to prevent recurrent UTI, with the modification of being an autovaccine since January 2018 [18].

During the last years, there have been different publications that demonstrate the high efficacy of Uromune® in preventing UTI without causing the side effects of antibiotics or increasing bacterial resistance. In 2013 Lorenzo-Gómez et al. showed that a group of 159 patients treated with Uromune® collection strain for 3 months had a four times lower risk of having a UTI, compared to 160 patients treated with trimethoprim/sulfamethoxazole 200/40 mg daily for 6 months. The same authors, 2 years later, with a larger sample of 360 patients who received the same vaccine for 3 months compared to 339 who received the same antibiotic treatment, confirmed that in the first group, the mean number of days until presenting a UTI was 180 days compared to 19 days in the second group.

To date, there are no published studies comparing the results of the Uromune® autovaccine with respect to antibiotics and collection strain Uromune®. In this study with a small sample of 377 patients, the great benefit of Uromune®, both autovaccine and collection strain, is demonstrated in terms of efficacy, with respect to continued treatment with antibiotics, at 3 and 6 months of follow-up. The best results were obtained in menopausal women because they constitute the majority group of the population studied.

Limitations of this study were the sample size and the follow-up only up to 6 months. On the other hand, cost analysis was not calculated.

Advantages of this study were the good results of the vaccines in terms of efficacy and improvement of quality of life, without presenting side effects or increasing bacterial resistance.

We recommend continuing to work on the prevention of UTI with vaccines and recording the results in a meticulous way in a longer sample with a follow-up period not less than 12 months, with the aim of improving the quality of life of our patients as well as being able to establish a re-vaccination schedule in the most refractory cases.

27.5 Conclusion

- Uromune® provided greater efficacy than continued treatment with antibiotics obtaining at 3 months 0–1 UTI in 86.4% with autovaccine and 86.7% with vaccine strain collection with respect to 66.5% with antibiotics.
- At 6 months of follow-up, the difference was even greater with 0–1 UTI in 72.8% with autovaccine and 71.1% with collection strain with respect to 50% with antibiotics.
- The results were similar between autovaccine and collection strain at 3 months but higher with autovaccine at 6 months.
- Whenever we have availability in our hospital, we recommend using Uromune® autovaccine as the first option to prevent recurrent UTI.

Acknowledgments No funds or financing have been necessary in the development of this work.

References

1. Foxman B. Epidemiology of urinary tract infections: incidence, morbidity and economics cost. Am J Med. 2002;113(Suppl 1A):5S–13S.
2. Palou J, Pigrau C, Molina I, Ledesma JM, Angulo J. Etiología y sensibilidad de los uropatógenos identificados en infecciones urinarias bajas no complicadas de la mujer (Estudio ARESC): implicaciones en la terapia empírica. Med Clin. 2011;136(1):1–7.
3. Hooton TM, Scholes D, Hughes JP, Winter C, Roberts PL, Stapleton AE, et al. A prospective study of risk factors for symptomatic urinary tract infection in young women. N Engl J Med. 1996;335:468–74.
4. Gomariz M, Vicente D, Pérez E. Infecciones no complicadas. Inf Ter Sist Nac Salud. 1998;22(6): 133–41.
5. Nicolle LE. Managing recurrent urinary tract infection in women. Women Health (Lond). 2005;1(1): 39–50.

6. Foxman B, Somsel P, Tallman P, Gillespie B, Raz R, Colodner R, et al. Urinary tract infection among women aged 40 to 65: behavioral and sexual risk factors. J Clin Epidemiol. 2001;54:710.
7. Nicolle LE. Asymptomatic bacteriuria in the elderly. Infect Dis Clin N Am. 1997;11:647.
8. Asociación Española de Urología. Cistitis no complicada en la mujer. Guía multidisciplinar. Editorial Zambón, Barcelona; 2008. https://portal.guiasalud.es/wpcontent/uploads/2018/12/GPC_506_Cistitis_mujer_2008.pdf.
9. Yang B, Foley S. First experience un the UK of treating women with recurrent urinary tract infections with the bacterial vaccine Uromune®. BJU Int. 2018;121(2):289–92.
10. Naber KG, Cho Y, Matsumoto T, Schaeffer AJ. Immunoactive prophylaxis of recurrent urinary tract infections: a meta-analysis. Int J Antimicrob Agents. 2009;33(2):111–9.
11. Bauer HW, Rahlfs VW, Lauener PA, Blessmann GSS. Prevention of recurrent urinary tract infections with immuno-active E. coli fractions: a meta-analysis of five placebo-controlled double-blind studies. Int J Antimicrob Agents. 2002;19(6):451–6.
12. Bauer HW, Alloussi S, Egger G, Blümlein HM, Cozma G, Schulman CC, et al. A long-term, multicenter, double-blind study of an Escherichia coli extract (OM-89) in female patients with recurrent urinary tract infections. Eur Urol. 2005;47(4):542–8.
13. Lorenzo-Gómez MF, Padilla-Fernández B, García-Criado FJ, Mirón-Canelo JA, Gil-Vicente A, Nieto-Huertos A, et al. Evaluation of a therapeutic vaccine for the prevention of recurrent urinary tract infections versus prophylactic treatment with antibiotics. Int Urogynecol J. 2013 Jan;24(1):127–34.
14. Lorenzo-Gómez MF, Padilla-Fernández B, García-Cenador MB, Virseda-Rodríguez ÁJ, Martín-García I, Sánchez-Escudero A, et al. Comparison of sublingual therapeutic vaccine with antibiotics for the prophylaxis of recurrent urinary tract infections. Front Cell Infect Microbiol. 2015;5:50.
15. Sihra N, Goodman A, Zakri R, Sahai A, Malde S. Nonantibiotic prevention and management of recurrent urinary tract infection. Nat Rev Urol. 2018;15(12):750–76. https://doi.org/10.1038/s41585-018-0106.
16. Beerepoot MAJ, Geerlings SE, Van Haarst EP, Mensing van Charante N, Ter Riet G. Nonantibiotic prophylaxis for recurrent urinary tract infections: a systematic review and meta-analysis of randomized controlled trials. J Urol. 2013;190:1981.
17. Pfau A, Sacks TG. Effective prophylaxis for recurrent urinary tract infections during pregnancy. Clin Infect Dis. 1992;14(4):810–4.
18. Prieto L, Esteban M, Salinas J, Adot JM, Arlandis S, Peri L, et al. Consensus document of the Spanish Urological Association on the management of uncomplicated recurrent urinary tract infections. Working group for the recommendations in the diagnosis and management of uncomplicated urinary tract infections. Carried out under the auspices of the Spanish Association of Urology 2013. Actas Urol Esp. 2015;39(6):339–48.

28 Immunoprophylaxis in Recurrent Urinary Tract Infection

Cristóbal Ramírez Sevilla, Esther Gómez Lanza, Juan Llopis Manzanera, Juan Antonio Romero Martin, and Miguel Ángel Barranco Sanz

28.1 Introduction

Urinary tract infections (UTI) are defined as symptoms secondary to the growth of bacteria in urine culture in units greater than >100,000 CFU/mL. They are a common reason for consultation in Primary Care centers and in the Emergency Departments. UTI affect 150 million people in the world each year, and in 2018 in the United Kingdom, 172,000 consultations were registered for this reason [1].

Thirty-three percent of women will have at least one UTI episode in their lifetime, and of these, up to 35% will recur within 3–6 months after infection. UTI are the second cause of hospitalization due to infectious disease in people over 65 years. The most frequent bacteria causing UTI in young women without risk factors is *Escherichia coli* in 80%, followed by *Proteus* spp., *Klebsiella pneumoniae*, and *Enterococcus faecalis* in this order [1].

Uncomplicated UTI are defined as urine infections that occur in the absence of functional or anatomical alterations of the urinary tract. In contrast, complicated UTI occur secondarily to functional or anatomical urinary disorders that facilitate the persistence, recurrence, and failure of treatment. The most prevalent location of UTI is the bladder, where they cause cystitis. Women can be up to 30 times more predisposed than men to suffer from them [2, 3].

Recurrences are classified as relapses (20%) and reinfections (80%). Relapses appear in the first weeks after the infection is cured and are usually caused by the same germ, indicating a treatment failure or the presence of an anatomical or functional alteration of the urinary tract. Reinfections consist of the appearance of two or more episodes in 6 months or of three or more in 12 months and are usually caused by different germs [4].

The high incidence and prevalence of urinary tract infections cause a very high health cost due to absenteeism from work, the increase in medical consultations, the performance of complementary tests, emergency room consultations, and the use of antibiotics. The cost of treating UTI in the United States was estimated in 2008 at more than 2.5 trillion dollars [5–7].

In addition to the increase in healthcare costs and the worsening of the secondary quality of life, patients with recurrent UTI are exposed to the side effects of antibiotics and increased bacterial resistance [8].

C. R. Sevilla (✉) · J. L. Manzanera · J. A. R. Martin · M. Á. B. Sanz
Urology Department, Hospital de Mataró, Barcelona, Spain
e-mail: jllopis@csdm.cat; jaromero@csdm.cat; mabarranco@csdm.cat

E. G. Lanza
Urology Department, Hospital Moisés Broggi de Sant Joan Despí, Barcelona, Spain

F. Dökmeci, D. E. E. Rizk (eds.), *Insights Into Incontinence and the Pelvic Floor*,
https://doi.org/10.1007/978-3-030-94174-1_28

The 2020 European Association of Urology (EAU) guidelines confirm that recurrent UTI risk factors are in young and premenopausal women: sexual intercourse, use of spermicide, a new sexual partner, a mother with history of UTI, history of UTI during childhood, and blood group antigen secretory status. These factors in older and postmenopausal women are history of UTI before menopause, urinary incontinence, atrophic vaginitis due to estrogen deficiency, cystocele, increased post-void urine volume, blood group antigen secretory status, and urine catheterization and functional status deterioration in elderly institutionalized women [9].

These are the AEU recommendations based on scientific evidence for the prevention of recurrent UTI in its 2020 guidelines: to use vaginal estrogen replacement in postmenopausal women with strength rating of weak (level of evidence 1b), to use immunoactive prophylaxis to reduce recurrent UTI in all age groups (level of evidence 1a), and to use continuous or post-coital antimicrobial prophylaxis to prevent recurrent UTI when non-antimicrobial interventions have failed (level of evidence 1b) [9].

The treatment with Uromune® is an authorized treatment in Spain since October 2010.

28.2 Literature Review

In 1986 Frey et al. prepared the first double-blind study on the efficacy of *Escherichia coli* extract in capsule form, taken orally for 3 months for the prevention of recurrent UTI. In a group of 27 patients, it showed a decrease in dysuria, bacteriuria, leukocyturia, and the need to take antibiotics compared to placebo [10].

Later, Tammenn et al. with a similar study observed a decrease in 12 episodes of UTI in the group treated with *Escherichia coli* extract (61 patients) compared to 41 in the placebo group (59 patients) at 3 months after treatment [11].

Two other studies in 1993 and 1994 reported by Schulman CC and Magasi P showed similar results regarding the reduction in the number of UTI and the consumption of antibiotics in patients treated with bacterial *Escherichia coli* extract versus placebo [12, 13].

In 2005 Bauer et al. published a study comparing 231 patients treated with *Escherichia coli* extract versus a placebo group of 222, demonstrating at 12 months of follow-up that the first group had 14.7% less UTI than the placebo group [14].

The study by Lorenzo-Gómez et al. compared 159 women treated for 3 months with Uromune® versus 160 women who followed daily treatment for 6 months with trimethoprim/sulfamethoxazole 40/200 mg orally. The group treated with Uromune® had a significant reduction in UTI 3 months after finishing treatment compared to the group treated with antibiotics, and this improvement was maintained at 9 and 15 months of follow-up. Three years later in 2015, the same authors corroborated these results with a larger sample of 360 women treated with the vaccine compared to 339 treated with the same antibiotic for 6 months, and they concluded that with the vaccine it is possible to reduce the consumption of antibiotics and thus not increase the bacterial resistance [15, 16].

28.3 Case Study

(a) **Aim and Scope**

To analyze the efficacy of Uromune® in reducing the episodes of UTI at 3, 6, and 12 months of follow up

We defined causes of exclusion of the study the presence of neurogenic bladder, symptomatic urinary lithiasis, ureteral catheter or nephrostomy, moderate-severe urinary incontinence defined as the presence of three or more 1-hour pad test equal to or greater than 50 cc, benign hyperplasia of prostate (BPH) in progression defined as patients with International Prostate Symptom Score (IPSS) greater than 15 despite medical treatment combined with alpha-blockers and inhibitors of 5-phosphodiesterase, BPH, and cystocele with post-void urine volume greater than 100 mL and patients with Bricker urinary diversion, neobladder, and cutaneous urostomy.

Table 28.1 Materials and methods

Materials and methods
n = 784 patients from 2 hospitals in Barcelona, Spain
3 or more uncomplicated UTI in the previous 12 months
Prospective evaluation along 74 months (2011–2017)
Uromune® sublingual with 2 pulsations on an empty stomach every 24 h for 3 months
Variables: number of UTI at the beginning, at 3, 6, and 12 months after treatment, sex, and menopause
Effectiveness was defined in the presence of 0–1 UTI after treatment at 3, 6, or 12 months
Menopause was defined as woman aged 50 or over

(b) **Study Design** (Table 28.1)

(c) **Results of the Study**

The mean age was 73 and the range 19–97. The female sex represented 83% and the male 17%. 90% of the women were menopausal (over 50 years old).

At the beginning of the treatment (0 months): 94.4% of the patients presented between 3 and 6 UTI. There were patients with 9 and 10 UTI. At 3 months after finishing treatment with Uromune®, 71% presented between 0 and 1 UTI (0 UTI 44% and 27% 1 UTI). At 6 months of follow-up, 64% presented 0-1 UTI (0 UTI 32% and 1 UTI 32%). Finally, at 12 months of follow-up, more than 60% had 0-1 UTI (0 UTI 14% and 1 UTI 46%).

The female sex presented better results than the male with 73%, 65%, and 61% of 0–1 UTI at 3, 6, and 12 months compared to 61%, 58%, and 57% in male.

Menopausal women, that is, over 50 years old, had a better response at 3, 6, and 12 months with 0–1 UTI in 74%, 66%, and 62% compared to premenopausal women with 64%, 56%, and 40%.

28.4 Discussion

In our study with a large sample of 784 patients, the reduction of the number of UTI episodes to zero or one was observed in 71.7% of the patients treated with Uromune® at 3 months, a percentage that remained at 64.7% at 6 months. These results were similar to those published by Lorenzo-Gómez et al. in 2015 with a 75% favorable response at 3 months with the vaccine. On the other hand, they are inferior to 78% of zero UTI at 3 months after finishing Uromune® published in February 2018 by Yang et al. although with a smaller sample of only 75 patients [17].

In October 2018, Sihrar et al. published their results and were superior to our study with 90.3% of a total of 360 patients with only up to one UTI 12 months after the end of the treatment with Uromune® [18].

The selection of a comparative group of patients, who had received antibiotic prophylaxis for uncomplicated recurrent UTI for 6 months, to be compared with respect to the group of patients of our study, who followed Uromune®, was rejected in the design of our study due to three reasons: the great difficulty in obtaining data in the medical records because before 2010 the medical records were not computerized in our hospital, the great variability in the data collection in terms of the antibiotic used as prophylaxis, and the fact that in many patients we could not obtain the results of the urine culture because the results had originated in different health centers of Primary Care.

28.5 Conclusion

- Uromune® obtained a high effectiveness reducing UTI to 0–1 in 71.7%, 64.7%, and 60.7% at 3, 6, and 12 months, respectively.
- Best results corresponded were observed in women over 50 years old.
- Uromune® could be considered the first choice in prevention of recurrent UTI according to the sample analyzed.

Acknowledgments No funds or financing have been necessary in the development of this work.

References

1. Foxman B. Epidemiology of urinary tract infections: incidence, morbidity and economic costs. Am J Med. 2002;113(Suppl1A):55–135.
2. Artero A, Inglada L, Gómez-Belda A, Capdevila JA, Diez LF, Arca A, et al. The clinical impact of bacteremia on outcomes in patients with pyelonephritis or urinary sepsis: a prospective multicenter study. PLoS One. 2018;13(1):1–9.
3. Benito-Villalvilla C, Cirauqui C, Diez-Rivero CM, Casanovas M, Subiza JL, Palomares O. MV140, a sublingual polyvalent bacterial preparation to treat recurrent urinary tract infections, human dendritic cells for generating Th1, Th17 and IL- 10 responses via Syk and MyD88. Mucosal Immunol. 2017;10(4):924–35.
4. Hooton TM, Scholes D, Hughes JP, Winter C, Roberts PL, Stapleton AE, et al. A prospective study of risk factors for symptomatic urinary tract infection in young women. N Engl J Med. 1996;335:468–74.
5. Nicolle LE. Managing recurrent urinary tract infection in women. Womens Health (Lond). 2005;1(1):39–50.
6. Rahn DD. Urinary tract infections: contemporary management. Urol Nurs. 2008;28(5):333–41.
7. Naber KG, Cho Y, Matsumoto T, Schaeffer AJ. Immunoactive prophylaxis of recurrent urinary tract infections: a meta-analysis. Int J Antimicrob Agents. 2009;33(2):111–9.
8. Andreu A, Planells I. Spanish cooperative group for the study of antimicrobial sensitivity of urological pathogens. Med Clin. 2008;130(13):481–6.
9. Grabe M, Bishop M, Bjerklund-Johansen T, Botto H, Cek M, Lobel B et al. Guidelines on urological infections. Eur Assoc Urol. 2009. http://www.uroweb.org/fileadmin/tx_aeuguidelines/2009/Full/Urological_Infections.pdf2009.
10. Frey C, Obolensky W, Wyss H. Treatment of recurrent urinary tract infections: efficacy of an orally administered biological response modifier. Urol Int. 1986;41:444–6.
11. Tammen H. Immunobiotherapy with Uro-Vaxom in recurrent urinary tract infection. The German Urinary Tract Infection Study Group. Br J Urol. 1990;65:6–9.
12. Schulman CC, Corbusier A, Michiels H, Taenzer HJ. Oral immunotherapy of recurrent urinary tract infections: a double-blind placebo-controlled multicentre study. J Urol. 1993;150:917–21.
13. Magasi P, Panovics J, Illes A, Nagy M. Uro-Vaxom and the management of recurrent urinary tract infection in adults: a randomized multicenter double blind trial. Eur Urol. 1994;26:137–40.
14. Bauer HW, Alloussi S, Egger G, Blumlein HM, Cozma G, Schulman CC, et al. A long-term, multicenter, double-blind study of an Escherichia coli extract (OM-89) in female patients with recurrent urinary tract infections. Eur Urol. 2005;47(4):542–8.
15. Lorenzo-Gómez MF, Padilla-Fernández B, García-Cenador MB, VirsedaRodríguez ÁJ, Martín-García I, Sánchez-Escudero A, et al. Comparison of sublingual therapeutic vaccine with antibiotics for the prophylaxis of recurrent tract infections. Front Cell Infect Microbiol. 2015;5:51–8.
16. Lorenzo-Gómez MF, Padilla-Fernández B, García-Criado FJ, Mirón-Canelo JA, Gil-Vicente A, Nieto-Huertos A. Evaluation of a therapeutic vaccine for the prevention of recurrent urinary tract infections versus prophylactic treatment with antibiotics. Int Urogynecol J. 2013;24(1):127–34.
17. Yang B, Foley S. First experience in the UK of treating women with recurrent urinary tract infections with the bacterial vaccine uromune. BJU Int. 2018;121(2):289–92.
18. Sihra N, Goodman A, Zakri R, Sahai A, Malde S. Nonantibiotic prevention and management of recurrent urinary tract infection. Nat Rev Urol. 2018;15(12):750–76. https://doi.org/10.1038/s41585-018-0106.

29 Impact of Recurrent Urinary Tract Infection on Renal Function

Bárbara Padilla-Fernández, Carlos Müller-Arteaga, Mónica Paola Coderque-Mejía, Misericordia Martínez-Huélamo, Filomena Herrera-Criado, Alfonso Sánchez-Escudero, Manuel José Vicente-Arroyo, Ignacio González-Casado, José María De Dios-Hernández, Emilio Blanco-Tarrío, María Begoña García-Cenador, and María Fernanda Lorenzo-Gómez

29.1 Introduction

Lower urinary tract infections (UTI) usually do not affect renal function [1], but it has been described a subclinical or silent damage of the renal parenchyma in 30% of the cases [2, 3], especially if the patient has had a UTI in the previous month or in lower UTI lasting more than 7 days [4]. Renal function alteration may carry important consequences and increase the risk of other complications, jeopardising the functionality of the renal unit.

Creatinine assessment has been the most used test for the diagnosis of acute renal insufficiency, the control of both its evolution and treatment, given the low cost of the test and the universal

B. Padilla-Fernández
Departamento de Cirugía, Facultad de Medicina, Universidad de La Laguna, Tenerife, Spain

C. Müller-Arteaga
Department of Urology, Hospital Universitario De Ourense, Ourense, Spain

M. P. Coderque-Mejía
Department of Urology, Complejo Asistencial Universitario de Salamanca, Salamanca, Spain

M. Martínez-Huélamo · F. Herrera-Criado · A. Sánchez-Escudero · M. J. Vicente-Arroyo · I. González-Casado · J. M. De Dios-Hernández · E. Blanco-Tarrío
Grupo De Investigación Multidisciplinar Urológico Renal (GRUMUR), Instituto de Investigación Biomédica De Salamanca (IBSAL), Salamanca, Spain

M. B. García-Cenador
Department of Surgery, University of Salamanca, Salamanca, Spain

M. F. Lorenzo-Gómez (✉)
Department of Urology, Complejo Asistencial Universitario de Salamanca, Salamanca, Spain

Grupo De Investigación Multidisciplinar Urológico Renal (GRUMUR), Instituto de Investigación Biomédica De Salamanca (IBSAL), Salamanca, Spain

Department of Surgery, University of Salamanca, Salamanca, Spain

F. Dökmeci, D. E. E. Rizk (eds.), *Insights Into Incontinence and the Pelvic Floor*, https://doi.org/10.1007/978-3-030-94174-1_29

availability. However, it increases when an important renal damage has been done and the glomerular filtration rate has drop by half. Furthermore, its concentration depends on changes in the muscle mass.

The measurement of the glomerular filtration rate (GF) is a sensitive indicator of renal excretory function, and a descent in GF corresponds to a decline in renal function. The magnitude of this drop depends on the changes in the glomerular functions, turning into a reduction in the excretion of liquids and solutes and the progressive increase of creatinine, urea, and other substances. However, the renal reserve allows the compensation of these elements until a given level, and that is the reason for the non-lineal relationship between the decrease of the glomerular filtration rate and the increase in the solutes' plasmatic levels [5].

29.2 Literature Review

It is well known that prolonged urinary tract infections in patients with anatomical or functional disorders (i.e., urinary lithiasis, obstructive uropathy, neurogenic bladder, etc.) develop renal scars that later may produce renal function disbalance and renal insufficiency [1].

Several risk factors for the development of subclinical pyelonephritis have been described: symptoms compatible with cystitis 1 week before the initiation of treatment, diabetes mellitus, immunocompromised patients, pregnancy, preexistent vesicoureteral reflux and other anatomical alterations of the urinary tract, history of pyelonephritis in the previous year, no symptomatic improvement after 3 days of treatment [6], children under 5 years old, and *Proteus* spp. infection [2]. However, bacterial colonisation of the renal parenchyma can be present without the existence of any of these factors.

Tubulointerstitial nephritis in the context of a UTI is usually related with drug treatment (70%), but it can also be associated with autoimmune, infectious, or neoplastic processes. Only a 10% of patients with drug-induced nephritis show the classical triad: fever, skin rash, and eosinophilia. If necessary, the diagnosis can be made with a kidney biopsy, but it usually disappears after drug withdrawal [7]. The extension of the damage is generally related with the host response: if it is excessive, acute damage develops with kidney failure; when it is less severe and becomes chronic, tubular atrophy, interstitial inflammation, and fibrosis may arise as a result of the injury of the pyelocaliceal system and the renal parenchyma [8].

Renal damage develops if the bacteria have the ability to infect kidney's medulla. Although the mechanism is not completely understood, specific virulence factors could help bacterial adhesion to host tissues, favouring an ascending infection even in the absence of vesicoureteral reflux [9]. On the other hand, bacteria's virulence is linked with surface factors (presence of fimbriae or pilli [1], K antigen [1], Gal and Gal-B adhesins [9]) or secreted factors (haemolysins, hydroxamate [1]) that are driven to the site of action [8].

29.3 Case Study: Variations in Renal Function in Patients with Recurrent Urinary Tract Infections: Solórzano Study

(a) **Aim and Scope**

There is a lack of studies showing renal function's variation in patients with recurrent urinary tract infections (RUTI). The aim of this study is to follow up patients with and without RUTI and compare their glomerular filtration rate (GF) at the beginning and at the end of this period (1 year).

(b) **Study Design and Material Methods**

A multicentre prospective observational study was conducted in 200 adult women who were divided in two groups:

- Group A (GA, n = 100): women with RUTI (case)
- Group B (GB, n = 100): women without RUTI (control)

Controls were women without RUTI followed by their Primary Care physicians after anti-incontinence surgery with suburethral sling performed by the urology department.

Patients under 18 years and/or with other urological disorders (including urinary tract lithiasis, intermediate-severe urinary incontinence, upper and lower urinary tract tumours) or immunosuppressive state that could favour infections were excluded.

A case report form (CRF) including the following variables was developed: age, personal and familiar medical background, toxic habits, disease-free interval, urine cultures, serum creatinine, proteinuria, initial (GF1) and final glomerular filtration rate (GF2), and abdominal ultrasound (focusing on kidney size, cortical thickness, corticomedullary differentiation). These variables were assessed at 1, 3, 6, 9, and 12 months. For statistical management of the data, an Excel worksheet was designed.

Glomerular filtration rate was calculated following the Cockcroft and Gault formula [10]:

[((140–age) × weight)/(72 × Serum Creatinine)] × 0.85 mL/min.

Data were analysed using the NCSS 2007/GESS 2007 statistical system (NCSS, LLC; Kaysville, Utah, USA). Descriptive statistics, student's t-test, chi-square distribution, Fisher's exact test, ANOVA (with Scheffé's method for normal samples and Kruskal-Wallis *H* test for other distributions), and Pearson and Spearman's correlation studies were applied. $p < 0.05$ was considered significant.

(c) **Results of the Study**

Two-hundred patients were included in the analysis. Average age of the whole sample was 59.83 years, without statistical differences between groups ($p = 0.08751$) (Table 29.1).

Table 29.1 Age in both groups

Group	Mean	SD	Median	Range
GA	60.48	0.2684	62	28–85
GB	59.54	0.7521	59	34–81

In Group A, GF1 was higher than GF2 (98.03 vs 80.97 mL/min). Younger patients had a higher GF both at the beginning and at the end of the study period compared to older patients (Fig. 29.1). For GF1, slope is −0.2401, correlation −0.3621, and coefficient of variation 0.2204. For GF2, slope is −0.3501, correlation −0.4109, and coefficient of variation 0.2206.

In Group B, GF2 was higher than GF1 (91.98 vs 88.03 mL/min). Younger patients had a higher GF both at the beginning and at the end of the study period compared to older patients (Fig. 29.1). For GF1, slope is −0.2402, correlation −0.4097, and coefficient of variation 0.02017. For GF2, slope is −0.1135, correlation −0.2019, and coefficient of variation 0.02014.

Regarding the study of secondary diagnoses in both groups, patients in GA were most frequently diagnosed with high blood pressure (HBP) than patients in GB, being this difference statistically significant. They also suffered more frequently diabetes mellitus (DM), and they took more frequently antiplatelet/anticoagulant treatment. On the other hand, significant differences were found in the incidence of allergies, osteoarticular diseases, chronic treatment with benzodiazepine/sedative/anxiolytic and anticholinergics, gyneco-obstetric interventions, and smoking habit that were more frequent in GB (Table 29.2).

HBP was more frequent in older patients in both groups (slope −0.0078, correlation −0.2102, coefficient of variation 0.04012 in GA; slope −0.0071, correlation −0.1821, coefficient of variation 0.0234 in GB).

In GA, mean GF1 was lower in those patients with HBP (92.34 mL/min) than without HBP (111.65 mL/min). The same trend was found regarding mean GF2 comparing patients with HBP (78.03 mL/min) towards those without HBP (95.62 mL/min). Differences in mean GF1 were not significant between patients with (87.03 mL/min) and without HBP (89.03 mL/min).

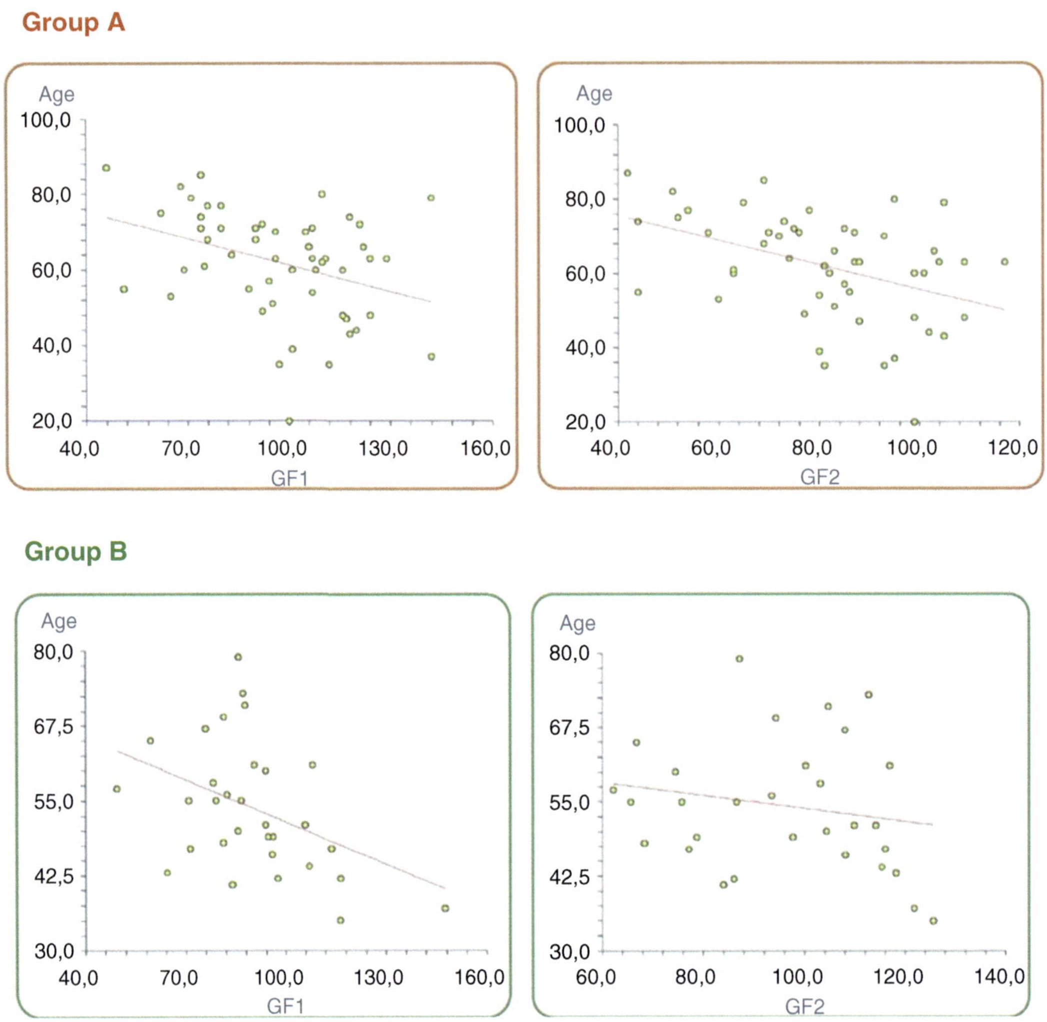

Fig. 29.1 Correlation of age and glomerular filtration rate at the beginning (GF1) and at the end (GF2) of the study period in patients with recurrent urinary tract infections (GA) and in control patients (GB, women without recurrent urinary tract infections)

Figure 29.2 shows the relationship between HBP and glomerular filtration rate at the beginning (GF1) and at the end (GF2) of the study period in both GA and GB.

29.4 Discussion

Following up the patients during a year, the decrease in GF is greater in patients with RUTI than in those treated for other reasons (in this case, stress urinary incontinence [SUI]). Although other comorbidities like high blood pressure could influence these results, we did not find significant differences in the group treated for SUI.

The Cockcroft-Gault formula was developed in 1973 using data from 249 men with creatinine clearance from approximately 30–130 mL/m^2 [10]. Given that it has not been expressed using standardized creatinine values and it is not adjusted for body surface area, this formula is

Table 29.2 Distribution of secondary diagnoses, concomitant drug treatment, gynaeco-obstetric background, and smoking habit in both groups

	GA, %	GB, %	p
Allergies	23.14	34.00	0.0022
Deliveries			
Eutocic	21.43	77.00	0.0001
Dystocic	2.86	8.67	0.0094
None	7.43	14.33	0.0049
Previous hysterectomy	18.57	17.33	0.2240
Previous curettage	3.14	29.33	0.0001
HBP	41.43	22.67	0.0001
DM	10.57	8.67	0.1862
Osteoarticular diseases	30.29	47.67	0.0001
Chronic treatment with benzodiazepine/sedative/anxiolytic	36.29	52.00	0.0001
Anticholinergic treatment	0.00	25.33	0.0001
Antiplatelet/anticoagulant treatment	20.86	14.33	0.0314
Smoker	10.57	51.33	0.0001

DM diabetes mellitus, *GA* group A, *GB* group B, *HBP* high blood pressure

used for research purposes only. The best way to determine drug dosing is with the CKD-EPI Creatinine Equation (2009) or the MDRD study [11, 12].

During usual renal ageing, nephrons are lost, and both glomerulosclerosis and tubulointerstitial fibrosis develop; in consequence, renal failure could result due to a minimal aggression by an inadequate compensation. Furthermore, this failure is greater in the elderly patients. Renal function decline is 3.5 times greater in patients over 70 years old, reaching 5 times in patients over 80 years old. This could explain the lower GF in older patients compared to younger patients in both groups (including patients without RUTI). In addition, all risk factors for renal function impairment are emphasised in the ageing kidney: drug-induced damage by antibiotics (i.e. aminoglycosides) and non-steroidal anti-inflammatory drugs (usually taken during UTIs) and hypovolemia (due to a low intake or an increased liquid loss) [13, 14].

Infection-induced renal damage can be explained in three stages [1, 15]:

- The bacteria stimulate the urothelium to produce inflammation mediators.
- The mediators (cytokines and interleukins) concentrate in the site of infection.
- The intensity of the inflammatory reaction influences the replacement of the damaged renal tissue.

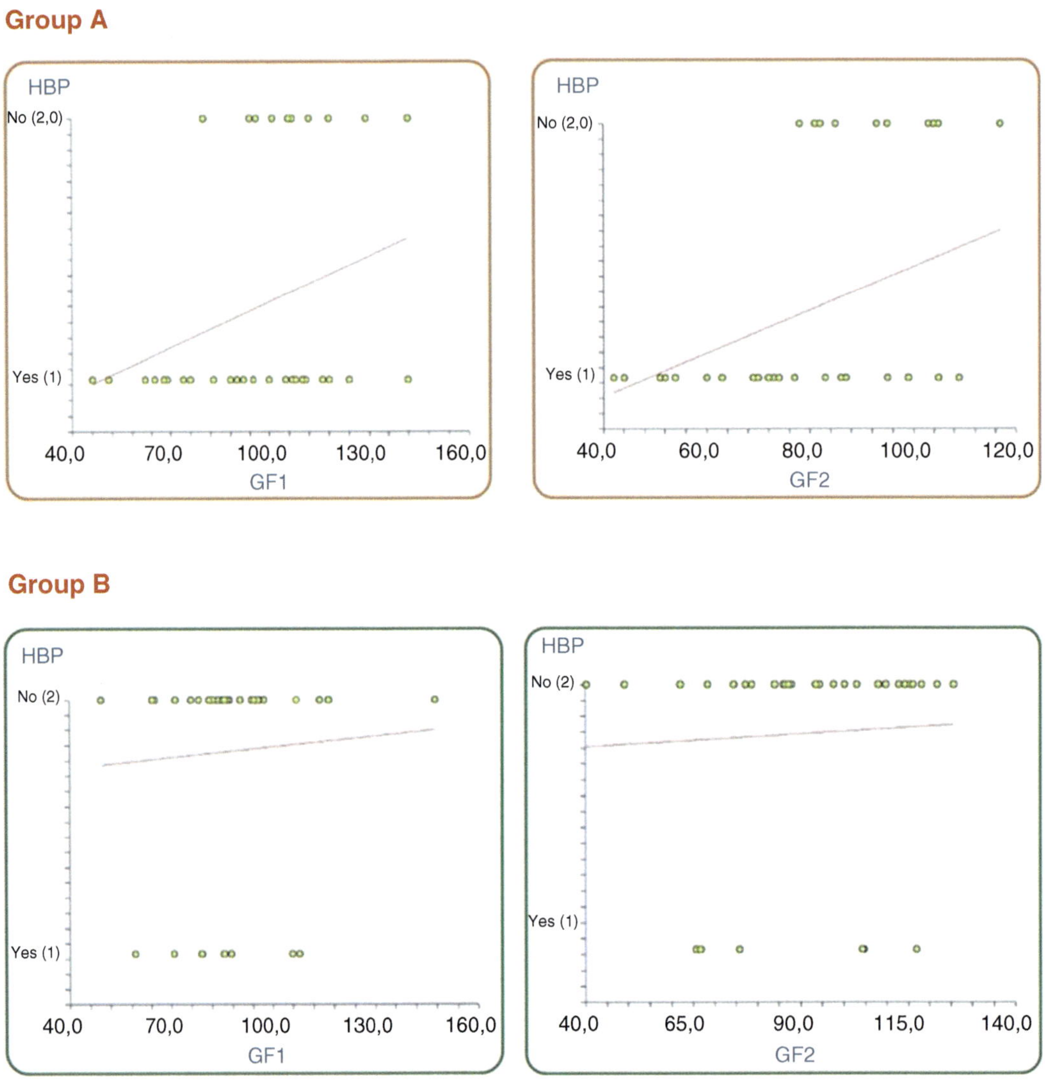

Fig. 29.2 Comparison of patient characteristics in both groups

29.5 Conclusion

Differences in renal function were found between patient with and without recurrent urinary tract infections. High blood pressure may act as an independent factor in both groups. Further study is needed to confirm these results.

Acknowledgment (Only of Funding) This study was developed thanks to the Solórzano grant 2016 of the *Fundación Memoria de Don Samuel Solórzano Barruso*, Universidad de Salamanca (Salamanca, Spain). Principal investigators: María Begoña García-Cenador and María Fernanda Lorenzo-Gómez.

References

1. Fünfstück R, Ott U, Naber KG. The interaction of urinary tract infection and renal insufficiency. Int J Antimicrob Agents. 2006;28(Suppl 1):S72–7. https://doi.org/10.1016/j.ijantimicag.2006.05.004.
2. Pigrau C, Horcajada JC, Cartón JA, Pujol M. Infección urinaria. In: Mensa J, editor. Protocolos clínicos SEIMC. SEIMC; 2006.
3. Ronald AR, Boutros P, Mourtada H. Bacteriuria localization and response to single-dose therapy in women. JAMA. 1976;235(17):1854–6.
4. Andreu Domingo A, Cacho J, Coira Nieto A, Lepe Jiménez JA. Diagnóstico microbiológico de las infecciones del tracto urinario Procedimientos en Microbiología clínica. Recomendaciones de la Sociedad española de Enfermedades Infecciosas y Microbiología Clínica. Madrid: SEIMC; 2010.
5. Müller Arteaga CA. Prevención de la afectación de la función renal en las infecciones del tracto urinario con profilaxis antibiótica frente a vacuna bacteriana. Salamanca; 2016.
6. Kurowski K. The women with dysuria. Am Fam Physician. 1998;57(9):2155–64, 69–70.
7. Tenorio Cañamás MT, Galeano Álvarez C, Rodríguez Mendiola N, Liaño García F. Diagnóstico diferencial de la insuficiencia renal aguda. Nefroplus. 2010;3(2):16–32. https://doi.org/10.3265/NefroPlus.pre2010.Jul.10548.
8. Bien J, Sokolova O, Bozko P. Role of uropathogenic Escherichia coli virulence factors in development of urinary tract infection and kidney damage. Int J Nephrol. 2012;2012:681473. https://doi.org/10.1155/2012/681473.
9. Nicolle LE. Uncomplicated urinary tract infection in adults including uncomplicated pyelonephritis. Urol Clin North Am. 2008;35(1):1–12, v. https://doi.org/10.1016/j.ucl.2007.09.004.
10. Cockcroft DW, Gault MH. Prediction of creatinine clearance from serum creatinine. Nephron. 1976;16(1):31–41. https://doi.org/10.1159/000180580.
11. Levey AS, Stevens LA. Estimating GFR using the CKD Epidemiology Collaboration (CKD-EPI) creatinine equation: more accurate GFR estimates, lower CKD prevalence estimates, and better risk predictions. Am J Kidney Dis. 2010;55(4):622–7. https://doi.org/10.1053/j.ajkd.2010.02.337.
12. Cockcroft-Gault Formula. National Kidney Foundation. https://www.kidney.org/professionals/KDOQI/gfr_calculatorCoc.
13. Himmelfarb J. Acute kidney injury in the elderly: problems and prospects. Semin Nephrol. 2009;29(6):658–64. https://doi.org/10.1016/j.semnephrol.2009.07.008.
14. Wang X, Bonventre JV, Parrish AR. The aging kidney: increased susceptibility to nephrotoxicity. Int J Mol Sci. 2014;15(9):15358–76. https://doi.org/10.3390/ijms150915358.
15. Kunin CM. Does kidney infection cause renal failure? Annu Rev Med. 1985;36:165–76. https://doi.org/10.1146/annurev.me.36.020185.001121.

Part VI

Pelvic Floor Physiotherapy

Connective Tissue Manipulation

30

Emel Sönmezer, Fulya Dökmeci,
Mehmet Murat Seval, and Ş. Esra Çetinkaya

Connective tissue manipulation (CTM) is a manipulative treatment method that differs from traditional massage in terms of technique and physiological effects [1, 2]. It includes many manipulative maneuvers for diagnosis and treatment. CTM is characterized by a strong pull applied to ligaments and subcutaneous tissues. This technique is used by physiotherapists to treat somatical and visceral diseases [2]. CTM was developed by Elizabeth Dicke, who had suffered from low back pain. Dicke felt tingling and warmth in her leg with endarteritis obliterans after an intense stroke. She applied CTM to her lower back area for the low back pain. She noticed that blood flow increased with regular treatment and improved and completely removed gangrene. In this manner, the technique was discovered, developed, and used today. Dicke shows that patients with visceral organ dysfunction have stiff connective tissue areas. It is accepted that treatment given to the visceral organs can be performed to treat these stiff areas [1, 3–5]. CTM, which is used with a pull stroke applied to connective tissue, is a reflex treatment technique to restore the balance of the autonomic nervous system and stimulate nerve endings [1].

Tractions of the skin should be performed in a special sequence and in accordance with its anatomical structure [2]. This stimulus created by tractions is applied to the reflex areas known as Head zones [1–3]. Henry Head defined Head zones as locations where pain, heat, cold, pressure, and extreme sensitivity to touch can occur within the dermatomes that are suitable for segmental innervation of the affected organ [1, 2, 5–7]. Head's Connective Tissue Zones share the same spinal segment as their related organ or physiological function [8]. It has been stated that these zones appear to be indrawn and feel tight or adherent between the dermis and fascia in a chronic condition and or are "puffy" and swollen between the dermis and hypodermis in acute conditions [2, 3].

They are zones that show hypersensitivity and increased tone, especially in the muscles of the thoracolumbar region, in accordance with the segment of the dysfunctional organ [1, 9].

30.1 Treatment Mechanism of Connective Tissue Manipulation

Although the therapeutic mechanism of CTM has not been fully clarified, the most common view on this issue has been associated with embryological

E. Sönmezer (✉)
Faculty of Health Science, Physiotherapy and Rehabilitation Department, Atılım University, Ankara, Turkey

F. Dökmeci · M. M. Seval · Ş. E. Çetinkaya
Obstetrics and Gynecology, Ankara University School of Medicine, Ankara, Turkey

F. Dökmeci, D. E. E. Rizk (eds.), *Insights Into Incontinence and the Pelvic Floor*,
https://doi.org/10.1007/978-3-030-94174-1_30

development. It is known that body parts innervated by the peripheral nervous system show a segmental distribution due to embryological development [1, 10]. Dermatomes and myotomes innervated at the same level of the medulla spinalis with the organ with the impaired function may reflect this disorder in the form of tension in the skin and subcutaneous tissues [1, 4, 10]. CTM application to the affected dermatome creates a reflex effect in the relevant organ innervated from the same segment as the dermatome [5, 11]. The therapeutic effects that are achieved occur as a result of blood flow changes in deep tissue or of the suppression of pain. This connection between deep and superficial tissue is provided by neural mechanisms known as cutaneo-visceral reflexes, including autonomic pathways and rich somatic sensory plexuses in the skin and subcutaneous tissues. CTM can be distinguished from traditional massage by this direct effect on the autonomic nervous system [10]. The goal is to treat somatic and visceral disorders with the local or reflex effects of CTM [10].

CTM is a reflex therapy in which pull strokes are applied to the connective tissue interfaces in the skin to stimulate autonomic nerve endings in order to regulate the balance between the sympathetic and parasympathetic parts of the autonomic nervous system [2]. These pulls are applied very specifically to the points of attachment of the fascia to the bone or to areas where the fascia is superficial. Following pulling, a characteristic "cutting sensation" occurs in that area, which is a sign that the fascial layer is stimulated. The intensity of the touch is modified in such a manner that it does not cause any discomfort such as pain in the patient [2]. Simultaneously, this strong cuteneal mechanoreceptor stimulation generated by CTM also activates the gate control mechanism [1, 2, 5].

30.2 Physiological Effects of Connective Tissue Manipulation

CTM has local and general effects. Stimulation applied to the skin creates friction effects in the superficial fascia, and mechanoreceptors are stimulated [2]. It is a method used to evaluate the changes in the Head zone objectively and to identify autonomic dysfunction and the factors that cause this dysfunction by associating them with any symptoms. These determined regional areas are then used as treatment areas [8]. It has been demonstrated that glycosaminoglycan formation increases through fibroblasts, which are responsible for soft tissue healing and remodeling. Connective tissue flexibility returns to normal, mobility increases, and responses to exercise improve [2, 4]. An increase in plasma myoglobin (transient) and β-endorphin concentration also occurs [2]. Pull strokes cause mast cells to release histamine and similar substances, which upon releasing from deep structures trigger axonal reflexes and increase the circulation in the skin locally. With increased circulation, recovery accelerates, collateral circulation increases, and muscle spasms decrease. Accordingly, pain is reduced and restoration of normal function is provided [2, 4–6]. When the skin is moved in a particular direction over the facial sublayer, a shear force is generated at the tissue interfaces. These stimulate the blood vessels innervated by the autonomic nerve endings. It is thought that the effect of CTM on the autonomic nervous system occurs through the autonomic nerve endings located at the level of capillary vessels underneath the submucosa. Its effect is postulated to be both segmental and supra-segmental. By providing a more balanced autonomic system, it may have a regulatory effect on sleep patterns, mood, energy levels, and endorphin release [12]. The effect of CTM is not only observed at the treatment site but also through the cutaneo-visceral reflex, as well as on the visceral organ which is reflexively innervated by the same spinal segment as the dermatome being manipulated. CTM treatment may improve the hydration and texture of the skin by increasing the capillary circulation of all related structures leading to an improved muscle tone and improved visceral function. Patients treated with CTM usually report a reduction in pain and tissue stiffness. Hence, in cases of persistent nerve root pain, stiff joints, chronic postoperative pain, and vaginal atrophy, CTM is thought to be an effective, alternative treatment option.

Clinical studies exist in the literature regarding the physiological effects of CTM on patients. Kisner and Taslitz [13] demonstrated that CTM produces an increase in sympathetic activity and this effect was found dominantly on diastolic blood pressure rather than systolic blood pressure. Horstkotte et al. [14] reported in their experimental study on peripheral blood flow that there was a sudden decrease in blood flow followed by an increase after 2 weeks. In another study, it was reported that there was a visible redness on the skin and a significant increase in skin temperature (measured by thermography) in the area where CTM was applied, lasting for at least 1 h and 15 min after the treatment [15]. Akbaş et al. [16] measured the acute effects of CTM in young adults without organic dysfunction on the respiratory rate (RR), heart rate, systolic and diastolic blood pressures (SP/DP), oxygen saturation (OS), and body temperature. It was observed that CTM initially maintained an acute suppression effect on the sympathetic nervous system in a young patient. In one case study, it was reported that in a patient who had developed facial paralysis after orthognathic surgery due to soft tissue compression, CTM improved the patient's venous-lymphatic circulation and increased the healing of nerve damage [17]. Castro-Sanchez et al. performed a study to investigate the effects of CTM in patients with peripheral arterial disease [18]. They concluded that CTM improved blood flow, foot temperature, and oxygen saturation as well as walking distances. The mechanism of the therapeutic effects of CTM is summarized as follows: CTM creates local mechanical effects on mast cells and fibroblasts in connective tissue and reveals reflex mechanisms that cause vasodilation by reducing sympathetic activity. As a result, circulation in related tissues increases, including in the parasympathetic ganglion, which increases circulation throughout the body [3]. Such an increase in circulation also accelerates wound healing, increases collateral circulation, normalizes or increases the flexibility of the connective tissue, improves the response to exercise, reduces muscle spasms, and ensures that there is balance in the autonomic nervous system [1, 10]. The most important feature that distinguishes CTM from other manual treatment methods is that it has a therapeutic effect by playing a balancing role in the autonomic nervous system [2].

30.3 Principles of Connective Tissue Manipulation Treatment

The pull force applied to the skin should be selected according to the underlying layer. This creates a shear force that stimulates mechanoreceptors at the tissue interfaces. In addition, this pull force stimulates mast cell secretion of histamine, nitric oxide, vasoactive intestinal polypeptide (a vasodilator), and heparin [19]. CTM application with an appropriate technique usually produces a triple reaction of swelling, or redness and swelling, without causing any skin irritation and discomfort.

Treatment starting from the top of the sacrum (bladder zone) is suggested to desensitize the skin area which is reflexively connected to the parasympathetic nervous system [1, 2, 10]. Hence, the effect of CTM begins to rebalance the autonomic nervous system in the desired direction. Commencing from this site is also assumed to reduce potential side effects, such as dizziness, sweating, fainting, extreme tiredness, irritability, and restlessness. With CTM application, tissue interfaces are targeted using an appropriate pattern to achieve fascial stimulation. It is applied to the deep fascia of the fascial stroke on the target tissue with a pull force that potentially affects the autonomic nervous system [1, 2]. The strokes are applied in places where the deep fascia lies under the skin instead of under muscle. This reduces any adverse reaction and also provides the best clinical effect in the fewest possible treatment sessions. If the stimulation has the correct effect, the patient should feel a painless but sharp (or "cutting") sensation [1, 2, 10].

Physiotherapists should be mindful regarding some conditions so as to provide the appropriate treatment effects of CTM strokes. The therapist's hand position is important to ensure sufficient and appropriately directed traction at the tissue. The pad of the longest (usually middle) finger should be used to provide the most effective stroke. Additionally, since the aim of the treatment is to reach the fascial interface, a special stroke pattern should be used [1, 10].

Another important issue is the correct determination of the treatment area. Once the symptomatic or asymptomatic Head zones are detected, they are linked to any symptoms to identify the dysfunction. Treatment should be planned considering any contraindications. If the patient has unstable blood pressure/heart conditions, acute inflammation, infection, hemorrhage, early or late stage pregnancy, malignancy, is menstruating or using anxiolytic drugs, CTM is contraindicated [1, 10].

The physiotherapist who performs this manipulation should have skilled training to provide safe and effective treatment. CTM activates the segmental reflexes through the traction of the skin and subcutaneous tissues in the same spinal zone. This manipulation ensures a balance between the sympathetic and parasympathetic nervous systems when these are overactive and hypersensitive. The end result is an improvement of conditions of organic dysfunction and circulation [1].

30.4 Literature Review

In the literature, there is only a limited number of well-designed studies providing consistent evidence regarding the objective outcomes of CTM treatment. Bakar et al. compared the short-term effects between classic massage and connective tissue massage on pressure pain threshold and muscle relaxation response in patients with chronic neck pain. This study showed that while one CTM treatment session had demonstrated a relaxation response, one classic massage session had also produced a decrease in pain [20].

In another study comparing CTM and abdominal massage in chronic constipation, it was observed that both techniques were effective, but one was not superior to the other [21]. Çelenay et al. showed that CTM applied in chronic lower back pain was superior to placebos in terms of pain, mobility, and well-being [22]. A similar result in pain relief with CTM was also revealed when applied to patients with migraine [6, 11]. Çıtak-Karakaya et al. compared the effects of combined ultrasound versus KDM in patients with fibromyalgia. Based on the short- and long-term results of this study, improvement in pain, which is the main symptom of fibromyalgia, was noted when applying CTM [6].

In another study investigating its effect on dysmenorrhea, it was concluded that CTM application improves menstrual pain and increases the quality of life of patients [23].

When the literature was searched, evidence was found such that autonomic dysfunction, particularly activation of the sympathetic nervous system, may play a role in the emergence of pressing urgency, one of the main complaints in an overactive bladder. Reduced sympathetic tone in women with OAB may explain the decrease in maximal bladder capacity. The decrease in sympathetic neural activity that accompanies the sensation of urgency may be related to the pathophysiology of OAB [24, 25]. However the efficacy of the treatment strategies for these alterations in patients with OAB syndrome is not studied. Besides there has been no research that examines the effects of applying CTM on autonomic innervation of the bladder.

Differences in sympathetic nervous system function have been demonstrated in OAB patients a few minutes after the onset of urgency and after voiding [26]. The lower urinary tract is innervated by complex integrated afferent and efferent peripheral neural circuits and somatic neurons, including the sympathetic and parasympathetic nervous system [27]. The sympathetic nervous system stimulates urethral sphincter closure and relaxation of the detrusor muscle during bladder filling. While the parasympathetic nervous system relaxes the urethral sphincter simultaneously, it is responsible for the contraction of the detrusor muscle during micturition [27].

Non-pharmacological treatment methods, such as lifestyle changes, bladder training, pelvic floor muscle exercises, electrical stimulation, and neuromodulation, have been proven to be effective methods in the treatment of OAB [28, 29]. Moreover, reflex manual treatment and somatic stimulation methods have been used to treat an overactive bladder [30, 31]. In a number of studies, somatic stimulation has been used for the treatment of dysfunctions of the urinary bladder. For example, acupuncture, transcutaneous electrical stimulation, and perineal massage therapies have successfully been used to treat an overactive bladder [30].

The first study aiming to influence bladder functions through the cutaneous-visceral reflex was carried out by Sato et al. [32]. In this study, the effects of mechanical or thermal stimulation of perineal skin on a full and empty bladder of cats were investigated. As a result of this study, it was shown that these stimulations activate the empty bladder but have an inhibitory effect in the full bladder. This effect has been attributed to noxious stimulation having had a stronger effect than non-noxious stimulation in this cutaneo-visceral reflex. Since the perineal area is the most effective area for stimulation among various areas of the skin, it was assumed that this effect created by somatic stimulation through the lumbosacral cord was stronger [32, 33].

In another study, the effect of smooth perineal massage with an elastic roller was investigated in patients with nocturia. According to the results of this study, gentle perineal stimulation produced an improvement of nocturia in elderly women with an overactive bladder [34].

Considering the effect of the autonomic nervous system on the pathogenesis of OAB, it can be assumed that CTM can have a therapeutic effect by playing a regulatory role in the autonomic nervous system, similar to somatic treatments. This therapeutic effect may occur as a result of a segmental effect, such as increasing circulation or improving bowel function, or a suprasegmental effect in which CTM modulates sympathetic background tone, such as relief or sympathetically sustained pain or anxiety, by stimulating the cutaneo-visceral reflexes via CTM.

30.5 Case Report: Connective Tissue Manipulation: Does It Have a Role in the Management of Women with Severe Urodynamic Urgency Urinary Incontinence? (Case Study)

Connective tissue manipulation can be used in many different pathological conditions, such as migraine, constipation, dysmenorrhea, and peripheral arterial disease [2, 6, 35, 36]. However, to date there has been no research that examines its efficacy on autonomic innervation of the bladder. We aimed to examine the acute effects of CTM on detrusor contractions during ambulatory urodynamic monitoring in women with severe urodynamic urgency urinary incontinence.

A 69-year-old female patient had eight pregnancies, three living children, with the highest birth weight of 3500 g. The cough test was negative in the patient with a muscle strength of 2 on the modified Oxford scale. The patient's PFDI total score was 79.16. The OAB-V8 score was 19 and the IIQ7 score was 9. The patient had been in menopause for 19 years, and her complaints continued for 5 years. She had been treated with several different pharmacological and non-pharmacological treatment agents. After these therapies, her complaints returned. Because she had a refractory overactive bladder, doctors made an ambulatory urodynamic evaluation decision. She was admitted with severe UUUI symptoms and underwent ambulatory urodynamic monitoring AUM (LUNA ambulatory monitoring recorder (MMS™)) with a standardized protocol [37]. At the end of the first voiding cycle during AUM, a case (pad test: 110, 230, 380 g) detected to have multiple phasic detrusor contractions led to the decision to perform CTM without removing the urodynamic catheters.

Connective tissue manipulation was performed on the patient's lumbosacral and lower abdominal region for approximately 15 min by the same physiotherapist without removing the urodynamic catheters.

CTM was applied to the basic, thoracic, and pelvic sections for dysfunctions involving the pelvic organs. The physiotherapist initiated CTM using the index and middle finger of one hand, alternating between the middle and ring fingers. The fingers were placed on the skin at an approximately 45-degree angle and moved to cause gentle mechanical fascial strokes [19].

Demographic variables and the results of the urodynamic evaluations of the case are shown in Table 30.1.

Although number of urgency did not change after CTM application, the number of detrusor contractions and incontinence had decreased remarkably. It was observed that the duration of the patient's maximum detrusor contraction and urgency incontinence episodes decreased after CTM during her second micturition cycle on AUM. Moreover, the number of detrusor overactivity amplitudes, the duration of detrusor overactivity, and pad weights decreased the CTM during the second micturition cycle on AUM (Fig. 30.1).

This case report demonstrates that a woman with severe urodynamic urgency urinary incontinence saw an improvement in OAB with CTM treatment without behavioral or pharmacologic therapy. The treatment given to the patient produced no side effects. Based upon the results of a literature search, this is the first report showing the acute physiological effects of CTM on patients with urgency incontinence. Additionally, the results of our study are very important to explain the mechanism of how CTM affects detrusor overactivity. In this study, every parameter evaluated with AUM significantly decreased with CTM treatment. This acute effect in detrusor overactivity can be explained in two possible ways. The first possible reason is the regulatory role in the autonomic nerve system of CTM. CTM performed on the skin stimulates autonomic reflexes via connective tissue interfaces. These reflexes are the mechanism through which CTM zones occur, and they are used to produce the powerful effects of CTM. Therefore, the treatment area played a critical role in the response to treatment.

In our study, treatment started at the apex of the sacrum. This zone is also the "bladder zone," which is reflexively linked to the parasympathetic nervous system [1]. This manipulative therapy technique utilizes connective tissue reflex zones to rebalance the parasympathetic and sympathetic systems in the desired direction with the aim of inducing segmental and supra-segmental reflex effects on the visceral and hormonal systems [8]. In our study, after applying CTM to the lumbosacral and pelvic regions, observed AUM findings during the second voiding cycle of the women after CTM highlights the apparent regulatory role of CTM on autonomic innervation of the bladder.

The second possible way in inhibited detrusor overactivity is the impact on the inner organs, which is caused by the awakening of the cutaneous visceral reflex. A cutaneous stimulus provides the releasing effect by going to the sympathetic ganglion and then to the spinal cord at the posterior nerve root of the spinal cord through the stimulus of sense nerves. Thus, the hyperactivity related to the visceral organ and being carried by small diameter nerve fibers is inhibited [31, 33]. The causes of overactive bladder have not been clarified. Theoretically, nevertheless, increased afferent nerve activity, decreased inhibitory control in the CNS, and increased sensitivity of the detrusor to efferent

Table 30.1 Demographic variables and AUM data of cases

Age	69	
BMI	26.5	
	Before CTM	After CTM
Number of urgency	5	5
Number of incontinence	7 (UI: 7, SI: 0)	2 (UI: 2, SI: 0)
Number of detrusor contraction:	10	2
Max. detrusor overactivity amplitude, cm H_2O	169	63
Mean detrusor overactivity amplitude, cm H_2O	101	43
Max. duration of detrusor overactivity, s	27	22
Mean duration of detrusor overactivity, s	20	14
Pad test, g	200	130
Test duration (min)	100	120

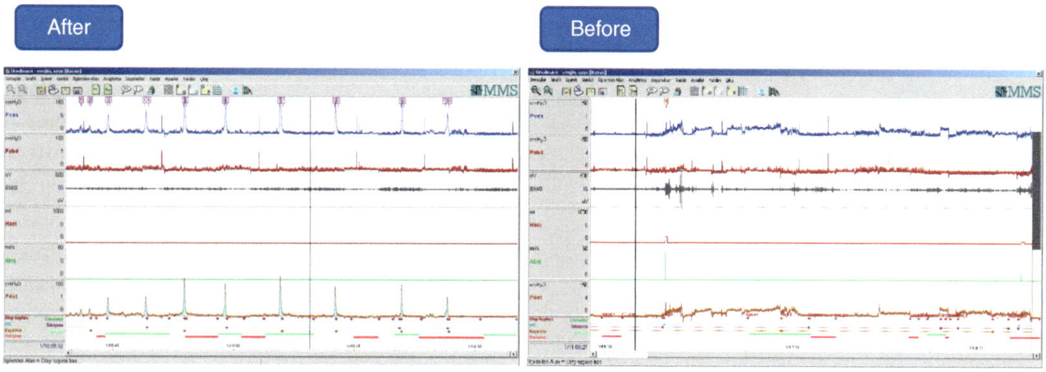

Fig. 30.1 Ambulatory urodynamic monitoring data before and after treatment protocol

stimulation may be involved [38]. In our study, the application of CTM to the pelvic and lumbosacral regions consists of mechanical somatic stimulation. This stimulation may stimulate the spinal opioidergic system and inhibit the micturition reflex. Therefore, CTM treatment may also relieve the sense of urgency as well as the sense of pain and pressure during urgency.

The results from this study are promising regarding the efficacy of the CTM approach on women with severe urodynamic urgency urinary incontinence. The results of the AUM findings after CTM show the emphasis on the apparent regulatory role of CTM in the autonomic innervation of the bladder. CTM provides a reflex effect on the autonomic nervous system by manipulating the fascial layers. Further randomized and controlled studies are needed to understand fully the physiological mechanisms and efficacy of CTM in patients with OAB.

References

1. Goats GC, Keir KA. Connective tissue massage. Br J Sports Med. 1991;25(3):131–3.
2. Holey EA. Connective tissue massage: a bridge between complementary and orthodox approaches. J Bodyw Mov Ther. 2000;4:72–80.
3. Dicke E, Schiliak H, Wolff A. A mannual of reflexive therapy of connective tissue. New York: Simon Publishers; 1978.
4. Reed V, Held M. Effects of sequential connective tissue massage on autonomic nervous system of middle-aged an elderly adults. Phys Ther. 1988;68:1231–4.
5. Ebner M. Connective tissue massage, theory and therapeutic application. Edinburgh; 1962.
6. Çıtak-Karakaya I, Akbayrak T, Demirtürk F, Ekici G, Bakar Y. Short and long-term results of connective tissue manipulation and combined ultrasound therapy in patients with fibromyalgia. J Manip Physiol Ther. 2006;29(7):524–8.
7. Ekici G, Bakar Y, Akbayrak T, Yuksel I. Comparison of manual lymph drainage therapy and connective tissue massage in women with fibromyalgia: a randomized controlled trial. J Manip Physiol Ther. 2009;32(2):127–33.
8. Holey LA. Connective tissue zones: an introduction. J Physiother. 1995;81(7):366–8.
9. Brattberg G. Connective tissue massage in the treatment of fibromyalgia. Eur J Pain. 1999;3:235.
10. Holey LA, Dixon J. Connective tissue manipulation: a review of theory and clinical evidence. J Bodyw Mov Ther. 2014;18(1):112–8.
11. Akbayrak T, Akarcalı I, Karabudak R, Demirturk F. The results of connective tissue manipulation in the treatment of tension type headache. Pain Clin. 2002;13:343–7.
12. Kaada B, Torsteinbo O. Increase of plasma betaendorphins in connective tissue massage. Gen Pharmacol. 1989;20:487–9.
13. Kisner CD, Taslitz N. Connective tissue massage: influence of the introductory treatment on autonomic functions. Phys Ther. 1968;48:107–19.
14. Horstkotte W, Klempien EJ, Scheppokat KD. Skin temperature and blood flow changes in occlusive arterial disease under physiological and pharmacological therapy. Angiology. 1967;18(1):1–5.
15. Holey LA, Dixon J, Selfe J. An exploratory thermographic investigation of the effects of connective tissue massage on autonomic function. J Manip Physiol Ther. 2011;34(7):457–62.
16. Akbaş E, Ünver B, Erdem EU. Acute effects of connective tissue manipulation on autonomic function in healthy young women. Complement Med Res. 2019;26(4):250–7.

17. Tsai PT, Chang YC, Chen YW. Connective tissue massage accelerates recovery of facial nerve palsy after orthognathic surgery. J Dent Sci. 2016;11(1):107.
18. Castro-Sánchez AM, Moreno-Lorenzo C, Matarán-Peñarrocha GA, Feriche-Fernández-Castanys B, Granados-Gámez G, Quesada-Rubio JM. Connective tissue reflex massage for type 2 diabetic patients with peripheral arterial disease: randomized controlled trial. Evid Based Complement Alternat Med. 2011;2011:804321. https://doi.org/10.1093/ecam/nep171.
19. Theoharides TC, Zhang B, Kempuraj D, et al. IL-33 augments substance P-induced VEGF secretion from human mast cells and is increased in psoriatic skin. Proc Natl Acad Sci U S A. 2010;107:4448–53.
20. Bakar Y, Sertel M, Öztürk A, Yümin ET, Tatarli N, Ankarali H. Short term effects of classic massage compared to connective tissue massage on pressure pain threshold and muscle relaxation response in women with chronic neck pain: a preliminary study. J Manip Physiol Ther. 2014;37(6):415–21.
21. Orhan C, Özgül S, Baran E, Üzelpasacı E, Akbayrak T. Comparison of connective tissue manipulation and abdominal massage combined with usual care vs usual care alone for chronic constipation: a randomized controlled trial. J Manipulative Physiol Ther. 2020;43(8):768–78. https://doi.org/10.1016/j.jmpt.2019.05.013.
22. Celenay ST, Kaya DO, Ucurum SG. Adding connective tissue manipulation to physiotherapy for chronic low back pain improves pain, mobility, and well-being: a randomized controlled trial. J Exerc Rehabil. 2019;15(2):308–15.
23. Sonmezer E, Düger T, Yosmaoglu HB, Akbyarak T. Comparison of effectiveness of connective tissue massage and kinesiotaping applications on pain and quality of life in primary dysmenorrhea. In: 31st kinesio taping research symposium.
24. Ben-Dror I, Weissman A, Leurer M, Eldor-Itskovitz J, Lowenstein L. Alterations of heart rate variability in women with overactive bladder syndrome. Int Urogynecol J. 2012;23(8):1081–6.
25. Hubeaux K, Deffieux X, Raibaut P, Le Breton F, Jousse M, Amarenco G. Evidence for autonomic nervous system dysfunction in females with idiopathic overactive bladder syndrome. Neurourol Urodyn. 2011;30(8):1467–72.
26. Homma Y. Hypersensitive bladder: towards clear taxonomy surrounding interstitial cystitis. Int J Urol. 2013;20(8):742–3.
27. Homma Y, Yamaguchi O, Hayashi K. Epidemiologic survey of lower urinary tract symptoms in Japan. Urology. 2006;68:560.
28. Wattanayingcharoenchai R, Manonai J, Vannatim N, Saritapirak S, Imsomboon C, Chittacharoen A. Impact of stress urinary incontinence and overactive bladder on quality of life in Thai women attending the urogynecology clinic. J Med Assoc Thail. 2007;90(1):26–31.
29. Lightner DJ, Gomelsky A, Souter L, Vasavada SP. Diagnosis and treatment of overactive bladder (non-neurogenic) in adults: AUA/SUFU guideline amendment 2019. J Urol. 2019;202(3):558–63.
30. Guo ZF, Liu Y, Hu GH, Liu H, Xu YF. Transcutaneous electrical nerve stimulation in the treatment of patients with poststroke urinary incontinence. Clin Interv Aging. 2014;9:851–6.
31. Mak HLJ, Cheon WC, Wong T, Liu YSJ, Tong WMA. Randomized controlled trial of foot reflexology for patients with symptomatic idiopathic detrusor overactivity. Int Urogynecol J. 2007;18(6):653.
32. Sato Y, Sato H, et al. Reflex changes in the urinary bladder after mechanical and thermal stimulation of the skin at various segmental levels in cats. Neuroscience. 1977;2:111–7.
33. Hotta H, Masunaga K, Miyazaki S, Watanabe N, Kasuya Y. A gentle mechanical skin stimulation technique for inhibition of micturition contractions of the urinary bladder. Auton Neurosci. 2012;167:12–20.
34. Hotta H, Watanabe N. Gentle mechanical skin stimulation inhibits micturition contractions via the spinal opioidergic system and by decreasing both ascending and descending transmissions of the micturition reflex in the spinal cord. PLoS One. 2015;10(8):0135185.
35. Reis CADAS, Hardy E, Sousa MHD. The effectiveness of connective tissue massage in the treatment of primary dysmenorrhea among young women. Rev Bras Saúde Mater Infant. 2010;10(2):247–56.
36. Bongi SM, Del Rosso A, Galluccio F, Sigismondi F, Miniati I, Conforti ML, Cerinic MM. Efficacy of connective tissue massage and Mc Mennell joint manipulation in the rehabilitative treatment of the hands in systemic sclerosis. Clin Rheumatol. 2009;28(10):1167–73.
37. Dokmeci F, Cetinkaya SE, Seval MM, Dai O. Ambulatory urodynamic monitoring of women with overactive bladder syndrome during single voiding cycle. Eur J Obstet Gynecol Reprod Biol. 2017;212:126–31.
38. Andersson KE. The overactive bladder: pharmacologic basis of drug treatment. Urology. 1997;50:74–84.

Interaction of Abdominal and Pelvic Floor Muscles

31

Alice Carvalhais, Thuane Da Roza, and Renato Natal Jorge

31.1 Introduction

Physical activity, from daily activities to sports or exercise practice, increases intra-abdominal pressure (IAP) and impact loading on the pelvic floor muscles (PFM) [1, 2]. The IAP is modulated by the muscles surrounding the abdominal-pelvic cavity, which is the diaphragm, the abdominals (Abd), multifidus, and the PFM [3, 4]. When the IAP is raised, the connective tissue of the ligaments and fascias and the PFM act to counteract the downward displacement of the organs and to ensure the necessary urethral closure to prevent urine leakage.

Synergetic activity between the PFM and the Abd muscles has been studied for more than two decades [5], and the issue is an ongoing discussion. Until now, the number of studies on this specific topic is small, and the sample size of the majority of them is also small. A systematic review performed by Bø et al. [6] aimed to investigate the scientific evidence for the effectiveness of transversus abdominis muscle (TrA) training alone or in combination with PFM training to treat urinary incontinence (UI) in women. Five studies [5, 7–10] were included, and all were conducted with healthy volunteers. The authors concluded that there is evidence that a co-contraction between TrA and the PFM occurs in asymptomatic women, but they believed that it can be lost or altered in women with UI. Ten years later, Ferla et al. [11] confirmed the results found by Bø et al. [6], where they also found scientific evidence of the synergetic contraction between the Abd and the PFM in healthy women. Recently, a systematic review with meta-analysis investigated the co-contraction between Abd and PFM including women with and without pelvic floor disorders [12]. Five of the 20 studies included were selected for the meta-analysis. The sensitive analysis showed that co-contraction between the TrA and PFM is higher in asymptomatic than in symptomatic women. Furthermore, women with pelvic floor disorders had increased co-contraction of the rectus abdominis muscle (RA), internal obliques muscle (IO), and external obliques muscle (EO), suggesting an altered muscle mechanism pattern.

Synergism between PFM and the diaphragm is less studied. Thompson et al. [13] measured the costal diaphragm and intercostal muscles in healthy continent women using EMG surface

A. Carvalhais (✉)
LAETA, INEGI, CESPU, Escola Superior de Tecnologias da Saúde do Tâmega e Sousa, Porto, Portugal
e-mail: alice.carvalhais@ipsn.cespu.pt

T. Da Roza
Laboratory of Biomechanics, Center for Health and Sports Sciences (CEFID), Universidade do Estado de Santa Catarina (UDESC), Florianópolis, Brazil

R. Natal Jorge
LAETA, INEGI, Faculdade de Engenharia, Universidade do Porto, Porto, Portugal
e-mail: rnatal@fe.up.pt

F. Dökmeci, D. E. E. Rizk (eds.), *Insights Into Incontinence and the Pelvic Floor*,
https://doi.org/10.1007/978-3-030-94174-1_31

electrodes and found a significant increase in Abd muscle activation with a voluntary PFM contraction. Since the diaphragm closes the pelvic cavity cranially, this muscle responds to changes in IAP through breathing patterns in step with PFM. During breathing and coughing, a parallel cranio-caudal movement was observed in healthy women [14]. Hodges et al. [15] reported that the PFM have a greater increase in activity during expiration, and Neumann et al. [9] demonstrated PFM activation during forced exhalations. In agreement with this data, Talasz et al. [16] found that women with stronger PFM were able to exhale more efficiently during forced expiration.

It is understood that muscle activation is different from muscle strength. While the PFM activation gives a qualitative description of the muscle activation pattern, the strength demonstrates the capacity of the PFM to generate force [17]. Data from transperineal EMG demonstrated a weak correlation with measures of PFM strength such as manometry and dynamometry [18]. To the best of the authors' knowledge, only two studies have looked at the correlation between the PFM with muscles of the abdominal cavity in terms of strength rather than muscle activation. Zachovajeviene et al. [19] carried out a study aimed to identify functional association between PFM, diaphragm, and trunk muscles. This study was conducted with 81 men before radical prostatectomy. While a positive and strong correlation between PFM and diaphragm strength was found (r = 0.79), the correlation between PFM with TrA was low (r = 0.31). However, no data regarding individual characteristics or continence status was provided. Recently, the same authors performed a prospective study analyzing the effect of three different interventions—(1) PFM training, (2) Abd muscle training, and (3) diaphragm muscle training – on PFM strength and endurance among incontinent men after radical prostatectomy [20]. The findings after a 6-month follow-up showed that the PFM training group had the greatest increase in PFM strength, and the diaphragm muscle training group had the best improvement in the PFM endurance. Unfortunately, despite having the same frequency and duration of the sessions for the three groups, only some sessions were supervised. Thus, it is not possible to guarantee that the protocol was completely respected by all individuals. Only one study was performed with female athletes (n = 20 continent and n = 20 incontinent), and the authors found a positive moderate association between PFM and Abd strength in both continent (r = 0.496) and incontinent athletes (r = 0.577) [21].

Besides having few studies regarding the relationship between PFM and Abd muscle strength, none of them performed an analysis to consider the PFM, the diaphragm, and the Abd muscles separately (superficial and deep). Therefore, to verify this relationship, we conducted this case study.

31.2 Case Study: Is There Any Relationship Between Pelvic Floor Muscles and Superficial and Deep Abdominal Muscle Strength?

(a) **Aim and Scope**

We aimed to analyze the association between the PFM strength with the strength of the respiratory diaphragm and superficial and deep Abd muscles, in continent and incontinent women.

(b) **Study Design and Materials and Methods**

This was a cross-sectional study in 32 continent and 16 incontinent women.

Selection criteria were nulliparous women aged more than 18 years old. The incontinent group presented symptoms of stress UI. Subjects were excluded if they reported back, pelvic, or hip pain, were diagnosed with neurological or respiratory disease, urinary tract or vaginal infection, or pelvic organ prolapse. Additional exclusion criteria were menstruation on the day of assessment, inability to perform a correct PFM contraction, and inability to insert or maintain the vaginal probe due to pain or discomfort.

The International Consultation on Incontinence (ICIQ-UI-SF) assessed the continence status and the type of urinary incontinence [22]. Stress UI was assigned to participants with positive responses to involuntary loss of urine associated with coughing, sneezing, effort, or physical exertion [23]. If no involuntary loss of urine was reported, the women was classified as continent. The ICIQ-UI-SF has been translated into the Portuguese language and validated by Tamanini et al [24].

PFM strength was assessed by manometry using the Peritron Perineometer 9300 (LABORIE Medical Technologies Canada ULC.), which has been found to be a reliable method of measuring PFM strength [25]. The vaginal probe was covered with a condom. Before insertion, the device was zeroed. The participant inserted the probe herself, until 2 cm remained outside the introitus [26]. An inward and posterior movement of the probe was monitored in all measurements to ensure the correct contraction of the PFM [27]. After insertion of the probe, the participants were instructed to relax the PFM, and a rest period was given. After zeroing, the women were asked to perform a maximal voluntary contraction (MVC) and hold it for 3 s, and the peak value was recorded (cmH_2O). This procedure was repeated three times, and the mean value was used as a measure of PFM strength [28]. To prevent muscle fatigue, a rest period was given after every contraction. Participants were instructed to breathe normally during the PFM contractions. We used standardized instructions for all participants: "Use your PFMs as if you want to stop urination and contract as hard as you can, hold for three seconds and then relax and breathe normally." We allowed a small visible in-drawing of the abdominal muscles, as long as the pelvis was not tilted [29]. Since SUI usually occurs in an upright position, all measurements except isokinetic measurements were performed while standing [30].

Maximal expiratory pressure (MEP) was used as a measure of TrA and IO strength [31]. Maximal inspiratory pressure (MIP) was used as a measure of the strength of the respiratory diaphragm [32]. MEP and MIP measures have been described as simple, noninvasive, and well-tolerated maneuvers of neuromuscular function of the respiratory muscles. MIP and MEP were measured (cmH_2O) using a handheld mouth pressure meter MicroRPM (CareFusion Micro Medical, Kent, UK), a one-way inspiratory or expiratory valve, with a single-use bacterial filter tube mouthpiece. Measurements were conducted according to the American Thoracic Society/European Respiratory Society standards [32]. A standard protocol was used including standardized, verbal instructions. Demonstration of the procedure and practice test was performed before obtaining the measures. The subjects were asked to not move the trunk in order to reduce the action of the RA and EO muscles. MIP was measured from residual volume after maximal expiration. MEP pressure was measured from total lung capacity after a maximal inspiration. There was a 1-min rest between each maneuver. The nose was closed with a nose clip throughout the effort. The maximum value of three maneuvers that varied less than 20% was used. High reliability for MIP measurement has been reported [33]. No reliability values for MEP have been found.

Isokinetic dynamometry evaluated the superficial Abd strength (RA and EO). Trunk flexor muscles strength was evaluated using a Biodex System 4 Pro dynamometer (Biodex Corp., Shirley, NY), coupled with the trunk extension-flexion component, a specific module moving in the sagittal plane. Isokinetic dynamometry has been shown to be a reliable method for measuring trunk muscles strength in healthy individuals [34]. Peak torque (Newton-meters (Nm)) of trunk muscle flexors was used as a surrogate measure of superficial Abd [34, 35].

Each subject was seated on a chair with her body strapped to the back of the chair. The fixed axis of the machine was aligned at the intersection point of the mid-axillary line and the lumbosacral junction (L5-S1), to isolate back movement [36]. The heels were placed against the footplate heel cups. The lower limbs and trunk were stabilized from top to bottom, in order to isolate back movement and to reduce potential movement of the pelvis and lower extremities, by (1) cervical pad at the posterior region of cervical spine, (2) scapular pad was positioned at the level of the scapula, (3) two pads stabilize the trunk anteriorly at the anterior part of the shoulder, (4) a pelvic belt was tightened across the top of the anterior superior iliac spines, and (5) the lower limbs were fixed with thigh and feet pads. Spinal range of motion 60° was set from −10° to 50°, 0° = vertical position. The angular velocity was set at 60°/s. The participants performed the test using two trials of ten consecutive repetitions [37].

All subjects performed a trial to familiarize and warm-up before formal testing. Starting position was the maximal extension position. Subjects were verbally encouraged during the test to move as fast as possible and to exert the maximal force through the entire range of motion for all repetitions.

All the evaluations were performed according to specific established guidelines, and the evaluator was blind to continence status.

For the statistical analysis, the Chi-square test and the Mann-Whitney test were used for comparison between continent and incontinent groups, as appropriate. The Spearman correlation test was applied to analyze the correlation between variables. A p-value <0.05 was considered for statistical significance.

(c) **Results of the Study**

The sample was composed of 48 young and nulliparous women. Two groups were formed, one with 32 continent women and another with 16 women reporting stress UI symptoms. The groups were similar in terms of age, body mass index (BMI), regular exercise practice, regular PFM contractions, and complaints of constipation. Incontinent women had stronger superficial Abd, deep Abd, and diaphragm. No differences were found on PFM strength between groups (Table 31.1).

Regarding the correlation analysis, a trend of a positive association between the PFM and the Abd muscles and the diaphragm can be observed in the continent group. However, the association was only statistically significant between the PFM and both superficial and deep Abd. The correlation between the PFM and superficial Abd was weak and moderate between PFM and deep Abd (Fig. 31.1).

Table 31.1 Sociodemographic characteristics and strength values of abdomino-pelvic muscles among continent and incontinent women

	Continent (n = 32)		Incontinent (n = 16)		p
	x (sd)	95% CI	x (sd)	95% CI	
Age (years)	24.6 (4.3)	23.06–26.19	23.3 (4.5)	20.12–26.50	0.390
BMI (kg/m^2)	21.3 (2.9)	20.27–22.38	23.1 (4.5)	20.69–25.46	0.120
	n (%)		n (%)		
Constipation (yes)	6 (18.8)		1 (6.3)		0.247
Regular exercise (yes) practice (yes)	23 (71.9)		11 (68.8)		0.824
Regular PFM contractions (yes)	5 (15.6)		3 (18.8)		0.784
Strength	x (sd)	95% CI	x (sd)	95% CI	
PFM (cmH_2O)	51.4 (19.14)	44.49–58.30	49.73 (23.17)	37.38–62.07	0.418
Superficial AbD (Nm)	109.19 (29.64)	98.50–119.88	133.73 (30.19)	117.64–149.81	0.008
Deep Abd (cmH_2O)	60.25 (19.88)	53.08–67.42	72.44 (17.08)	63.34–81.54	0.043
Diaphragm (cmH_2O)	60.59 (21.51)	52.84–68.35	75.44 (21.34)	64.07–86.81	0.024

Abd abdominals, *BMI* body mass index, *CI* confidence interval, *Nm* Newton-meters, *PFM* pelvic floor muscle, *X* mean, *sd* standard deviation

31.3 Discussion

Our results show that while a positive correlation was found between the strength of PFM with the strength of superficial and deep Abd among continent women, no associations were found in incontinent women. To the best of the authors knowledge, until now only one study verified the association between PFM and Abd strength among continent and incontinent female athletes [21]. Their findings showed a positive association between PFM and superficial Abd muscles in both continent and incontinent athletes, with the correlation among incontinent being stronger.

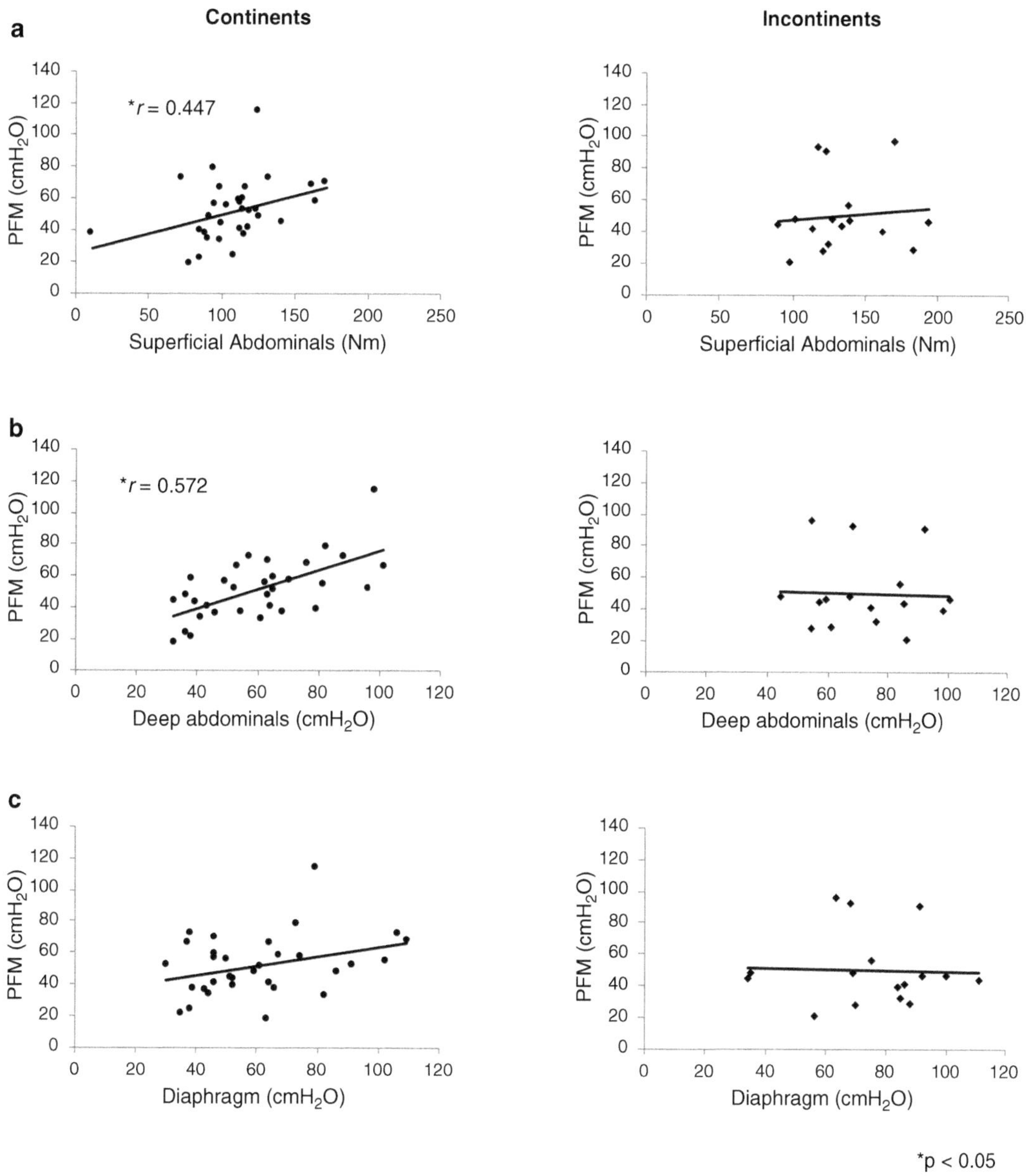

Fig. 31.1 Distribution plot of Spearman's correlation coefficients between pelvic floor muscle (PFM) strength and the strength of the muscles of the abdominal cavity. (**a**) PFM/superficial abdominals; (**b**) PFM/deep abdominals; (**c**) PFM/diaphragm

This data is different from our findings. One possible explanation for this contradictory result is the sample. Dos Santos et al. [21] studied athletes, and we studied women from the general population. Although about one-third of our sample practiced regular physical exercise, they were not involved in high-intensity training, which involves high-load physical and technical training. Both studies used isokinetic evaluation of the Abd muscle strength and a manometer for PFM strength assessment. Since the present study found a positive correlation only in continent women, this might also reflect that among female athletes the pathophysiology of UI is different from women in the general population, or the coordinated activity (between Abd and PFM) can be disrupted in incontinent women of the general population. Further research is warranted to investigate this relationship.

Studies in healthy continent women found a co-contraction of the PFM and the Abd [9, 38]. In the literature, a PFM contraction results in a co-contraction of the Abd and vice versa [1, 8, 9, 13, 39], suggesting that this synergetic activity is a normal function in nulliparous women without pelvic floor dysfunction symptoms. Some studies investigated the activation pattern and have been found that the PFM contraction precedes the elevation of IAP [7] and raising the arms [15], which can support a feedforward mechanism for this pattern of activity. Looking for a pattern activity between the Abd and the PFM, Verelst et al. [40] show that PFM contracted 160 ms before the Abd muscles in both continent and incontinent women. Although this pattern was found in the majority of the sample, a reverse direction of activity was observed in 24% and 30% of continent and incontinent women, respectively. Also, Neumann et al. [9] found different recruitment patterns between the PFM and each of the Abd muscles in healthy nulliparous women and noted different patterns of activation between but not within subjects. We do not know if this activation can result in a training effect on the PFM. Further studies are needed in this population with results that may contribute to a better understanding of pathophysiology of UI and thus outline more appropriate interventions.

The AbD muscles comprise four different muscles (TrA, IO, EO, and RA) grouped in two layers, a superficial and a deep layer. The former comprises the EO and the RA, and the deep layer comprehends the TrA and the IO. A closer relationship has been found between the PFM with the TrA and the IO than the RA and EO in healthy women [1, 7, 13, 41]. Confirming that, another study has shown that contraction of the TrA was associated with an ascending movement of the bladder neck in women without pelvic floor dysfunction [1]. However, a downward movement of the PFM has also been reported with the same task [42]. This could reflect, in part, the stronger correlation between the PFM and the deep Abd than between the PFM and the superficial Abd found in our study. The diaphragm and the PFM are functionally linked through a pressure relationship, meaning that when the diaphragm descends, the pelvic floor follows this movement [14]. Whether this descending movement, rather than a passive elongation can be an eccentric contraction of the PFM is not known. In the current study, no association was found between PFM and diaphragm strength. Only one study investigates this relationship in men, and in contrast to our results, the authors found a strong and positive association [19]. Whether or not anatomy differences between man and woman can explain this difference is not possible to determine, since no studies were found that have explored this subject, and thus our results cannot be compared with previous studies.

During functional tasks, the IAP was raised [1, 43]. The diaphragm [3] the trunk muscles [44] and the PFM [1] are involved in the modulation of IAP. Since it has been demonstrated that in continent women PFM activates in response to IAP increase [1], it could be expected that, in line with the correlation between PFM and both superficial and deep Abd found in the current study, the same result would be obtained with the diaphragm. Despite not having statistical significance, it was noted that in continent women the PFM and diaphragm had a linear relationship, and among the incontinent, this relationship almost does not exist. This study revealed no difference in PFM strength between continent and incontinent women. Comparison of PFM strength between continent and incontinent women has been a topic of debate in recent years. Several studies have focused on this issue, and contradictory results have been shown. Numerous studies found that continent women have higher PFM strength than incontinent ones [40, 45–52]. However, no differences have also been reported [53–56], and even higher PFM strength was reported on incontinent female athletes compared to continent ones [21]. Verelst et al. [52] also found no differences in PFM strength between parous continent and incontinent women. However, when the absolute force was adjusted for body weight, the values were lower in the incontinent group. The authors suggested that this result could be associated with obesity. In our sample, the BMI was higher, and the PFM strength was lower in incontinent women; however, the difference does not reach statistical significance. This inconsistency in the results reported by the different studies seems to indicate that, in addition to the strength of the PFM, other variables should be taken into account. The comparison focused only on the evaluation of the PFM so it considers only one of the structures that surround the abdominal cavity. For a more comprehensive view, the remaining structures should also be considered.

In the current study, incontinent women present higher Abd muscles and diaphragm strength, while no difference in PFM strength was observed. Interestingly, contrary to our findings, Dos Santos et al. [21] verified no difference in Abd muscles strength between groups and stronger PFM among the incontinent women. These results may reflect the fact that athletes need a different response to the IAP changes and the UI in this population had other physiopathology. It remains unclear whether associations between these three structures occur with increasing IAP. The relationship between incontinence and IAP should be further explored in a longitudinal cohort study.

Similar to the investigations regarding PFM and Abd, the relationship between Abd and IAP has been studied using muscle activity, and it has been demonstrated that both are linked [44]. Considering the different Abd muscles, it has been mentioned that RA did not contribute to IAP development in females and males judo athletes [57]. TrA has been more consistently related to IAP changes in men [58, 59]. Studies regarding the relationship between Abd strength and IAP are scarce, but results suggest that increasing Abd strength generates higher IAP [60]. Our data suggest that a more comprehensive and integrated view of pelvic floor assessment should be considered and may be important to delineate treatment interventions. However, more studies are needed to clarify this assumption.

Based on the synergistic activity between the Abd and the PFM, interventions focused on abdominal exercises have been suggested to improve the PFM function and, therefore, to improve UI. Despite several studies already carried out on this subject, many questions need to be clarified. Co-activation between the Abd of the deepest layer seems to be a common finding among continent women. This fact may show one of the mechanisms through which regular exercise is associated with a beneficial effect on the pelvic floor function, as opposed to the effect of a sedentary lifestyle [61]. In women where this coordination integrates, exercising the abdominals in order to improve or maintain PFM function makes perfect sense. Indeed, this was suggested many years ago by Bø et al. [5] who hypothesized that abdominal curls may strengthen the PFM in subjects without pelvic floor dysfunction. But, as for incontinent individuals can the same be expected? Since studies on incontinent women are practically non-existent, we have no data to support this hypothesis. Further, adding to the fact that we do not know whether this co-activation, even if it occurs in women with pelvic floor dysfunction, will have the potential to promote sufficient changes in PFM to treat UI symptoms. Until now, the number of well-designed RCTs is scarce which makes further research necessary in order to assess the effectiveness of such interventions.

Regarding prospective studies, some previous investigations have been performed. Kamel et al. [62] implemented a randomized controlled trial to compare two types of interventions, implemented for 12 weeks, to treat stress UI in a sample of obese women. One group performed Abd exercises (TrA and IO) and the other group PFM exercises using a perineometer for feedback. At the end of the intervention, vaginal pressure and leak point pressure improved significantly only in the Abd group. All the women received dietary modification instructions, but a decreased in waist-hip ratio was only observed in the Abd group. The physical activity level was not monitored. Since obesity is a well-known risk factor for UI [63], it is not possible to determine the extent to which the improvement observed was due to the Abd exercises or the alterations in nutrition and lifestyle. To better understand the effects of the Adb muscle, PFM training, and diaphragm muscle training in PFM strength and endurance among men with UI after radical prostatectomy, a prospective 6-month follow-up study was performed [20]. The findings demonstrated that PFM strength and PFM endurance increased in all training groups in comparison with those at baseline. Furthermore, the group who performed PFM training got significantly higher PFM strength, and the PFM endurance was highest in the diaphragm group. The exact role of PFM strength and endurance in continence is still unknown and should be investigated.

Resende et al. [64] performed a randomized control trial comparing two different protocols in a sample of 61 women with pelvic organ prolapse stage II. The duration of interventions was 3 months. One group underwent a hypopressive exercise program, and the other group did PFM training. At the end of the study, women from the PFM training group had greater improvement in PFM activation, PFM strength, and pelvic organ prolapse symptoms. Stüpp et al. [39] investigated the activation of the PFM and Abd when performing voluntary PFM contraction and an abdominal hypopressive maneuver (TrA activation). The results showed that TrA and PFM coactivate synergically, but the activation of the PFM is more effective with a voluntary PFM contraction than an abdominal hypopressive maneuver. Also, Bø et al. [42] found that instruction to contract the PFM was more effective in lifting the pelvic floor than the contraction of the TrA or a combination of both structures, measured by ultrasonography. This finding is in line with the study of Junginger et al. [1] Recently, Kruger et al. [65] assessed the increase in PFM strength, measured by a novel intravaginal pressure sensor, in a sample of 21 women. The results showed that the contraction of PFM develops higher pressure than the pressure raised with the contraction of different muscle groups as the Abd, hip, and also during deep inspiration and expiration. The increments observed in PFM strength varied between 30 and 50% of a PFM contraction.

This study had several limitations. First, the cross-sectional design of our study prevents determination of the causal relationships between Abd and PFM. Second, although many factors were included in our study, there could be other unobserved confounding factors that we have neither considered nor controlled. Although we have a small sample, all participants are nulliparous. Finally, this study used indirect measurements for the diaphragm and Abd muscles, but these techniques are validated and widely used in the literature.

31.4 Conclusions

In conclusion, PFM strength appears to be associated with Abd strength only in continent women. These findings are in line with ICS recommendation that in incontinent women PFM training should be used to improve PFM function. Further studies into the effectiveness of conservative management addressing modifiable risk factors in community-dwelling older adults are clearly needed.

Acknowledgments AC was involved in planning the study and data collection and reviewed and analyzed the literature, wrote the paper, and approved the final version. TR was involved in reviewing and analyzing the literature and wrote the paper and approved the final version. RNJ was involved in planning the study and critically revised the article and approved the final version.

Funding The authors truly acknowledge the funding provided by Ministério da Ciência, Tecnologia e Ensino Superior - Fundação para a Ciência e a Tecnologia (Portugal), through LAETA, under project UIDB/50022/2020.

References

1. Junginger B, Baessler K, Sapsford R, Hodges PW. Effect of abdominal and pelvic floor tasks on muscle activity, abdominal pressure and bladder neck. Int Urogynecol J. 2010;21:69–77.
2. Shaw JM, Hamad NM, Coleman TJ, Egger MJ, Hsu Y, Hitchcock R, et al. Intra-abdominal pressures during activity in women using an intra-vaginal pressure transducer. J Sports Sci. 2014;32(12):1176–85.
3. Hodges PW, Gandevia SC. Changes in intra-abdominal pressure during postural and respiratory activation of the human diaphragm. J Appl Physiol. 2000;89:967–76.
4. Cresswell AG. Responses of intra-abdominal pressure and abdominal muscle activity during dynamic trunk loading in man. Eur J Appl Physiol. 1993;66: 315–20.
5. Bø K, Stien R. Needle EMG registration of striated urethral wall and pelvic floor muscle activity patterns during cough, valsalva, abdominal, hip adductor, and gluteal muscles contractions in nulliparous healthy females. Neurourol Urodyn. 1994;13(1):35–41.
6. Bø K, Mørkved S, Frawley H, Sherburn M. Evidence for benefit of transversus abdominis training alone or in combination with pelvic floor muscle training to treat female urinary incontinence: a systematic review. Neurourol Urodyn. 2009;28:368–73.
7. Sapsford RR, Hodges PW. Contraction of the pelvic floor muscles during abdominal maneuvers. Arch Phys Med Rehabil. 2001;82:1081–8.
8. Sapsford R, Hodges PW, Richardson CA, Cooper DH, Markwell SJ, Jull GA. Co-activation of the abdominal and pelvic floor muscles during voluntary exercises. Neurourol Urodyn. 2001;20:31–42.
9. Neumann P, Gill V. Pelvic floor and abdominal muscle interaction: EMG activity and intra-abdominal pressure. Int Urogynecol J. 2002;13:125–32.
10. Sapsford R, Markwell SJ, Clarke B. The relationship between urethral pressure and abdominal muscle activity. In: 7th National CFA conference on incontinence, Australia; 1998.
11. Ferla L, Darski C, Paiva LL, Sbruzzi G, Vieira A. Synergism between abdominal and pelvic floor muscles in healthy women: a systematic review of observational studies. Fisioterapia em Movimento. 2016;29(2):399–410.
12. Vesentini G, El Dib R, Righesso LAR, Piculo F, Marini G, Ferraz GAR, et al. Pelvic floor and abdominal muscle co-contraction in women with and without pelvic floor dysfunction: a systematic review and meta-analysis. Clinics. 2019;74:e1319.
13. Thompson JA, O'Sullivan PB, Briffa NK, Neumann P. Differences in muscle activation patterns during pelvic floor muscle contraction and valsalva manouevre. Neurourol Urodyn. 2006;25(2):148–55.
14. Talasz H, Kremser C, Kofler M, Kalchschmid E, Lechleitner M, Rudisch A. Phase-locked parallel movement of diaphragm and pelvic floor during breathing and coughing—a dynamic MRI investigation in healthy females. Int Urogynecol J. 2011;22(1):61–8.
15. Hodges PW, Sapsford R, Pengel LHM. Postural and respiratory functions of the pelvic floor muscles. Neurourol Urodyn. 2007;26:362–71.
16. Talasz H, Kofler M, Kalchschmid E, Pretterklieber M, Lechleitner M. Breathing with the pelvic floor? Correlation of pelvic floor muscle function and expiratory flows in healthy young nulliparous women. Int Urogynecol J. 2010;21(4):475–81.
17. Bø K, Frawley HC, Haylen BT, Abramov Y, Almeida FG, Berghmans B, et al. An International Urogynecological Association (IUGA)/International Continence Society (ICS) joint report on the terminology for the conservative and nonpharmacological management of female pelvic floor dysfunction. Neurourol Urodyn. 2017;36:221–44.
18. Brazález BN, Lacomba MT, de la Villa P, Sánchez BS, Gómez VP, Del Barco ÁA, et al. The evaluation of pelvic floor muscle strength in women with pelvic floor dysfunction: a reliability and correlation study. Neurourol Urodyn. 2018;37(1):269–77.
19. Zachovajeviene B, Siupsinskas L, Zachovajevas P, Milonas D, Lapinskaite L. Functional interaction of pelvic floor, diaphragm and trunk muscles among men with prostate cancer. Baltic J Sport Health Sci. 2012;3(86):107–14.
20. Zachovajeviene B, Siupsinskas L, Zachovajevas P, Venclovas Z, Milonas D. Effect of diaphragm and abdominal muscle training on pelvic floor strength and endurance: results of a prospective randomized trial. Sci Rep. 2019;9:19192.
21. Santos KM, Da Roza T, Mochizuki L, Arbieto ER, Luz SC. Assessment of abdominal and pelvic floor muscle function among continent and incontinent athletes. Int Urogynecol J. 2019;30(5):693–9.
22. Avery K, Donovan J, Peters TJ, Shaw C, Gotoh M, Abrams P. ICIQ: a brief and robust measure for evaluating the symptoms and impact of urinary incontinence. Neurourol Urodyn. 2004;23:322–30.
23. Haylen BT, De Ridder D, Freeman RM, Swift SE, Berghmans B, Lee J, et al. An International Urogynecological Association (IUGA)/International Continence Society (ICS) joint report on the terminology for female pelvic floor dysfunction. Int Urogynecol J. 2010;21:5–26.
24. Tamanini JT, Dambros M, D'Ancona CA, Palma PC, Netto NR. Validation of the "International Consultation on Incontinence Questionnaire—Short Form" (ICIQ-SF) for Portuguese. Rev Saude Publica. 2004;38(3):438–44.
25. Ferreira CH, Barbosa PB, de Oliveira SF, Antônio FI, Franco MM, Bø K. Inter-rater reliability study of the modified Oxford Grading Scale and the Peritron manometer. Physiotherapy. 2011;97(2):132–8.
26. Quartly E, Hallam T, Kilbreath S, Refshauge K. Strength and endurance of the pelvic floor mus-

cles in continent women: an observational study. Physiotherapy. 2010;96:311–6.
27. Bø K, Kvarstein B, Hagen R, Larsen S. Pelvic floor muscle exercise for the treatment of female stress urinary incontinence: II. Validity of vaginal pressure measurements of pelvic floor muscle strength and the necessity of supplementary methods for control of correct contraction. Neurourol Urodyn. 1990;9:4 79–87.
28. Frawley H, Galea M, Phillips B, Sherburn M, Bø K. Reliability of pelvic floor muscle strength assessment using different test positions and tools. Neurourol Urodyn. 2006;25:236–42.
29. Bø K, Sherburn M. Evaluation of female pelvic-floor muscle function and strength. Phys Ther. 2005;85:269–82.
30. Bø K, Finckenhagen HB. Is there any difference in measurement of pelvic floor muscle strength in supine and standing position? Acta Obstet Gynecol Scand. 2003;82:1120–4.
31. Ito K, Nonaka K, Ogaya S, Ogi A, Matsunaka C, Horie J. Surface electromyography activity of the rectus abdominis, internal oblique, and external oblique muscles during forced expiration in healthy adults. J Electromyogr Kinesiol. 2016;28:76–81.
32. ATS/ERS statement on respiratory muscle testing. Am J Respir Crit Care Med. 2002;166(4):518–624.
33. Maillard JO, Burdet L, van Melle G, Fitting JW. Reproducibility of twitch mouth pressure, sniff nasal inspiratory pressure, and maximal inspiratory pressure. Eur Respir J. 1998;11:901–5.
34. Guilhem G, Giroux C, Couturier A, Maffiuletti NA. Validity of trunk extensor and flexor torque measurements using isokinetic dynamometry. J Electromyogr Kinesiol. 2014;24:986–93.
35. Hildenbrand K, Noble L. Abdominal muscle activity while performing trunk-flexion exercises using the Ab Roller, ABslide, FitBall, and conventionally performed trunk curls. J Athl Train. 2004;39(1):37–43.
36. Karatas GK, Göğüs F, Meray J. Reliability of isokinetic trunk muscle strength measurement. Am J Phys Med Rehabil. 2002;81(2):79–85.
37. den Hartog D, Eker HH, Tuinebreijer WE, Kleinrensink GJ, Stam HJ, Lange JF. Isokinetic strength of the trunk Xexor muscles after surgical repair for incisional hernia. Hernia. 2010;14:243–7.
38. Madill SJ, McLean L. Relationship between abdominal and pelvic floor muscle activation and intravaginal pressure during pelvic floor muscle contractions in healthy continent women. Neurourol Urodyn. 2006;25:722–30.
39. Stüpp L, Resende APM, Petricelli CD, Nakamura MU, Alexandre SM, Zanetti MRD. Pelvic floor muscle and transversus abdominis activation in abdominal hypopressive technique through surface electromyography. Neurourol Urodyn. 2011;30(8):1518–21.
40. Verelst M, Leivseth G. Are fatigue and disturbances in pre-programmed activity of pelvic floor muscles associated with female stress urinary incontinence? Neurourol Urodyn. 2004;23:143–7.
41. Madill SJ, McLean L. Quantification of abdominal and pelvic floor muscle synergies in response to voluntary pelvic floor muscle contractions. J Electromyogr Kinesiol. 2008;18:955–64.
42. Bø K, Sherburn M, Allen T. Transabdominal ultrasound measurement of pelvic floor muscle activity when activated directly or via a transversus abdominis muscle contraction. Neurourol Urodyn. 2003;22(6):582–8.
43. Cresswell AG, Thorstensson A. The role of the abdominal musculature in the elevation of the intra-abdominal pressure during specified tasks. Ergonomics. 1989;32(10):1237–46.
44. Tayashiki K, Takai Y, Maeo S, Kanehisa H. Intra-abdominal pressure and trunk muscular activities during abdominal bracing and hollowing. Int J Sports Med. 2016;37(2):134–43.
45. Hahn I, Milsom I, Ohlsson BL, Ekelund P, Uhlemann C, Fall M. Comparative assessment of pelvic floor function using vaginal cones, vaginal digital palpation and vaginal pressure measurements. Gynecol Obstet Invest. 1996;41(4):269–74.
46. Mørkved S, Salvesen KA, Bø K, Eik-Nes S. Pelvic floor muscle strength and thickness in continent and incontinent nulliparous pregnant women. Int Urogynecol J Pelvic Floor Dysfunct. 2004;15(6):384–9.
47. Amaro JL, Moreira EC, De Oliveira Orsi Gameiro M, Padovani CR. Pelvic floor muscle evaluation in incontinent patients. Int Urogynecol J. 2005;16:352–4.
48. Thompson JA, O'Sullivan PB, Briffa NK, Neumann P. Assessment of voluntary pelvic floor muscle contraction in continent and incontinent women using transperineal ultrasound, manual muscle testing and vaginal squeeze pressure measurements. Int Urogynecol J Pelvic Floor Dysfunct. 2006;17(6):624–30.
49. Chamochumbi CCM, Nunes FR, Guirro RRJ, Guirro ECO. Comparison of active and passive forces of the pelvic floor muscles in women with and without stress urinary incontinence. Braz J Phys Ther. 2012;16(4):314–9.
50. Peng Q, Jones R, Shishido K, Omata S, Constantinou CE. Spatial distribution of vaginal closure pressures of continent and stress urinary incontinent women. Physiol Meas. 2007;28:1429–50.
51. Shishido K, Peng Q, Jones R, Omata S, Constantinou CE. Influence of pelvic floor muscle contraction on the profile of vaginal closure pressure in continent and stress urinary incontinent women. J Urol. 2008;179(5):1917–22.
52. Verelst M, Leivseth G. Force and stiffness of the pelvic floor as function of muscle length: a comparison between women with and without stress urinary incontinence. Neurourol Urodyn. 2007;26:852–7.
53. Morin M, Bourbonnais D, Gravel D, Dumoulin C, Lemieux M-C. Pelvic floor muscle function in continent and stress urinary incontinent women using

dynamometric measurements. Neurourol Urodyn. 2004;23:668–74.
54. Bø K, Stien R, Kulseng-Hanssen S, Kristofferson M. Clinical and urodynamic assessment of nulliparous young women with and without stress incontinence symptoms: a case-control study. Obstet Gynecol. 1994;84(6):1028–32.
55. Madill SJ, Harvey MA, McLean L. Women with SUI demonstrate motor control differences during voluntary pelvic floor muscle contractions. Int Urogynecol J. 2009;20:447–59.
56. Da Roza T, Brandão S, Oliveira D, Mascarenhas T, Parente M, Duarte JA, et al. Football practice and urinary incontinence: relation between morphology, function and biomechanics. J Biomech. 2015;48(9):1587–92.
57. Essendrop M, Bente S. Intra-abdominal pressure and activation of abdominal muscles in highly trained participants during sudden heavy trunk loadings. Spine (Phila Pa 1976). 2004;29(21):2445–51.
58. Cresswell AG, Grundström H, Thorstensson A. Observations on intra-abdominal pressure and patterns of abdominal intra-muscular activity in man. Acta Physiol Scand. 1992;144(4):409–18.
59. Cresswell AG, Thorstensson A. Changes in intra-abdominal pressure, trunk muscle activation and force during isokinetic lifting and lowering. Eur J Appl Physiol Occup Physiol. 1994;68(4):315–21.
60. Cresswell AG, Blake PL, Thorstensson A. The effect of an abdominal muscle training program on intra-abdominal pressure. Scand J Rehabil Med. 1994;26(2):79–86.
61. Nygaard IE, Shaw JM. Physical activity and the pelvic floor. Am J Obstet Gynecol. 2016;214(2):164–71.
62. Kamel DM, Thabet AA, Tantawy SA, Radwan MM. Effect of abdominal versus pelvic floor muscle exercises in obese Egyptian women with mild stress urinary incontinence: a randomised controlled trial. Hong Kong Physiother J. 2013;31(1):12–8.
63. Subak LL, Richter HE, Hunskaar S. Obesity and urinary incontinence: epidemiology and clinical research update. J Urol. 2009;182(6 Suppl):S2–7.
64. Resende APM, Bernardes BT, Stüpp L, Oliveira E, Castro RA, Girão MJBC, et al. Pelvic floor muscle training is better than hypopressive exercises in pelvic organ prolapse treatment: an assessor-blinded randomized controlled trial. Neurourol Urodyn. 2019;38(1):171–9.
65. Kruger J, Budgett D, Goodman J, Bø K. Can you train the pelvic floor muscles by contracting other related muscles? Neurourol Urodyn. 2019;38(2):677–83.

32 Physiotherapy in Women for Pelvic Floor and Sexual Dysfunction

Emel Sönmezer, Mehmet Murat Seval, Ş. Esra Çetinkaya, and Fulya Dökmeci

Pelvic floor dysfunction includes involuntary leakage of urine, increased urinary frequency, pelvic organ prolapses, and defecation problems. Although pelvic floor dysfunction is not a medical condition that leads to mortality, it is common in every age group and especially common in women, causing biopsychosocial changes in women and adversely affecting quality of life [1]. It has been reported that women diagnosed with pelvic floor dysfunction have poorer quality of life and body image perceptions and are affected not only physically but also in terms of their sexual health [1].

"Sexual health is a state of physical, emotional, mental and social well-being in relation to sexuality; it is not merely the absence of disease, dysfunction or infirmity. Sexual health requires a positive and respectful approach to sexuality and sexual relationships, as well as the possibility of having pleasurable and safe sexual experiences, free of coercion, discrimination and violence" [2].

Sexual health is an integral component of general health; in fact, sexual function is a complex process that depends on the integrity of neurological, vascular, and endocrine systems and is influenced by numerous psychosocial and individual factors, including family background, sexual partner, self-concept, and self-esteem [3]. Mood seriously affects quality of life, self-confidence, and well-being, and it causes emotional and relational problems [4–8]. Sexuality is a concept that includes emotional, intellectual, and sociocultural components in addition to being desirable for women, childbearing ability, and body image.

Treatment of sexual health problems with physiotherapy may be available in many areas of rehabilitation. Current guidelines show that pelvic floor rehabilitation is an effective treatment for pelvic floor and sexual dysfunction. The treatments applied can also have a positive effect on anxiety and depression, which can indirectly affect sexual health positively [9].

In the literature, the relationship between the musculoskeletal system and sexual dysfunction is generally established on the pelvic floor. Although the pelvic floor is one of the important structures for sexual function, a broader perspective is required to examine the impact of musculoskeletal problems on both physiological and psychological aspects of sexual function [10–14].

Patients with chronic pain face physical function difficulties, such as joint stiffness and difficulty in sexual activity due to pain [14]. In fact,

E. Sönmezer (✉)
Faculty of Health Science, Physiotherapy and Rehabilitation Department, Atılım University, Ankara, Turkey

M. M. Seval · Ş. E. Çetinkaya · F. Dökmeci
Obstetrics and Gynecology, Ankara University School of Medicine, Ankara, Turkey

F. Dökmeci, D. E. E. Rizk (eds.), *Insights Into Incontinence and the Pelvic Floor*,
https://doi.org/10.1007/978-3-030-94174-1_32

they must feel comfortable to touch and have a physical function to move for satisfied sexual activity. Thus, a decrease in pain and mobility of the neck, trunk, and extremities as well as changes in sensation limits comfortable sexual activity [15].

Chronic musculoskeletal disorders cause fatigue, pain, depression, decreased physical capacity and function, decreased joint mobility, and muscle strength [14, 16–18]. All of which may negatively affect sexual function and lead to decreased quality of life [5]. Poor quality of life may cause sexual health to deteriorate, just as deterioration of sexual health may lead to poor quality of life.

Musculoskeletal problems are related to chronic pain and disability, and fear of increased pain and fatigue during sex may decrease sexual desire, frequency, and satisfaction [14, 17, 18]. Studies on women with fibromyalgia have found decreased sexual desire and frequency of sexual activity compared to normal controls [19]. Sexual difficulties in women with musculoskeletal disorders are similar to those found in patients with chronic pain, including cancer pain and neuropathic conditions. These difficulties are both physical and psychosocial and are affected by factors such as pharmacologic agents, fatigue and emotional stress, depression, and anxiety, as well as changes in body image.

Keeping these in mind, patients with musculoskeletal pain require a treatment plan that addresses specific factors such as pain, stiffness, and fatigue to reduce and eliminate sexual problems. While these factors are often taken into account in measuring the parameters of sexual function, such as frequency, desire, arousal, orgasm, and sexual pain, there has been limited research into the effectiveness of treatment techniques of musculoskeletal problems for sexual health [14, 20–23].

32.1 Literature Review

Physiotherapy improves physical function, and it may promote good sexual health both directly and indirectly [15]. There are several areas where physiotherapy programs affect sexual health, one of which is teaching pelvic floor rehabilitation to patients with gynecological and/or urological problems [24, 25]. There is evidence that pelvic floor rehabilitation administered by physiotherapists not only directly improves sexual health [13, 26, 27] but also treats lower urinary tract problems, indirectly lowering sexual anxieties [28, 29]. It has been shown that pelvic floor rehabilitation in women with stress urinary incontinence improves quality of life as well as sexual function [1, 30]. Studies have also shown that women receiving pelvic floor rehabilitation see an improvement in sexual function, desire, and orgasm stages [30]. Additionally, it has also been reported that physiotherapy methods improve sexual function in women with pelvic pain [1, 30].

An individual physiotherapy program tailored to a disease contributes to satisfactory treatment results and functional recovery of patients. Physiotherapy prepares the tissues and body for physical activities. It is used to reduce pain and inflammation and regulate muscle tone. Among the physiotherapeutic methods used, local and whole body thermotherapy methods, transcutaneous electrical nerve stimulation (TENS), and other electrotherapy methods, such as magnetic field and laser therapy, are also useful. Hydrotherapy treatments, such as whirlpool and underwater massage, also play a role in reducing pain. Exercise therapy following all these applications is also an essential element of improving the locomotor system, which endeavors to restore the tension balance in the ligament-tendon-muscular system [31].

Therapeutic exercise therapy, prescribed regularly by physical therapists as part of rehabilitation, is beneficial in reducing pain, improving joint mobility, and increasing strength, stability, and endurance [32]. Moreover, it improves the patient's performance during activity of daily living [33]. In order to improve sexual function in women with musculoskeletal pain, exercises should include range of motion, strengthening, and endurance exercises. In addition, assisted devices, splints, and position recommendations specially designed to increase joint mobility and strength reduce fatigue and increase endurance, improve disability in patients, and increase the quality of activity of daily living [14].

The reduced mobility, inflammation, and dysfunction of the back, hip, sacroiliac, spine, and symphysis pubis and surrounding muscles also contribute to pain during sexual activity. The pelvic floor muscles should relax comfortably during deep breathing to allow painless sexual function. Special exercises and positional techniques can be taught to patients to ensure that they enjoy sexual activity comfortably and painlessly [26].

Regular exercise reduces fatigue and improves physical fitness, strength, balance, flexibility, and endurance of the muscles. Therefore, it can be assumed that systematic exercise training not only improves the physical performance of patients but also positively affects the quality of sexual health. It should be noted that women who exercise regularly have greater desire for sexual activity. The reason for this increase in desire is that exercise increases testosterone secretion during training. This hormone leads to an increase in sexual desire and reduces the occurrence of erectile dysfunction [29].

The treatments being applied can have a positive effect on anxiety and depression, which can indirectly affect sexual health positively [9]. Physiotherapy can also increase the possible position choices for sexual intercourse by improving joint mobility, increasing muscle strength and patients' knowledge of their own physical abilities [34]. Different exercise positions included in physiotherapy programs help patients to choose different and comfortable positions while engaging in sexual activity [35]. A number of exercise positions used in physiotherapy are also used during sexual intercourse. The joint and muscle tension that the patient feels while in these positions can provide insight into how the patient will feel in such a position while engaging in sexual activity, and it can be a guide for position choices. For example, in patients who have had hip replacement surgery and/or shoulder surgery, the operation may also affect the patient's coitus positions. Physiotherapists should advise on positions to prevent dislocation, especially for patients who have undergone joint replacement surgery [36].

In addition to reducing pain and improving muscular function, physiotherapy technically helps sexuality in a field beyond the physical, including the development of a therapeutic relationship between the patient and the therapist. Successful treatment facilitates greater self-awareness, self-confidence, improved body image, a reduction in anxiety, and feelings of empowerment, all of which improve sexual health [20]. In addition, physiotherapists can answer questions from patients about how injured joints are affected during sexual activity [24, 25, 37].

Physiotherapy interventions aimed at improving sexual health should not only target patients with traumatic injuries or chronic diseases, they should also be addressed as a general health problem. Healthy living habits positively affect sexual health. A physically active lifestyle has positive effects on sexual health. Physiotherapists often encourage physical activity to improve on a healthy lifestyle and prevent illnesses [38, 39]. Physical activity interventions are an essential and important part of physiotherapy to improve overall health and physical capacity in both ill and healthy people. Increased participation in leisure activities that include physical exercise reduces pain and fatigue and may indirectly improve sexual function [40, 41]. Studies examining the relationship between the frequency of sexual activity and physical activity levels show that exercise interventions are required to improve both physical fitness and sexual health [38, 42–45]. Regular physical activity positively affects sexual health, as increased physical activity is associated with sexual function [38, 43, 46, 47]. Thus, physical activity coaching and exercise interventions can improve both physical fitness and sexual health [38, 42–45]. Exercise may directly affect overall sexual health in terms of erectile function, sexual desire, function, and satisfaction [5]. Additionally, patients reported that they experienced positive emotions during physiotherapy, which could positively affect sexual health together with increased self-esteem [35].

As emotions such as stress and anxiety may negatively affect sexual health, stress-reducing physiotherapy interventions that include relaxation techniques may also help improve sexual health [47]. In addition, physiotherapy applications have positive effects on body image and body appreciation, again improving sexual function [35, 48–50]. Physical activity interventions and body awareness therapies aimed at improving physical capacity and physical function have been shown to have more positive effects on sexual health than weight loss by improving body image [51].

In summary, individual and tailored physiotherapy programs alleviate pain and disability, increase physical function, reduce depression, and improve quality of life. All these positive effects create a healthier sex life. Therefore, it can be recommended to be used as a treatment option in the treatment of sexual dysfunction in patients with chronic pain.

32.2 Case Study: Effects of Conventional Physiotherapy on Sexual Function in Women with Chronic Musculoskeletal Pain

(a) **Introduction and Aim of the Study**

The negative effects of chronic pain syndromes on sexual function have been reported in several studies. The aim of this study was to evaluate the effects of conventional physiotherapy without pelvic floor muscle exercises on sexual function in women with chronic musculoskeletal pain.

(b) **Methods**

Fifty women with chronic musculoskeletal pain (mean age 43 ± 8 years) were enrolled in this study (Table 32.1). The volunteer subjects provided written informed consent. The Declaration of Helsinki was strictly followed throughout the study.

Patients with a history of cardiovascular disease, medical complications (cardiac rhythm problems, unstable angina, thrombosis, etc.), and/or cognitive disorders, as well as patients with contraindications for physical exercise or physiotherapy programs, and patients who were still being actively investigated or treated elsewhere for their chronic pain diseases were excluded from this study.

Table 32.1 Baseline characteristics of patients

Patient characteristics (*n* = 50)	
Age (years), mean ± SD	43 ± 8
Median (min-max)	42 (28–58)
Diagnosis of musculoskeletal disease	
– Fibromyalgia, *n* (%)	14 (28)
– Osteoarthritis, *n* (%)	4 (8)
– Low back pain, *n* (%)	11 (22)
– Neck pain, *n* (%)	7 (14)
– Impingement, *n* (%)	12 (24)
– Myofascial pain syndrome, *n* (%)	2 (4)
Postmenopausal status, *n* (%)	11 (22)
Parity, mean ± SD	1.5 ± 1.4
Body mass index (kg/m^2), mean ± SD	24.2 ± 2.2

The baseline demographics and clinical characteristics were recorded at admission.

The patients received conventional physiotherapy five times per week for 3 weeks. This program included 20 minutes of heat therapy and TENS for painful localization and exercise for postural alignments. Ergonomic education was also given during the program. Sexual function was assessed with the Female Sexual Function Index (FSFI) before and after treatment. This questionnaire had six subscales: desire, arousal, lubrication, orgasm (three items), satisfaction, and pain [52, 53].

Every variable was analyzed using a paired t-test.

(c) **Results**

The participants presented with a wide variety of pain conditions, including fibromyalgia 28%, osteoarthritis 8%, low back pain 22%, neck pain 14%, impingement 24%, and myofascial pain syndrome 4% (Table 32.1). Significant improvements were observed in all subscales and the total scores of the FSFI after 15 physiotherapy treatment sessions (Table 32.2).

32.3 Discussion

In this study, an investigation was made into the effect of chronic pain syndrome on women's sexual function and how physiotherapy and rehabili-

Table 32.2 Comparison of pre- and post-treatment total scores of the Female Sexual Function Index

FSFI	Before the treatment ($n = 50$)	After the treatment ($n = 50$)	P
Desire	5.5 ± 2.3	5.8 ± 2.1	0.003[a]
Arousal	12.8 ± 5.4	13.5 ± 4.9	< 0.001[a]
Lubrication	14.7 ± 4.2	15.3 ± 3.7	0.005[a]
Orgasm	10.8 ± 3.9	11.5 ± 3.2	0.001[a]
Satisfaction	11.3 ± 3.7	11.9 ± 3.1	0.005[a]
Pain	11.1 ± 3.1	12.1 ± 2.3	<0.001[a]
Total score	66.4 ± 21.1	70.3 ± 17.7	<0.001[a]

FSFI Female Sexual Function Index
[a]$p < 0.05$, Wilcoxon

tation being applied change their sexual function.

As a result of our study, it has been shown that conventional physiotherapy has a positive effect on the sexual functioning of women with chronic pain syndrome. This is a clinically important finding because when the literature was reviewed, it was found that the sexual dysfunction score, especially the parameters of sexual intercourse frequency, satisfaction, avoidance, and orgasm disorder, is significantly higher in patients with chronic pain syndrome compared to healthy individuals [54]. The reason for this may be that chronic pain and the resulting disability, depression, and low quality of life negatively affect sexual function [54]. Batmaz et al. reported that chronic pain leads to a decrease in all physical activities, including sexual activity [55]. However, to date no study has been found in the literature investigating the effects of treatment methods for chronic pain syndrome on sexual dysfunction. The findings of this study show that physiotherapy programs improve sexual function in women with chronic pain syndrome.

When the literature was reviewed, sexual dysfunction was found to be associated with depression, especially in patients with chronic pain syndrome. However, it was reported that characteristic symptoms, such as widespread pain, stiffness, weakness, poor quality sleep, depression, and decreased quality of life, may be associated with sexual dysfunction [56, 57]. Therefore, it can be predicted that any application that can improve these symptoms can have a positive effect on sexual function [58]. Physiotherapy approaches that reduce pain and increase mobility have been shown in the literature to have a positive effect on sexual health. According to the results of previous studies, conventional physiotherapy treatments improve pain and mobility. This may explain the improvement in sexual health created by conventional physiotherapy without any additional sexual therapy or pelvic floor rehabilitation.

Another important marker affecting sexual health is physical function. Chronic pain syndromes may affect the patient's willingness or ability to engage in sexual activity by causing physical function problems, such as muscle spasms, stiffness, and flexibility and mobility problems. Healthy living habits and exercise approaches are another physiotherapy method that improves physical function. Conventional physiotherapy programs, including exercise programs for postural alignments, improve the physical function of patients with chronic musculoskeletal pain, and the improvements that ensue create positive effects on these patients' sexual function [28].

32.4 Conclusion

Conventional physiotherapy programs significantly improve not only physical function but also sexual function in women with chronic musculoskeletal pain. Therefore, conventional physiotherapy should be advised as a treatment option to improve the sexual life of women with chronic pain syndrome.

References

1. Bo K, Frawley HC, Haylen BT, Abramov Y, Almeida FG, Berghmans B, et al. An International Urogynecological Association (IUGA)/International Continence Society (ICS) joint report on the terminology for the conservative and nonpharmacological management of female pelvic floor dysfunction. Int Urogynecol J. 2017;28(2):191–213.
2. World Health Organisation. https://www.who.int/reproductivehealth/topics/sexual_health/sh_definitions/en/. Accessed 20 Nov 2020.
3. Nusbaum MR, Hamilton C, Lenahan P. Chronic illness and sexual functioning. Am Fam Physician. 2003;67(2):347–54.
4. Anastasiadis AG, Davis AR, Ghafar MA, Burchardt M, Shabsigh R. The epidemiology and definition of female sexual disorders. World J Urol. 2002;20: 74–8.
5. Cormie P, Newton RU, Taaffe DR, Spry N, Galvao DA. Exercise therapy for sexual dysfunction after prostate cancer. Nat Rev Urol. 2013;10:731–6.
6. Davison SL, Bell RJ, Lachina M, Holden SL, Davis SR. The relationship between self-reported sexual satisfaction and general wellbeing in women. J Sex Med. 2009;6:2690–7.
7. Lamont J. Female sexual health consensus clinical guidelines. J Obstet Gynaecol Can. 2012;34:769–75.
8. Moin V, Duvdevany I, Mazor D. Sexual identity, body image, and life satisfaction among women with and without physical disability. Sex Disabil. 2009;27:83–95.
9. Khan ZA, Whittal C, Mansol S, Osborne LA, Reed P, Emery S. Effect of depression and anxiety on the success of pelvic floor muscle training for pelvic floor dysfunction. J Obstet Gynaecol. 2013;33:710–4.
10. Reissing ED, Brown C, Lord MJ, Binik YM, Khalife S. Pelvic floor muscle functioning in women with vulvar vestibulitis syndrome. J Psychosom Obstet Gynaecol. 2005;26:107–13.
11. Reissing ED, Binik YM, Khalife S, Cohen D, Amsel R. Vaginal spasm, pain and behaviour: an empirical investigation of the diagnosis of vaginismus. Arch Sex Behav. 2004;33:5–17.
12. Goldfinger C, Pukall CF, Gentilcore-Saulnier E, McLean L, Chamberlain S. A prospective study of pelvic floor physical therapy: pain and psychosexual outcomes in provoked vestibulodynia. J Sex Med. 2009;6:1955–68.
13. Rivalta M, Sighinolfi MC, De Stefani S, Micali S, Mofferdin A, Grande M, Bianchi G. Biofeedback, electrical stimulation, pelvic floor muscle exercises, and vaginal cones: a combined rehabilitative approach for sexual dysfunction associated with urinary incontinence. J Sex Med. 2009;6:1674–7.
14. Rosenbaum TY. Musculoskeletal pain and sexual function in women. J Sex Med. 2010;7:645–53.
15. Matthias RE, Lubben JE, Atchison KA, Schweitzer SO. Sexual activity and satisfaction among very old adults: results from a community-dwelling Medicare population survey. Gerontologist. 1997;37:6–14.
16. Dzierzanowski M, Dzierzanowski M, Wrzecion K, Slomko W, Radziminska A, Kazmierczak U, Strojek K, Srokowski G, Zukow W. Discopathy of the lumbar-sacral segment and its influence on sexual dysfunction. Adv Clin Exp Med. 2013;22:93–100.
17. Josefsson KA, Gard G. Sexual health in patients with rheumatoid arthritis: experiences, needs and communication with health care professionals. Musculoskeletal Care. 2012;10:76–89.
18. Tajar A, O'Neill TW, Lee DM, O'Connor DB, Corona G, Finn JD, Bartfai G, Boonen S, Casanueva FF, Forti G, Giwercman A, Han TS, Huhtaniemi IT, Kula K, Lean ME, Pendleton N, Punab M, Purandare N, Silman AJ, Vanderschueren D, Wu FC, McBeth J. The effect of musculoskeletal pain on sexual function in middle-aged and elderly European men: results from the European male ageing study. J Rheumatol. 2011;38:370–7.
19. Baldini GR, Andrade PA, Alqualo-Costa R, et al. Assessment of sexual activity in patients with fibromyalgia—a controlled study. Arthritis Rheum. 2003;48:305.
20. Rosenbaum T, Owens A. The role of pelvic floor physical therapy in the treatment of pelvic and genital pain related sexual dysfunction. J Sex Med. 2008;5:513–23.
21. Guess MK, Connell K, Schrader S, Reutman S, Wang A, LaCombe J, Toennis C, Lowe B, Melman A, Mikhail M. Genital sensation and sexual function in women bicyclists and runners: are your feet safer than your seat? J Sex Med. 2006;3:1018–27.
22. Popeney C, Ansell V, Renney K. Pudendal entrapment as an etiology of chronic perineal pain: diagnosis and treatment. Neurourol Urodyn. 2007;26:820–7.
23. Stay K, Dwyer PL, Roberts L, Pudendal neuralgia. Fact or fiction? Obstet Gynecol Surv. 2009;64:190–9.
24. Reissing ED, Armstrong HL, Allen C. Pelvic floor physical therapy for lifelong vaginismus: a retrospective chart review and interview study. J Sex Marital Ther. 2013;39:306–20.
25. Rosenbaum TY. Addressing anxiety in vivo in physiotherapy treatment of women with severe vaginismus: a clinical approach. J Sex Marital Ther. 2011;37:89–93.
26. Rosenbaum TY. Pelvic floor involvement in male and female sexual dysfunction and the role of pelvic floor rehabilitation in treatment: a literature review. J Sex Med. 2007;4:4–13.
27. Zahariou AG, Karamouti MV, Papaioannou PD. Pelvic floor muscle training improves sexual function of women with stress urinary incontinence. Int Urogynecol J. 2008;19:401–6.
28. Martinez CS, Ferreira FV, Castro AA, Gomide LB. Women with greater pelvic floor muscle strength have better sexual function. Acta Obstet Gynecol Scand. 2014;93:497–502.
29. Areskoug-Josefsson K, Gard G. Physiotherapy as a promoter of sexual health. Physiother Theory Pract. 2015;31(6):390–5.

30. Abrams P, Andersson KE, Apostolidis A, Birder L, Bliss D, Brubaker L, Cotterill N. 6th International Consultation on Incontinence. Recommendations of the International Scientific Committee: evaluation and treatment of urinary incontinence, pelvic organ prolapse and faecal incontinence. Neurourol Urodyn. 2018;37(7):2271–2.
31. Zuk B, Maslinska M. The importance of physiotherapy in the sexuality of patients with rheumatic diseases. Reumatologia. 2017;55(5):237.
32. Kuukkanen T, Malkia E, Kautiainen H, Pohjolainen T. Effectiveness of a home exercise program in low back pain: a randomized five-year follow-up study. Physiother Res Int. 2007;12:213–24.
33. Morris DM, Taub E, Macrina DM, Cook EW, Geiger BF. A method for standardizing procedures in rehabilitation: use in the extremity constraint induced therapy evaluation multisite randomized controlled trial. Arch Phys Med Rehabil. 2009;90:663–8.
34. Moreno JA, Arango Lasprilla JC, Gan C, McKerral M. Sexuality after traumatic brain injury: a critical review. NeuroRehabilitation. 2013;32:69–85.
35. Josefsson KA, Gard G. Women's experiences of sexual health when living with rheumatoid arthritis: an explorative qualitative study. BMC Musculoskelet Disord. 2010;11:240.
36. Meiri R, Rosenbaum TY, Kalichman L. Sexual function before and after total hip replacement: narrative review. J Sex Med. 2014;2:159–67.
37. Rosenbaum TY. Pelvic floor physiotherapy for women with urogenital dysfunction: indications and methods. Minerva Urol Nefrol. 2011;63:101–7.
38. Bortz WM, Wallace DH. Physical fitness, aging, and sexuality. West J Med. 1999;170:167–9.
39. Sharma R, Biedenharn KR, Fedor JM, Agarwal A. Lifestyle factors and reproductive health: taking control of your fertility. Reprod Biol Endocrinol. 2013;11:66.
40. Monga TN, Tan G, Ostermann HJ, Monga U, Grabois M. Sexuality and sexual adjustment of patients with chronic pain. Disabil Rehabil. 1998;20:317–29.
41. Reinseth L, Uhlig T, Kjeken I, Koksvik HS, Skomsvoll JF, Espnes GA. Performance in leisure-time physical activities and self-efficacy in females with rheumatoid arthritis. Scand J Occup Ther. 2011;18:210–8.
42. Baillot A, Mampuya WM, Comeau E, Meziat-Burdin A, Langlois MF. Feasibility and impacts of supervised exercise training in subjects with obesity awaiting bariatric surgery: a pilot study. Obes Surg. 2013;23:882–91.
43. Hsiao W, Shrewsberry AB, Moses KA, Johnson TV, Cai AW, Stuhldreher P, Dusseault B, Ritenour CW. Exercise is associated with better erectile function in men under 40 as evaluated by the international index of erectile function. J Sex Med. 2012;9:524–30.
44. La Vignera S, Condorelli R, Vicari E, D'agata R, Calogero AE. Physical activity and erectile dysfunction in middle-aged men. J Andrology. 2012;33:154–61.
45. Speck RM, Gross CR, Hormes JM, Ahmed RL, Lytle LA, Hwang WT, Schmitz KH. Changes in the body image and relationship scale following a one-year strength training trial for breast cancer survivors with or at risk for lymphedema. Breast Cancer Res Treat. 2010;121:421–30.
46. Post MW, Gianotten WL, Heijnen L, Lambers EJ, Willems M. Sexological competence of different rehabilitation disciplines and effects of a discipline-specific sexological training. Sex Disabil. 2008;26:3–14.
47. Rosman L, Cahill JM, McCammon SL, Sears SF. Sexual health concerns in patients with cardiovascular disease. Circulation. 2014;129:313–6.
48. Pujols Y, Meston CM, Seal BN. The association between sexual satisfaction and body image in women. J Sex Med. 2009;7:905–16.
49. Hedlund L, Gyllensten AL. The experiences of basic body awareness therapy in patients with schizophrenia. J Bodyw Mov Ther. 2010;14:245–54.
50. Jorge RT, Brumini C, Jones A, Natour J. Body image in patients with rheumatoid arthritis. Mod Rheumatol. 2010;20:491–5.
51. Satinsky S, Reece M, Dennis B, Sanders S, Bardzell S. An assessment of body appreciation and its relationship to sexual function in women. Body Image. 2012;9(1):137–44.
52. Rosen R, Brown C, Heiman J, Leiblum S, Meston C, Shabsigh R, Ferguson D, D'Agostiona R. The female sexual function index (FSFI): a multidimensional self-report instrument for the assessment of female sexual function. J Sex Marital Ther. 2000;26:191.
53. Oksuz E, Malhan S. Reliability and validity of the female sexual function index in Turkish population. Sendrom. 2005;17:54.
54. Williams AC, Hill P, Gunary R, Cratchley G. Sexual difficulties of chronic pain patients. Clin J Pain. 2001;17(2):138–45.
55. Batmaz I, Sarıyıldız MA, Dilek B, Inanır A, Demircan Z, Hatipoglu N, Atar M, Cevik R. Sexuality of men with fibromyalgia: what are the factors that cause sexual dysfunction? Rheumatol Int. 2013;33(5):1265–70.
56. Woertman L, Prins MA, Van Middendorp H, Geenen R. Low relationship satisfaction and high partner involvement predict sexual problems of women with fibromyalgia. J Sex Marital Ther. 2006;32(5):409–23.
57. Blake DJ, Maisiak R, Alarcon GS, Brown S. Sexual quality of life of patients with arthritis compared to arthritis-free control. J Rheumatol. 1987;14:570–6.
58. Lipe H, Longstreth WT, Bird TD, Linde M. Sexual function in married men with Parkinson's disease compared to married men with arthritis. Neurology. 1990;40:1347–9.

GPSR Compliance

The European Union's (EU) General Product Safety Regulation (GPSR) is a set of rules that requires consumer products to be safe and our obligations to ensure this.

If you have any concerns about our products, you can contact us on ProductSafety@springernature.com

In case Publisher is established outside the EU, the EU authorized representative is:

Springer Nature Customer Service Center GmbH
Europaplatz 3
69115 Heidelberg, Germany

Batch number: 09224018

Printed by Printforce, the Netherlands